BENZODIAZEPINES IN CLINICAL PRACTICE

Benzodiazepines in Clinical Practice

DAVID J. GREENBLATT, M.D.

Clinical Fellow in Medicine (Clinical Pharmacology),
Massachusetts General Hospital;
Research Fellow in Pharmacology, Harvard Medical School;
Research Fellow of the Medical Foundation, Inc., Boston

RICHARD I. SHADER, M.D.

Director, Psychopharmacology Research Laboratory,
Massachusetts Mental Health Center;
Director of Clinical Psychiatry,
Massachusetts Mental Health Center;
Associate Professor of Psychiatry,
Harvard Medical School

Raven Press • New York

International Standard Book Number 0-911216-52-9

Library of Congress Catalog Card Number 73-83887

Printed in U.S.A. by
NOBLE OFFSET PRINTERS, INC.
New York, N.Y. 10003

Preface

Published surveys show that no less than one in ten adult Americans takes a benzodiazepine tranquilizer or hypnotic in a year's time. Physicians prescribe benzodiazepines to treat neurotic anxiety, depression, insomnia, muscle spasm, and countless functional disorders ranging from headaches to dyspareunia. Tens of thousands more patients receive benzodiazepines in the hospital setting for treatment of alcohol withdrawal, intractable seizures, tetanus, or strychnine poisoning; as premedication for endoscopic or surgical procedures; or as induction agents prior to general anesthesia. It is no surprise that thousands of papers have been published on the pharmacologic properties and clinical uses of these drugs. Yet there has been no "distillation" of this voluminous literature into a guide to rational therapeutics for the practicing physician.

This book is written for the clinician who uses benzodiazepine tranquilizers and hypnotics in the daily practice of medicine. At the same time, it will serve as a reference source for investigators in clinical research and basic science. More than 2,000 papers have been reviewed in critical fashion. Our interpretations of the published findings are presented in a format useful to clinicians. Although a large amount of nonclinical data is presented, we have stressed the possible relevance (or lack of relevance) of the experimental findings to clinical medicine.

Only books, monographs, chapters, and articles published in the English language are cited in this volume. To the best of our knowledge, however, we have completely reviewed the English language literature, including publications appearing through mid-1973. Each paper has been studied by the authors to determine its scientific validity. Our conclusions emphasize the results of well-designed investigations in which the stated interpretations of the data are justified and reasonable. Anecdotal reports, uncontrolled studies, and other papers of lower quality are stressed less strongly, but in no case are papers omitted from the bibliography. When the literature on a given topic is particularly voluminous, the bibliography has been listed as an appendix to the text. Appendix 6 is devoted to an alphabetical bibliography of review articles, most of which were cited elsewhere in the volume.

We are indebted to a number of physicians and investigators whose constructive comments and suggestions lead to many improvements in the manuscript. These individuals are: Donald Green, Ramon Greenberg, Jerold S. Harmatz, Samuel Irwin, Turan M. Itil, Ken M. Janis, Anthony Kales, Stanley A. Kaplan, Jan Koch-Weser, Allen A. Mitchell, Grace Mushrush, Chester

Pearlman, Martin B. Scharf, J. Arthur F. deSilva, Chester Swett, and Robert I. Taber.

Mr. James A. Donahue of R.A. Gosselin and Co., Inc., kindly granted permission for publication of parts of the data cited in Chapter 13. Figure 13-1 was furnished by Dr. Mitchell Balter. Mrs. Margaret Jonah and Ms. Teri Silken contributed secretarial assistance. Ms. Eveline Morrissette was responsible for rapid, accurate typing of most of the manuscript as well as for layout of tabular material. Her expertise allowed prompt preparation of the book and minimized the inevitable delays between writing and publication.

DAVID J. GREENBLATT
RICHARD I. SHADER

Boston, Massachusetts
September, 1973

Contents

Chapter 1
Introduction

The "tranquilizer decade" was coined in the mid-1960's to describe the remarkable era into which pharmacotherapeutics had passed over the preceding 10 or so years.[1] During this period, the treatment of mental illness with drugs became a reality—one so complex and perplexing that many physicians and laymen were unable to separate pharmacologic fact from conjecture. Countless volumes of clinical and experimental literature appeared within a very few years, much of which was irrelevant, premature, or misleading. Yet, more than enough sound evidence was made available to document that the mentally ill could be successfully treated and their rehabilitation facilitated by drugs.

The tranquilizer decade began "insidiously" rather than suddenly during the early 1950's as the use of the phenothiazine tranquilizers and reserpine became widespread. It had taken 200 years for the psychotropic effects of *Rauwolfia serpentina* to reappear in the Western literature. In 1755 Rumpf had described its tranquilizing properties "...valet contra anxietatum..." in a Dutch publication entitled *Herbari Amboinensis Auctuarium*.[2] By 1956, the antipsychotic efficacy of the phenothiazines was an epidemiologic as well as a scientific fact. At this time, statistics emerged showing a decline in the total mental hospital inpatient population—a reversal of an incessant yearly increase dating from the mid-1920's.[3] Thousands of previously disabled, hospitalized schizophrenics were sufficiently improved on drug therapy to return to their homes and communities as functional citizens.

For those with neurotic anxiety, the prospects of new, effective pharmacotherapy were equally bright. Meprobamate was introduced in 1955, acclaimed as a drug which specifically reduced anxiety and tension without producing drowsiness and sleep—the drug which would do for neurotic outpatients what the phenothiazines were doing for hospitalized schizophrenics.[4,5] In the years that followed, millions of Americans were treated with meprobamate, and testimony of effectiveness filled both lay and medical press. Yet, by 1958 it became clear to critical observers that the excessive enthusiasm was unjustified.[6] Nearly all the favorable reports were based on uncontrolled trials, and the few controlled studies showed that meprobamate added little if any therapeutic benefit to that available from the barbiturates. Meprobamate, in retrospect, may have been an opportunist of the tranquilizer decade,[7] and the ironic fact remained that those with the least severe illness were least helped by drugs. The disordered thinking of the schizophrenic

1

could be radically altered by phenothiazines, and the "black cloud" of the depressed patient could be lifted by pharmacologic antidepressants. Even by 1960, however, individuals with distressing anxiety symptoms could be offered only nonspecific sedation.

DEVELOPMENT OF THE BENZODIAZEPINES

The tranquilizer decade did not end after 10 years, but rather has continued as an era of psychopharmacology. The continuing efficacy of the major tranquilizers and antidepressants is one reason that the decade became an era. The development of new agents for the treatment of neuroses is another.

The synthesis of chlordiazepoxide, the first benzodiazepine tranquilizer, was a fortuitous one.[8-12] Leo H. Sternbach, while working on benzophenone structures in Cracow, Poland, during the mid-1930's, had synthesized several compounds known as heptoxdiazines, having seven-membered rings. His interest in these compounds remained dormant until 1954 when he and his associates at Roche Laboratories studied a number of heptoxdiazines in their search for psychopharmacologically active compounds. In doing so, Sternbach found that the designated structure of these heptoxdiazines was incorrect: they were not seven-membered but rather six-membered ring compounds known as quinazoline-3-oxides. Of some 40 derivatives screened for pharmacologic activity, all proved to be inert.

In late 1955, Sternbach elected to treat one of these quinazolines with

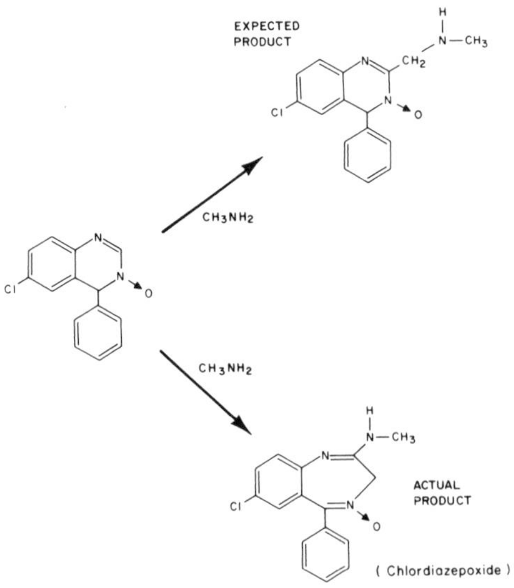

FIG. 1-1. Chlordiazepoxide: unexpected product following methylamine treatment of quinazoline 3-oxide.

methylamine, a primary amine. The other 40 derivatives had been treated with secondary and tertiary amines. The new compound, Ro 5-0690, was also assumed to be inert and was put aside without being screened. Testing was not undertaken until May 1957 when Roche's Lowell O. Randall found Ro 5-0690 to have entirely unexpected "hypnotic, sedative, and antistrychnine effects in mice similar to meprobamate. In cats it is about twice as potent in causing muscle relaxation and ten times as potent in blocking the flexor reflex."[13] Chemical analysis in 1958 showed that methylamine treatment of the precursor quinazoline-3-oxide had not yielded the expected derivative. Instead, a rearrangement and enlargement of the heterocyclic ring occurred, yielding a substituted 1,4-benzodiazepine, specifically, 2-methylamino-7-chloro-5-phenyl-3H-1,4-benzodiazepine 4-oxide (Fig. 1-1), a seven-membered ring structure. Thus, Ro 5-0690 was not a quinazoline-3-oxide compound like its 40 inert predecessors. The new drug received the trivial designation methaminodiazepoxide, later changed to chlordiazepoxide (CDX). The pure preparation is a water-soluble, colorless crystalline material existing as a hydrochloride conjugate. When exposed to ultraviolet light, isomerization of the N-oxide occurs, forming an oxaziridine with a higher melting point and different pharmacologic properties[14] (Fig. 1-2). Although the original structure can be restored by heating or treatment with acid, the clinical implication is that the drug must be protected from light. Chlordiazepoxide is likewise unstable in solution, and preparations for parenteral administration must be freshly mixed and used immediately.

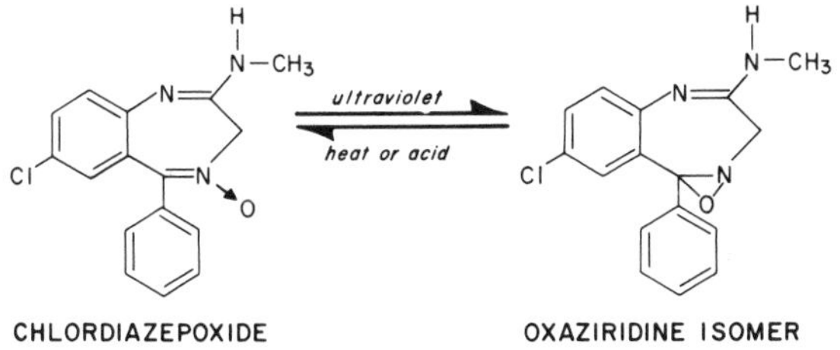

CHLORDIAZEPOXIDE   OXAZIRIDINE ISOMER

FIG. 1-2. Photoisomerization of chlordiazepoxide.

Detailed accounts of the pharmacology of chlordiazepoxide appeared in 1960.[13,15] The most striking effects were the behavioral changes induced in aggressive animals. Vicious Macaque monkeys given chlordiazepoxide (1 mg/kg orally) became calm and tame; 10 times that dose could be given before ataxia and somnolence were observed. Similar taming could be produced by meprobamate, chlorpromazine, and phenobarbital, but with these three drugs the taming dose produced ataxia and somnolence. In rats made aggressive and irritable by stereotactic septal brain lesions, chlordiazepoxide reduced irritability in doses (11 mg/kg intraperitoneally) 10 times smaller than those which reduced locomotor activity. "Quieting" and muscle relaxation in cats were noted with 10 mg/kg orally; after 3 mg/kg intravenously, objective depression of spinal reflexes could be demonstrated. In rats without brain lesions, shock-motivated avoidance and escape behavior were suppressed by chlordiazepoxide, as if the animals no longer feared the punishment.

Anticonvulsant effects were also prominent. The incidence of pentylenetetrazol-induced convulsions in mice (125 mg/kg subcutaneously) was reduced by 50% in animals pretreated with chlordiazepoxide (18 mg/kg orally). Chlordiazepoxide was also effective, although less strikingly so, against shock-induced seizures. In rats, anti-inflammatory and analgesic effects of chlordiazepoxide were shown after 12.5 mg/kg orally. A final interesting property was appetite stimulation seen with chronic administration in rats and dogs. Daily oral doses of 60 mg/kg produced increased food consumption in rats as well as a statistically significant enhancement of weight gain in comparison to controls. Similar effects occurred in dogs given 10 to 15 mg/kg per day for 3 months.

Toxicity was minimal. In mice the 50% lethal dose (LD_{50}) was 720 mg/kg by the oral route and 268 mg/kg intraperitoneally; chronic administration of large doses to rats and dogs produced no evidence of hematologic or hepatic toxicity. Teratogenic effects were also absent. Acute intravenous administration to dogs (1 mg/kg) caused no significant alteration of heart rate or blood pressure. The remarkable taming and seizure-preventing properties of chlordiazepoxide seemed unaccompanied by significant toxicity in these animal studies.[16]

EARLY CLINICAL STUDIES

In November 1959, a group of investigators gathered at the University of Texas Medical Branch in Galveston to present the results of early clinical trials with chlordiazepoxide. The proceedings of the symposium appeared in March 1960, as a supplement to *Diseases of the Nervous System*, and have been summarized and discussed in several publications.[17-20] Later in 1960, papers by other investigators, both American and European, began to appear in the medical and psychiatric literature.

Most of these papers dealt with the use of chlordiazepoxide in anxious nonpsychotic patients seen by psychiatrists, internists, and general practitioners. Twenty articles described the results of treatment in a total of 1,137 patients.[21-40] Of these, 810 (71%) were considered meaningfully improved with chlordiazepoxide. None of these studies was controlled. Several other authors studied chlordiazepoxide in schizophrenic patients. Frain[41] treated 169 acutely psychotic females with chlordiazepoxide, 75 mg/day. Seventy-nine percent became quieter and more cooperative, but in none was an improvement in thought disorder or other schizophrenic manifestations noted; the other 21% deteriorated. Smith[42] noted similar effects in an uncontrolled trial in 143 psychotic patients. However, in a smaller placebo-controlled study in this same chronic schizophrenic population, chlordiazepoxide produced no significant benefit. Weckowicz and Ward[43] also reported that high doses of chlordiazepoxide (150 mg/day) were not significantly different from placebo in a study involving hospitalized schizophrenic females. Accounts of the use of chlordiazepoxide in affective disorders were also published in 1960. Pignataro and Hoffmann[44] recommended combining chlordiazepoxide and isocarboxazide in the treatment of depressed and anxious patients. In an uncontrolled trial, English[45] treated 87 depressed individuals with chlordiazepoxide. Although the drug did not seem to have a mood-elevating or antidepressant effect, reduction in anxiety was noted in all patients.

Preliminary results in other disorders were also promising. Three groups were encouraged by the effects of chlordiazepoxide in acute and chronic alcoholism.[46–48] Two others described the first trials of chlordiazepoxide in convulsive disorders.[49,50] Robinson used the drug in a large number of patients with various dermatologic conditions exacerbated by emotion.[51] The results were good. McGovern and associates[52] conducted a crossover trial in patients with allergic disorders, including rhinitis, eczema, and asthma. Chlordiazepoxide was effective in reducing overt anxiety and dermatologic complaints in 80% of patients, whereas only 8% improved on placebo.

These early investigators were alert to the toxic effects of chlordiazepoxide. Nearly all described manifestations of central nervous system depression: drowsiness, somnolence, lethargy, dysarthria, or ataxia. The incidence is impossible to estimate, since the effects were dose-dependent. Of patients receiving 50 to 75 mg/day or more, oversedation occurred in a significant proportion.[53] In most cases, manifestations disappeared when dosage was lowered. Lemere[54] described four cases in which chlordiazepoxide produced an ethanolic-like state of intoxication. One patient fell asleep at meals, his head dropping onto his plate of food; another fell and fractured her sacrum while "Libriumized." Murray[55] claimed that chlordiazepoxide produced an insidious deterioration of mood and motor function. Of 68 automobile drivers taking the drug over a 3-month period, 16 were involved in automobile accidents—a 10-fold increase over the expected incidence. Impaired motor function caused by chlordiazepoxide was presumed to be the basis for this increase. Most of these early observations of drowsiness were uncontrolled or anecdotal, but it was obvious that high doses of chlordiazepoxide could produce central depression similar to other sedative-hypnotics.

Other side effects were less common. A number of authors noted weight gain during chlordiazepoxide therapy,[21,29,32,50,51] consistent with the appetite-stimulating effects seen in animal studies. Another interesting finding in a number of cases was an increase in hostility or rage.[21,27,29,35,37,42] This effect was considered paradoxical because of chlordiazepoxide's reputation as a taming agent. One taciturn schoolteacher struck his wife of 20 years for the first time shortly after beginning chlordiazepoxide therapy.[36] This release of hostility has subsequently been noted by others in controlled animal and human experiments and will be described in later chapters. The phenomenon probably represents a drug-induced release of anxiety-bound hostility, or a dose-dependent disinhibition similar to that seen with ethanol.

Other side effects are nonspecific and are reported to some degree in all drug trials, whether the agents being tested are pharmacologically active or inert. These include headache, constipation, diarrhea, nausea, palpitations, rash, increased sexual potency, decreased sexual potency, tremor, and blurring of vision. Kaebling[56] described an episode of nonfatal granulocytopenia in a young female occurring shortly after chlordiazepoxide therapy was begun. The association may have been a fortuitous one, but the report nevertheless raised for the first time the possibility of hematologic toxicity in humans.

Published clinical studies of chlordiazepoxide in 1960 were encouraging. The drug seemed to be sufficiently beneficial for anxious neurotic individuals to warrant widespread controlled trial. Toxicity was generally mild and could be handled by adjustment of dosage; in very few instances were adverse effects disabling. Although psychotic patients seemed to benefit little from the drug, other studies suggested that chlordiazepoxide might be of use in convulsive disorders and in alcoholism. Carrying the brand name of Librium®, chlordiazepoxide was approved for marketing by the Food and Drug Administration (FDA) on February 24, 1960. Each year since, the literature describing the treatment of anxiety and other disorders with this agent has become more massive. Industry chemists, meanwhile, turned to synthesizing structural analogues of chlordiazepoxide in the hope of finding compounds with enhanced pharmacologic activity and reduced toxicity.

MORE BENZODIAZEPINES

Much of the further tedious work of synthesis, purification, and pharmacologic screening of 1,4-benzodiazepines also took place at Roche Laboratories. Diazepam was synthesized by Sternbach in 1959 and its pharmacology was described in 1961.[57] Chemically, diazepam differs from chlordiazepoxide in several ways (Fig. 1-3). The 1,2 double bond is reduced, and the methamino group in position 2 is replaced by a ketone. N-1 is methyl-substituted, and the N-4 oxide is omitted. Diazepam has the same order of toxicity as chlordiazepoxide, but it is five to 10 times more potent in muscle-relaxant, antidecerebrate rigidity, and anticonvulsant effects. Diazepam was marketed as Valium® and released by the FDA for use in December 1963. Further work yielded a third compound, nitrazepam, which has a nitro- instead of a chloro- in position 7 and is unsubstituted at position 1. This alteration greatly increased anti-pentylenetetrazol activity while simultaneously reducing toxicity.[58] Much of the pharmacologic data on

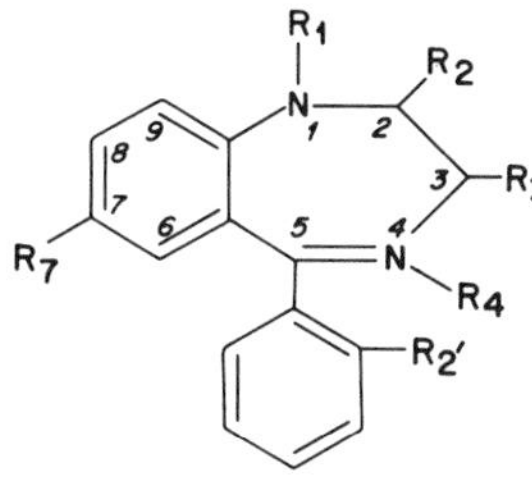

FIG. 1-3. 1,4-Benzodiazepine nucleus.

nitrazepam appear in French and German. The drug at present is not available for clinical use in the United States, but it has been widely used in Europe since 1965 as a nonbarbiturate hypnotic under the trade name Mogadon®. The N-1 methyl derivative of nitrazepam has been screened and described by Japanese pharmacologists.[59]

Several other benzodiazepines originating from investigators at Roche are of some significance. Flurazepam has a 2´-fluoro substitution and a novel diethylaminoethyl group at position 1, while retaining the 2-ketone.[60] This agent was introduced in the United States in 1970 as Dalmane® and has proved to be a safe and effective hypnotic. Medazepam (Nobrium®) is a diazepam analogue with the 2-ketone omitted, and is used abroad as an antianxiety agent of potency close to that of chlordiazepoxide.[61,62] Demoxepam, formed by removal of the 2-methamino group from chlordiazepoxide, is in fact an *in vivo* metabolite of chlordiazepoxide which possesses pharmacologic activity of its own.[63] Likewise, the metabolites of diazepam formed by 1-demethylation and 3-hydroxylation are pharmacologically active.[63] The 3-hydroxy derivative of diazepam (Ro 5-5345) is in fact marketed as a psychotropic drug (temazepam) by an Italian pharmaceutical firm.[64] Flunitrazepam (Ro 5-4200) and clonazepam (Ro 5-4023) are nitrazepam analogues with potent sedative properties currently under investigation as hypnotic and anticonvulsant agents, respectively.

Wyeth Laboratories has produced another important group of 1,4-benzodiazepines. These investigators have worked primarily with 3-hydroxy derivatives. Oxazepam, synthesized in 1961 by S. C. Bell, was of intermediate potency between chlordiazepoxide and diazepam, but seemed to be less toxic than either of these two drugs.[65] Wyeth researchers attributed this to the 3-hydroxy group, necessary for conjugation to glucuronide and detoxification, which was already present, thus obviating the need for further biotransformation before detoxification. They correctly point out that oxazepam glucuronide is a major metabolite of diazepam in most *in vivo* systems. Oxazepam has been available since 1965 in the United States, marketed as Serax®. 2´-Chloro substitution of oxazepam produces a marked increase in potency.[66,67] This analogue (lorazepam) is among the benzodiazepines with the greatest milligram potency.

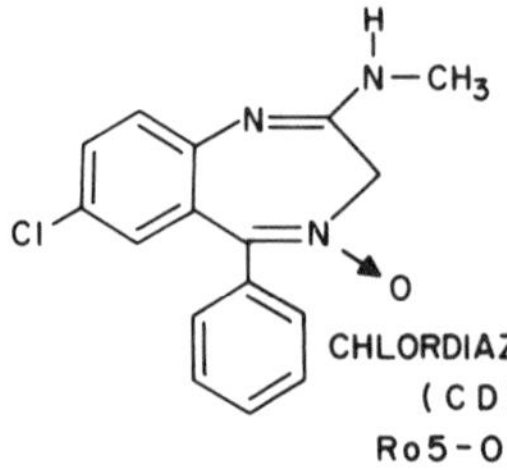

CHLORDIAZEPOXIDE
(C D X)
Ro5 - 0690

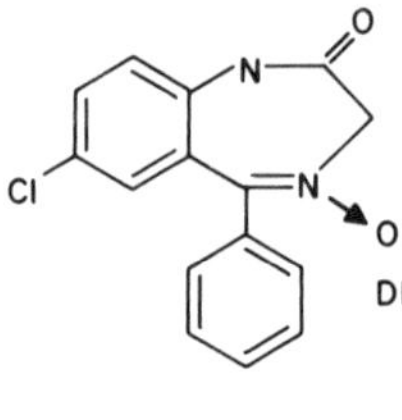

DEMOXEPAM (DMX)
LACTAM
Ro 5 - 2092

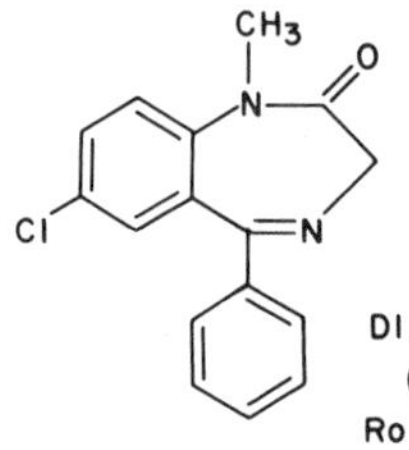

DIAZEPAM
(D Z)
Ro 5 - 2807

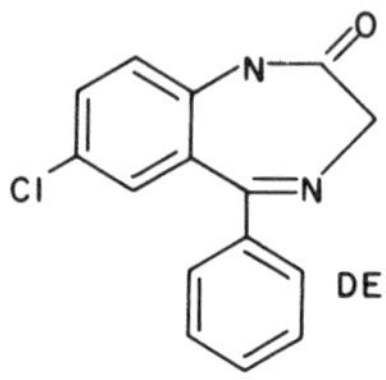

DESMETHYLDIAZEPAM
(DMDZ)
Ro 5 - 2180

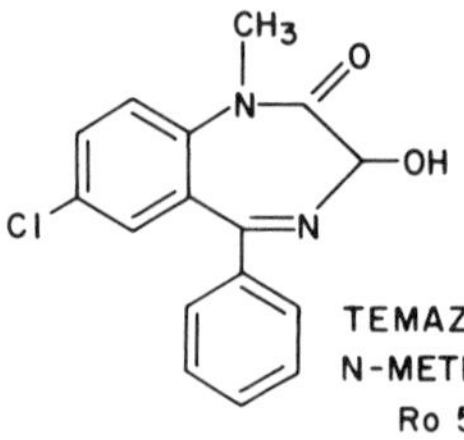

TEMAZEPAM (T M Z)
N-METHYLOXAZEPAM
Ro 5 - 5 3 4 5
Wy 2 9 1 7

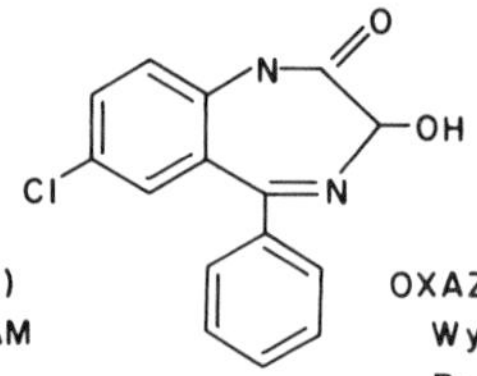

OXAZEPAM (OXZ)
Wy 3498
Ro5 - 6789

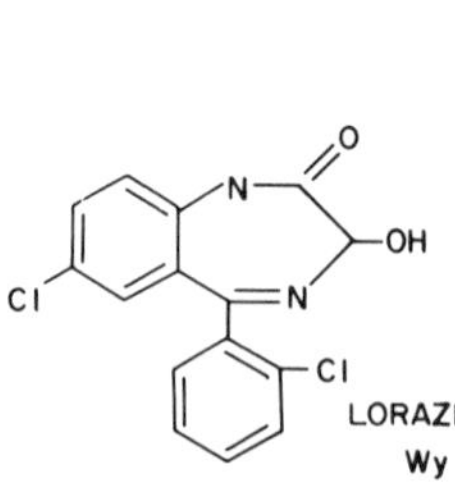

LORAZEPAM (L R Z)
Wy 4036

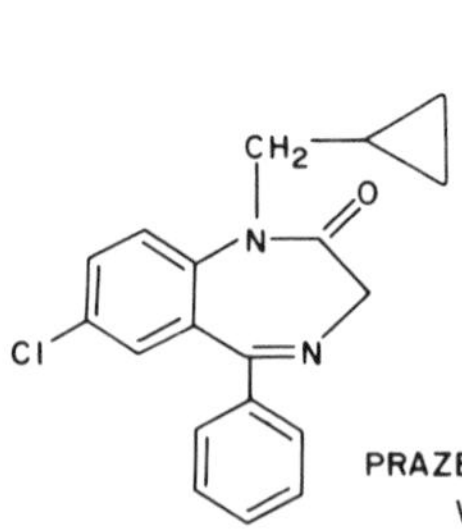

PRAZEPAM (PRZ)
W 4020

FIG. 1-4. Structural formulas of important benzodiazepine derivatives.

NITRAZEPAM
(NTZ)
Ro 4-5360
Ro 5-3059

CLONAZEPAM
(CNZ)
Ro 5-4023

FLURAZEPAM
(FLZ)
Ro5-6901

NIMETAZEPAM
(NMTZ)
S-1530

MEDAZEPAM
(MDZ)
Ro 5-4556

CHLORAZEPATE
(CZP)
4306-SB
AB35616

BROMAZEPAM
(BMZ)
Ro5-3350

FLUNITRAZEPAM
(FNTZ)
Ro5-4200

Prazepam, a product of the Warner-Lambert Research Institute, has an N-1 cyclopropylmethyl group in place of the N-1 methyl of diazepam.[68] The large alkyl side chain imparts resistance to metabolic degradation, such that prazepam may have promise as a long-acting benzodiazepine tranquilizer. Dipotassium chlorazepate[69] (Tranxene®) has been marketed in France since 1968 and in the United States since October 1972, by Abbott Laboratories. A number of other benzodiazepines have been described and are currently under investigation.[70-77]

Figure 1-4 shows the chemical structures, generic names, and code designations of some of the more important benzodiazepine derivatives. Also included are the abbreviations used in this volume. A discussion of the synthetic methods and chemical properties of these compounds is beyond the scope of this book, but in Appendix 1 an extensive bibliography is provided for chemists and other investigators who may find these references helpful.

STRUCTURE-ACTIVITY RELATIONSHIPS

Intensive pharmacologic screening of hundreds of 1,4-benzodiazepines has generated a great deal of information regarding the relationship of chemical structure to pharmacologic activity in animals. At the present time a number of important generalizations are possible.[10-12,78-80]

The benzodiazepines appear to fall into two subcategories: the 2-amino-4-oxides and the 1,3-dihydro-2-ketones (Fig. 1-5). Chlordiazepoxide belongs to the first group and is among the most active. The 2-methylamino substitution ($R_N = CH_3$, $R'_N = H$) seems to be optimal: activity is reduced with no substitution ($R_N = R'_N = H$) or with larger acyl groups. Any substitution in position 3 also lowers potency. An electronegative group in position 7 is essential for psychopharmacologic activity. 7-Chloro substitution

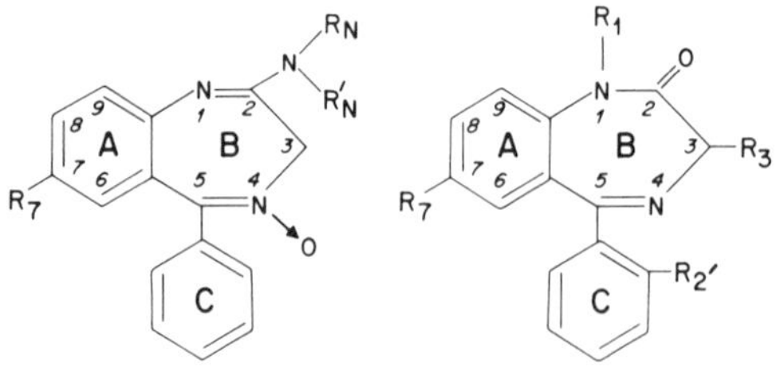

2-amino-4-oxides   1, 3-dihydro-2-ketones

FIG. 1-5. Structural skeletons of pharmacologically active benzodiazepines.

is among the best; 7-trifluoromethyl (R_7 = CF_3) substitution increases anticonvulsant properties. 7-Bromo and 7-nitro compounds are pharmacologically active, but less so than the 7-chloro compound. Replacement at R_7 with hydrogen or a methyl group markedly reduces activity. The phenyl substitution at position 5 is essential for optimal activity; all other substitutions reduce potency.

Nearly all of the other clinically useful benzodiazepines belong to the 1,3-dihydro-2-ketone group and in general have greater overall potency per milligram than the chlordiazepoxide analogues. Again, electronegativity is necessary in position 7, with greater electron "draw" enhancing potency. 7-Trifluoromethyl substitution produces greatest potency. 7-Nitro, -bromo, -chloro, and -fluoro analogues have decreasing potency in the order indicated. 7-Cyano and 7-nitro substitutions are approximately equivalent. Other analogues (R_7 = H, CH_3, SCH_3, or $SOCH_3$) are far less active. Phenyl groups, although strongly electronegative, appear to reduce activity when substituted at position 7, as do other substituents of larger size. The effect of replacement at other positions on ring A is uniform: any and all substitutions at positions 6, 8, or 9 reduce activity.

The 5-phenyl group on ring B produces optimal activity. 5-Pyridyl derivatives are less active, and activity is markedly reduced by any other 5-substitution. 2′-Halogenation enhances overall potency; large 2′-substitutions, whether electronegative or electropositive, interfere with activity as do any substitutions other than *ortho* in the 5-phenyl ring. Reduction of the 4,5 double bond also adversely influences pharmacologic activity.

N-1 substitution is beneficial, with 1-methyl being optimal. 1-Ethyl, 1-allyl ($-CH_2-CH=CH_2$), 1-acetonyl ($-CH_2COCH_3$), and 1-cyclopropyl analogues are less active. Longer substituents reduce potency considerably. The 1-acetamido compound [R_1 = ($CH_2-CO-NH_2$)] has decreased muscle-relaxing and taming properties, but anticonvulsant effects in animals are equivalent to those of diazepam. Of substitutions in position 3, a methyl group or no substitution seems optimal. Electronegative groups (hydroxy or methoxy) reduce potency somewhat but also appear to reduce toxicity, possibly due to greater ease of conjugation. Larger groups reduce activity considerably. 2-Thio analogues are of low potency compared to the 2-keto compounds. Replacement of the 2-ketone by hydrogen atoms also reduces activity but to a lesser degree.

Table 1-1 presents data depicting basic pharmacologic properties of a number of benzodiazepines. For purposes of comparison, phenobarbital is also listed. These data are derived from a number of reviews and original sources. [78,81–84] The first column designates the dose which is lethal to 50% of treated mice (LD_{50}). The dose which causes 50% of treated mice to slide off a 70-degree inclined screen is given in the second column and is representative of sedative and/or muscle-relaxing effects. Taming properties are represented by the foot shock test in which mice are stimulated to fight with

Table 1-1. *Pharmacologic properties of certain 1,4-benzodiazepines**

Drug	Mice LD_{50}	Inclined screen ED_{50}	Foot shock	Cat	Anticonvulsant ED_{50} PTZ	MaxES	MinES
Chlordiazepoxide	720	100	40	2.0	8.0	30	92
Demoxepam	1,950	100	40	5.0	6.0	52	400
Diazepam	620	30	10	0.2	1.4	6	64
Desmethyldiazepam	2,750	75	20	1.0	6.0	25	130
Temazepam	1,160	20	5	0.7	0.7	12	89
Oxazepam	> 4,000	225	40	1.0	0.7	28	233
Nitrazepam	1,550	15	5	0.1	0.7	31	357
Nimetazepam	750	10	2.5	0.1	0.7	15	140
Clonazepam	> 4,000	250	2.5	0.1	0.2	400	800
Flurazepam	870	200	20	2.0	1.6	82	84
Prazepam	> 2,000	100	10	0.5	4.1	62	300
Medazepam	1,070	150	20	4.0	1.6	38	> 800
Lorazepam	> 3,000				0.1	2	
Chlorazepate	700				1.7	5	
Bromazepam	2,350	30	10	0.2	0.7	34	122
Flunitrazepam	1,380	1	0.8	0.02	0.1	10	135
Phenobarbital	242	120	80	50	26.0	12	90

*All doses are in mg/kg body weight orally. See text for explanation of parameters depicted.

other animals by electric shock delivered to the cage floor. The minimum effective dose to prevent fighting is given in the third column. The minimum effective dose producing sedation and muscle relaxation in unanesthetized cats is shown in the next column. The final three columns depict anticonvulsant effects in mice, given as the dose effective in preventing induced seizures in 50% of the animals (ED_{50}). Convulsions were induced by three methods which are standard in animal testing: subcutaneous pentylenetetrazol (PTZ), 125 mg/kg; maximal electroshock (MaxES); and minimal electroshock (MinES).

Many of the structure-activity relationships previously described are illustrated in the table. The difficulties in predicting effects in humans on the basis of the animal data are monumental[85,86] and will be discussed in subsequent chapters.

COMMENT

The 1,4-benzodiazepines displayed remarkable sedative and anticonvulsant properties in animal studies. Early published clinical results seemed to underscore the wide range of utility of these compounds, but reports appearing in 1960 were suggestive rather than conclusive. Many years and numerous controlled studies were necessary before the psychotropic efficacy of chlordiazepoxide and its analogues was firmly established.

REFERENCES

1. Berger FM: The tranquilizer decade. J Neuropsychiat 5:403-410, 1964
2. Rumpf GE: *Herbari Amboinensis Actuarium.* Amsterdam; Mynard, Uytwerf et al; 1755
3. Klerman GL: Historical baselines for the evaluation of maintenance drug therapy of discharged psychiatric patients. In, *Mental Patients in Transition.* Edited by M Greenblatt, DJ Levinson, GL Klerman. Springfield, Illinois, Charles C. Thomas, 1961, pp 287-302
4. Berger FM: The pharmacological properties of 2-methyl-2-n-propyl-1,3-propanediol dicarbamate (Miltown), a new interneuronal blocking agent. J Pharmacol Exp Ther 112:413-423, 1954
5. Berger FM: The chemistry and mode of action of tranquilizing drugs. Ann NY Acad Sci 67:685-700, 1957
6. Laties VG, Weiss B: A critical review of the efficacy of meprobamate (Miltown, Equanil) in the treatment of anxiety. J Chronic Dis 7:500-519, 1958
7. Greenblatt DJ, Shader RI: Meprobamate: a study of irrational drug use. Amer J Psychiat 127:1297-1303, 1971
8. Cohen IM: The benzodiazepines. In, *Discoveries in Biological Psychiatry.* Edited by FJ Ayd, B Blackwell. Philadelphia, JB Lippincott, 1970, pp 130-141
9. Sternbach LH: The discovery of Librium®. Agents and Actions 2:193-196, 1972
10. Sternbach LH: Chemistry of 1,4-benzodiazepines and some aspects of the structure-activity relationship. In, *The Benzodiazepines.* Edited by S Garattini, E Mussini, LO Randall. New York, Raven Press, 1973, pp 1-26
11. Sternbach LH: 1,4-Benzodiazepines. Chemistry and some aspects of the structure-activity relationship. Agnew Chem (Internat Edit) 10:34-43, 1971
12. Sternbach LH, Randall LO: Some aspects of the structure-activity relationship in psychotropic agents of the 1,4-benzodiazepine class. In, *CNS Drugs.* Edited by GS Sidhu et al. New Delhi, Council of Scientific Research, 1966, pp 53-69
13. Randall LO, Schallek W, Heise GA, Keith EF, Bagdon RE: The psychosedative properties of methaminodiazepoxide. J Pharmacol Exp Ther 129:163-171, 1960
14. Sternbach LH, Koechlin BA, Reeder E: Quinazolines and 1,4-benzodiazepines. (VIII). The photoisomerization of 7-chloro-2-methylamino-5-phenyl-3H-1,4-benzodiazepine 4-oxide. J Org Chem 27:4671-4672, 1962
15. Randall LO: Pharmacology of methaminodiazepoxide. Dis Nerv Syst 21 (March supp):7-10, 1960
16. Randall LO: Pharmacology of chlordiazepoxide (Librium). Dis Nerv Syst 22(July supp):7-15, 1961
17. Marks J: Methaminodiazepoxide (Librium): a new psychotropic drug. Chemother Rev 1:141-144, 1960
18. Harris TH: Methaminodiazepoxide. JAMA 172:1162-1163, 1960
19. Hines LR: Methaminodiazepoxide (Librium): a psychotherapeutic drug. Curr Ther Res 2:227-236, 1960
20. Hayman M: The effects of Librium in psychiatric disorders. Dis Nerv Syst 22 (July supp):60-69, 1961
21. Tobin JM, Lewis NDC: New psychotherapeutic agent, chlordiazepoxide. JAMA 174:1242-1249, 1960
22. Sussex JN: The use of Librium in office treatment of mixed neurotic states. Dis Nerv Syst 21 (March supp):53-56, 1960

23. Thomas LJ: Preliminary observation on the use of Librium (Ro 5-0690) in internal medicine. Dis Nerv Syst 21 (March supp):40-42, 1960

24. Constant GA: Preliminary report on the use of a new agent in depression and tension states. Dis Nerv Syst 21 (March supp):37-39, 1960

25. Breitner C: Drug therapy in obsessional states and other psychiatric problems. Dis Nerv Syst 21 (March supp):31-35, 1960

26. Farb HH: Experience with Librium in clinical psychiatry. Dis Nerv Syst 21 (March supp):27-30, 1960

27. Kinross-Wright J, Cohen IM, Knight JA: The management of neurotic and psychotic states with Ro 5-0690 (Librium). Dis Nerv Syst 21 (March supp):23-26, 1960

28. Bowes HA: The role of Librium in an out-patient psychiatric setting. Dis Nerv Syst 21 (March supp):20-22, 1960

29. Tobin JM, Bird IF, Boyle DE: Preliminary evaluation of Librium (Ro 5-0690) in the treatment of anxiety reactions. Dis Nerv Syst 21 (March supp):11-19, 1960

30. Darling HF: Use of Librium in 100 private patients. Dis Nerv Syst 21:691-694, 1960

31. Toll N: Librium as an adjunct to psychotherapy in private psychiatric practice. Dis Nerv Syst 21:264-266, 1960

32. Hirshleifer I: The use of chlordiazepoxide in cardiovascular disorders. Curr Ther Res 2:501-508, 1960

33. Pernikoff M: Clinical results with Librium in a private nonpsychiatric practice. Clin Med 67:2313-2318, 1960

34. Pignataro FP: Clinical experience with Librium in private psychiatric practice. Clin Med 67:1133-1143, 1960

35. Walzer RS, Kurland ML, Braun M: Clinical trial of methaminodiazepoxide (Librium). Amer J Psychiat 117:456-457, 1960

36. Ingram IM, Timbury GC: Side-effects of Librium. Lancet 2:766, 1960

37. Denham J: Side-effects of Librium. Lancet 2:875, 1960

38. Berkwitz NJ: Clinical experience with Librium in private practice. Minnesota Med 43:463-465, 1960

39. Usdin GL: Preliminary report on Librium, a new psychopharmacologic agent. J Louisiana State Med Soc 112:142-147, 1960

40. Kagan G: Side-effects of Librium. Lancet 2:876, 1960

41. Frain MK: Physical, mental, and emotional effects of Librium in hospitalized psychotic patients. Dis Nerv Syst 21:453-457, 1960

42. Smith ME: A comparative controlled study with chlordiazepoxide. Amer J Psychiat 117:362-363, 1960

43. Weckowicz TE, Ward T: Clinical trial of Ro 5-0690 and chlorpromazine on disturbed chronic schizophrenic patients. Dis Nerv Syst 21:527-528, 1960

44. Pignataro FP, Hoffmann GT: Bipolar management of neuropsychiatric disorders. Dis Nerv Syst 21:629-634, 1960

45. English DC: Librium, a new non-sedative neuroleptic drug: a clinical evaluation. Curr Ther Res 2:88-91, 1960

46. Lawrence FE, Johnson JM, Webster AP, Schwartz L: Chlordiazepoxide in the treatment of alcoholism. J Neuropsychiat 2:93-101, 1960

47. Speight PH: Notes on the use of "Librium" in the treatment of alcoholism. Med J Aust 2:741-742, 1960

48. Ticktin HE, Schultz JD: Librium, a new quieting drug for hyperactive alcoholic and psychotic patients. (Preliminary study). Dis Nerv Syst 21 (March supp):49-52, 1960

49. Rosenstein IN: A new psychosedative (Librium) as an anticonvulsant in grand mal type convulsive seizures. Dis Nerv Syst 21 (March supp):57-60, 1960

50. Kaim SC, Rosenstein IN: Anticonvulsant properties of a new psychotherapeutic drug. Dis Nerv Syst 21 (March supp):46-48, 1960

51. Robinson RCV: Adjunctive therapy of dermatoses with Librium. Dis Nerv Syst 21 (March supp):43-45, 1960

52. McGovern JP, Ozkaragoz K, Barkin G, Haywood T, McElhenny T, Hensel AE: Studies of chlordiazepoxide in various allergic diseases. Ann Allergy 18:1193-1199, 1960

53. Fullerton AG, Bethell MS: Side-effects of Librium. Lancet 2:875, 1960

54. Lemere F: Toxic reactions to chlordiazepoxide. JAMA 174:893, 1960

55. Murray N: Methaminodiazepoxide. JAMA 173:1760-1761, 1960

56. Kaebling R, Conrad FG: Agranulocytosis due to chlordiazepoxide hydrochloride. JAMA 174:1863-1865, 1960

57. Randall LO, Heise GA, Schallek W, Bagdon RE, Banziger R, Boris A, Moe RA, Abrams WB: Pharmacological and clinical studies on Valium®, a new psychotherapeutic agent of the benzodiazepine class. Curr Ther Res 3:405-425, 1961

58. Hernandez-Peon R, Rojas-Ramirez JA: Central mechanisms of tranquilizing, anticonvulsant, and relaxant actions of Ro 4-5360. Int J Neuropharmacol 5:263-267, 1966

59. Sakai S, Kitagawa S, Yamamoto H: Pharmacological studies on 1-methyl-7-nitro-5-phenyl-1,3-dihydro-2H-1,4-benzodiazepin-2-one (S-1530). Arzneim-Forsch 22:534-539, 1972

60. Randall LO, Schallek W, Scheckel CL, Stefko PL, Banziger RF, Pool W, Moe RA: Pharmacological studies on flurazepam hydrochloride (RO 5-6901), a new psychotropic agent of the benzodiazepine class. Arch Int Pharmacodyn 178:216-241, 1969

61. Randall LO, Scheckel CL, Pool W: Pharmacology of medazepam and metabolites. Arch Int Pharmacodyn 185:135-148, 1970

62. Schallek W, Kovacs J, Kuehn A, Thomas J: Some observations on the neuropharmacology of medazepam hydrochloride (Ro 5-4556). Arch Int Pharmacodyn 185:149-158, 1970

63. Randall LO, Scheckel CL, Banziger RF: Pharmacology of the metabolites of chlordiazepoxide and diazepam. Curr Ther Res 7:590-606, 1965

64. Mille T, Pastorino G, Arrigo A: A new benzodiazepine: electroencephalographic studies of its anticonvulsant activity in non-anesthetized, non-curarized rabbits. Arzneim-Forsch 19:730-735, 1969

65. Gluckman MI: Pharmacology of oxazepam (Serax), a new antianxiety agent. Curr Ther Res 7:721-740, 1965

66. Owen G. Hatfield GK, Pollock JJ, Steinberg AJ, Tucker WE, Agersborg HPK: Toxicity studies of lorazepam, a new benzodiazepine, in animals. Arzneim-Forsch 21:1065-1073, 1971

67. Gluckman MI: Pharmacology of 7-chloro-5-(o-chlorophenyl)-1,3-dihydro-3-hydroxy-2H-1,4-benzodiazepin-2-one (Lorazepam; Wy 4036). Arzneim-Forsch 21:1049-1055, 1971

68. Robichaud RC, Gylys JA, Sledge KL, Hillyard IW: The pharmacology of prazepam, a new benzodiazepine derivative. Arch Int Pharmacodyn 185:213-227, 1970

69. Brunaud M, Navarro J, Salle J, Siou G: Pharmacological, toxicological, and teratological studies on dipotassium-7-chloro-3-carboxy-1,3-dihydro-2,2-dihydroxy-5-phenyl-2H-1,4-benzodiazepine—chlorazepate (dipotassium chlorazepate, 4306 CB), a new tranquillizer. Arzneim-Forsch 20:123-125, 1970

70. Rudzik AD, Hester JB, Tang AH, Straw RN, Friis W: Triazolobenzodiazepines, a new class of central nervous system-depressant compounds. In, The Benzodiazepines. Edited by S Garattini, E Mussini, LO Randall. New York, Raven Press, 1973, pp 285-297

71. Gordon M, Pachter IJ, Wilson JW: A trifluoromethyl benzodiazepine derivative. Arzneim-Forsch 13:802-804, 1963

72. Nakajima R, Take Y, Moriya R, Saji Y, Yui T, Nagawa Y: Pharmacological studies on new potent central depressants, 8-chloro-6-phenyl-4H-s-triazolo[4,3a][1,4] benzodiazepine (D-40TA), and its 1-methyl analogue (D-65 MT). Jap J Pharmacol 21:497-519, 1971

73. Nakajima R, Hattori C, Nagawa Y: Structure-activity relationship of s-triazolo-1,4-benzodiazepines in central nervous depressant action. Jap J Pharmacol 21: 489-495, 1971

74. Nakanishi M, Tsumagari T, Takigawa Y, Shuto S, Kenjo T, Fukuda T: Studies on psychotropic drugs. XIX. Pharmacological studies of 1-methyl-5-o-chlorophenyl-7-ethyl-1,2-dihydro-3H-thieno [2,3-e] [1,4] diazepin-2-one (Y-6047). Arzneim-Forsch 22:1905-1914, 1972

75. Kamioka T, Takagi H, Kobayashi S, Suzuki Y: Pharmacological studies on 10-chloro-11b-(2-chlorophenyl)-2, 3, 5, 6, 7, 11b-hexahydrobenzo-[6, 7]-1,4-benzodiazepino [5,4-b]-oxazol-6-one (CS-370), a new psychosedative agent. Arzneim-Forsch 22:884-891, 1972

76. Itil TM, Saletu B, Marasa J, Mucciardi AN: Digital computer analyzed awake and sleep EEG (sleep prints) in predicting the effects of a triazolobenzodiazepine (U-31,889). Pharmacopsychiat Neuro-Psychopharmacokol 5:225-240, 1972

77. Itil T, Gannon P, Cora R, Polvan N, Akpinar S, Elveris F, Eskazan E: SCH-12,041, a new anti-anxiety agent (Quantitative pharmaco-electroencephalography and clinical trials). Behav Neuropsychiat 4:15-24, (Aug-Sept) 1972

78. Sternbach LH, Randall LO, Banziger R, Lehr H: Structure-activity relationships in the 1,4-benzodiazepine series. In, *Drugs Affecting the Central Nervous System*, vol 2. Edited by A Burger. New York, Marcel Dekker, Inc., 1968, pp 237-264

79. Childress SJ, Gluckman MI: 1,4-benzodiazepines. J Pharmaceut Sci 53:577-590, 1964

80. Moffett RB, Rudzik AD: Central nervous system depressants. 10. 1-Carbamoyl-benzodiazapines. J Med Chem 15:1079-1081, 1972

81. Randall LO, Schallek W: Pharmacological activity of certain benzodiazepines. In, *Psychopharmacology: A Review of Progress 1957-1967.* Edited by DH Efron. Washington, D.C., USPHS publication #1836, 1968, pp 153-184

82. Sternbach LH, Randall LO, Gustafson SR: 1,4-benzodiazepines (chlordiazepoxide and related compounds). In, *Psychopharmacological Agents*, vol I. Edited by M Gordon. New York, Academic Press, 1964, pp 137-224

83. Jindal MN, Doctor RB, Kelkar VV, Choksey HK: Certain aspects of pharmacological profiles of chlordiazepoxide and diazepam. Indian J Physiol Pharmacol 12:141-152, 1968

84. Randall LO, Kappell B: Pharmacological activity of some benzodiazepines and their metabolites. In, *The Benzodiazepines*. Edited by S Garattini, E Mussini, LO Randall. New York, Raven Press, 1973, pp 27-51

85. Loew DM: Methods of evaluation of anxiolytics. In, *Advances in Neuro-Psychopharmacology.* Edited by O Vinar, Z Votava, PB Bradley. Amsterdam, North-Holland Publishing Co., 1971, pp 155-166

86. Loew DM, Taeschler M: Profiles of activity of psychotropic drugs. A way to predict therapeutic effects. Int Pharmacopsychiat 1:1-20, 1968

Chapter 2
Detection and Quantitation

With the development of highly precise techniques of analytical chemistry, a great deal has been learned in recent years about the pharmacokinetics and metabolism of the benzodiazepines.[1,2] The field is an inherently difficult one to study. Due to extensive biotransformation and/or extensive tissue distribution, benzodiazepines are present in body fluids only in trace amounts after usual therapeutic doses, requiring the most sensitive methods for reliable quantitation. Moreover, the major metabolic products of benzodiazepines administered in therapeutic doses cannot be distinguished from the parent compounds in many analytical systems. This problem is compounded by the pharmacologic activities of the metabolites themselves, which often mimic those of the precursor drugs in intensity and duration of action. Finally, in some methods, the benzodiazepines may undergo drastic chemical alteration in the process of analysis.

In general, *qualitative* detection is easier than *quantitation*. A variety of screening procedures exist whereby blood or urine may be analyzed to detect poisons or drugs of abuse. Similar screening techniques are used in pharmaceutical analysis. Most utilize either thin-layer chromatography (TLC), gas-liquid chromatography (GLC) (with or without mass spectrometry), or spectrophotofluorometry. In many of these systems (see Appendix 2), benzodiazepine tranquilizers are detectable if present, but precise quantitation of levels in blood or urine cannot be achieved without more specific methods. This fact is important to the clinician who may not be aware of the lack of sensitivity and specificity of drug screens which are commercially available.

Some investigators have attempted quantitative analyses of benzodiazepines by liquid-solid chromatography and polarography,[3–6] but these methods have never been sufficiently sensitive for determinations of levels in body fluids after therapeutic doses. At the present time GLC is considered the most useful approach, but numerous problems are encountered. At the high column temperatures used in GLC, 3-hydroxy and N-oxide derivatives, in particular chlordiazepoxide (CDX), demoxepam (DMX), and oxazepam (OXZ), become thermolyzed to form benzophenones or rearrange to form quinazolines.[7] Only recently have GLC techniques been adapted for determinations of these benzodiazepines. Other analogues [diazepam (DZ), temazepam (TMZ), desmethyldiazepam (DMDZ), medazepam (MDZ)] are thermally stable, but in some GLC systems assay of the intact drugs does not yield optimal sensitivity.[8–11] Acid hydrolysis of the benzodiazepines to form benzophenones, together with use of the electron-capture detector, increases the sensitivity of the procedure considerably. However, the preparatory hydrolysis is time consuming; additionally, some specificity may be lost (Fig. 2-1). Diazepam and temazepam, for example, produce the same hydrolysis product (2-methamino-5-chlorobenzophenone; MACB); similarly, desmethyldiazepam

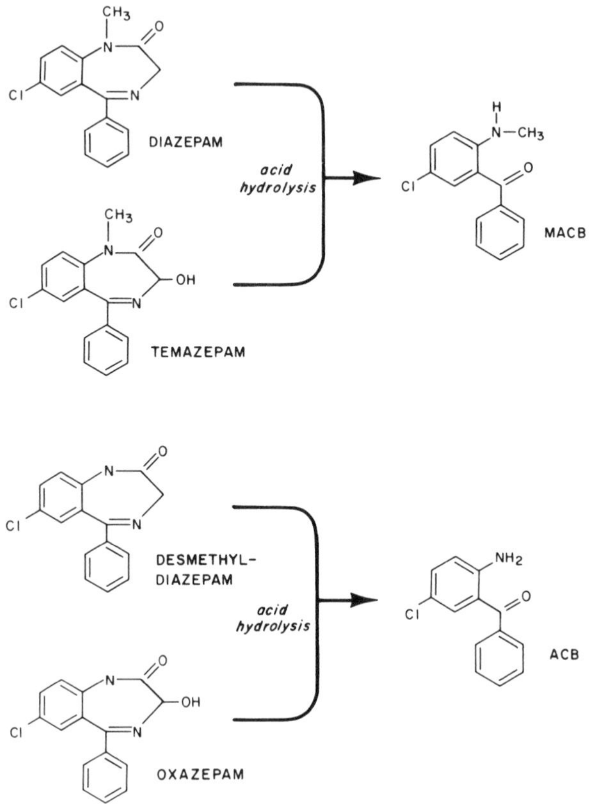

FIG. 2-1. Acid hydrolysis products of diazepam and its metabolites.

and oxazepam, when hydrolyzed, yield 2-amino-5-chlorobenzophenone (ACB). Since intact temazepam and oxazepam are only minor metabolites of diazepam in man, acid hydrolysis is acceptable for human studies of diazepam pharmacokinetics. In animal or *in vitro* studies in which these metabolites must be distinguished, sacrifice of specificity to achieve sensitivity obviously is unacceptable.

Adequate quantitative assays are now available for most or all of the benzodiazepines and their metabolites. The following sections present descriptions of these methods and their application in pharmacokinetic studies.

CHLORDIAZEPOXIDE

As described in Chapter 1, chlordiazepoxide is water soluble and sensitive to light. It has an acidic pK (4.8) and is bound to plasma protein. There are no studies of protein-binding in humans, but *in vitro* and *in vivo* investigations using dog plasma suggest that chlordiazepoxide is approximately 87 to 88% protein bound, predominantly to albumin, over a wide range of concentrations.[12]

Early studies of chlordiazepoxide pharmacokinetics in retrospect yielded somewhat misleading results, since the available quantitative assays did not distinguish chlordiazepoxide from its major metabolites desmethylchlordiazepoxide (DMCDX; Ro 5-0883) and demoxepam. Smyth and associates in 1963 described a quantitative spectrophotometric assay using the products of acid hydrolysis.[13,14] Administration of a single, large oral dose (100 mg) of chlordiazepoxide to nine volunteers resulted in average maximum total drug blood concentrations (chlordiazepoxide plus metabolites) of 5 μg/ml 5 hr following ingestion.[14] The subjects were profoundly sedated after this dose. Blood levels fell slowly, and less than 2% of the total dose was excreted unchanged in the urine in the next 48 hr. Koechlin and D'Arconte,[15] also in 1963, reported a more specific spectrofluorometric micro method sensitive to blood levels as low as 0.25 μg/ml. This assay distinguished chlordiazepoxide from demoxepam, the ultimate metabolite, but not from desmethylchlordiazepoxide, the intermediate metabolite.

Koechlin and D'Arconte estimated the half-life of chlordiazepoxide in humans (after a single oral dose of 30 mg) to be 20 to 24 hr, whereas that in dogs was 12 to 20 hr. Studies using ¹⁴C-labeled chlordiazepoxide yielded similar results (see Table 2-1).[16] Demoxepam was noted to be the major metabolite in man and dog, but desmethylchlordiazepoxide was not identified as an intermediate. Because of the nonspecificity of the assays available to these investigators, the half-life of chlordiazepoxide *per se* was

TABLE 2-1. *The metabolic fate of radiolabeled chlordiazepoxide in various animal species**

Variable	Rat	Dog	Man
Dose of ¹⁴C-CDX	4 mg/kg	4 mg/kg	15 mg
Half-life of total radioactivity	4 hr	14 hr	20-24 hr
% of total dose appearing in urine	40-45%	44%	34-60%
% of total dose appearing in feces	50-55%	44%	20%

*Koechlin et al.: J Pharmacol Exp Ther 148:399-411, 1965

overestimated. This, however, is of little clinical consequence since both metabolites of chlordiazepoxide are pharmacologically active.

In 1966, Schwartz and Postma,[17] adapting the method of Koechlin and D'Arconte,[15] first identified desmethylchlordiazepoxide as a metabolite of chlordiazepoxide during *in vitro* studies on rat liver homogenates. After a single intravenous dose of 100 mg in humans, chlordiazepoxide alone had a half-life of 14 hr, and both desmethylchlordiazepoxide and demoxepam were found in the plasma. Desmethylchlordiazepoxide was then postulated

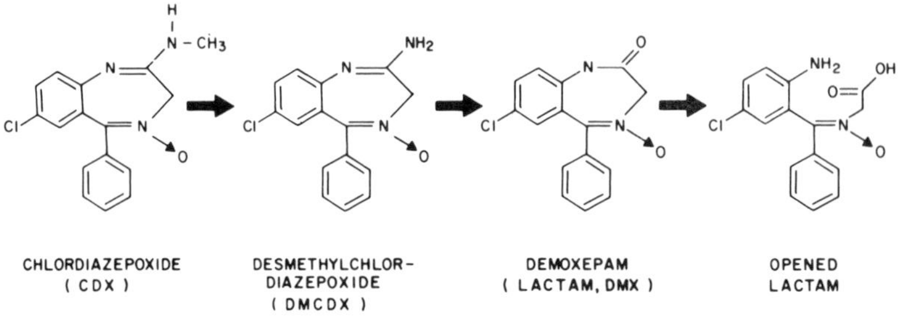

FIG.2-2. Metabolic transformations of chlordiazepoxide.

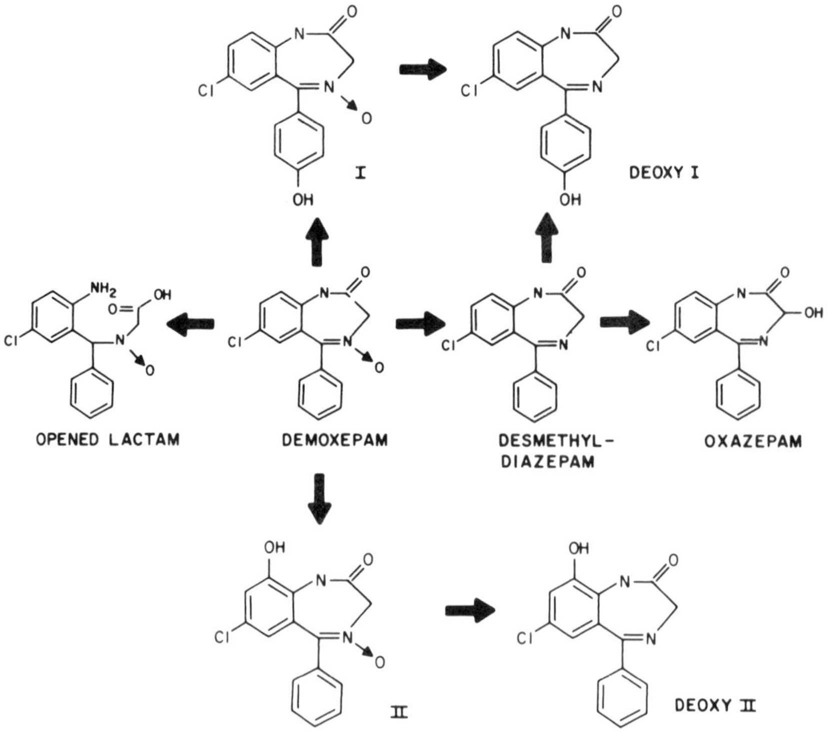

FIG. 2-3. Metabolic transformations of demoxepam.

TABLE 2-2. *Chlordiazepoxide: Pharmacokinetic scheme in the dog**

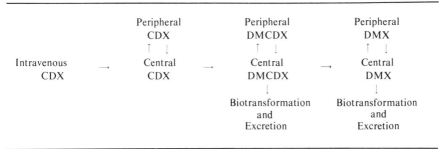

*Kaplan SA et al.: J Pharmaceut Sci 59:1569-1574, 1970

as a metabolic intermediate in humans. In subsequent studies, Schwartz and associates have elucidated the metabolic pathway of chlordiazepoxide which is currently understood as correct. A 20-mg oral dose in six human subjects produced a maximum blood level of 0.78 to 1.24 μg/ml from 2 to 6 hr after the dose.[18] Chlordiazepoxide levels then declined slowly, but with a highly variable half-life ranging from 6.6 to 28 hr. In five of the six subjects, however, the half-life was between 6.6 and 15 hr, and it would appear from this small sample that a half-life of greater duration is uncommon. Desmethyl-chlordiazepoxide can be detected in plasma at levels as high as 0.46 μg/ml anywhere from 8 to 24 hr after the dose. Demoxepam appears even later and at lower levels (Fig. 2-2). Metabolism is far from complete after the appearance of demoxepam, as can be illustrated by administration of demoxepam alone (20 mg orally).[19] This drug has a half-life in humans ranging from 14 to 95 hr, with a variety of metabolites identified, including oxazepam (Fig. 2-3). After 7 days, 60 to 64% of the total dose has appeared in the urine and 12 to 18% in the feces. Free demoxepam makes up approximately 25% of total urinary excretion, and the opened lactam another 3 to 5%. Some 15% of urinary metabolites are conjugated to glucuronide, primarily oxazepam, with lesser amounts of 5-parahydroxyphenyl and 9-hydroxy derivatives, identified as compounds I and II in Fig. 2-3. In dogs, the metabolic pattern differs slightly.[20,21] More of the total dose appears in the feces, whereas in the urine the glucuronide derivative of compound I and free demoxepam appear in approximately equal quantities. Kaplan and associates[22] have devised a pharmacokinetic model for chlordiazepoxide in the dog, summarized in Table 2-2, which has been shown to predict accurately the actual experimental results.

Gottschalk and Kaplan[23] used the fluorometric assay technique to investigate the relation between plasma levels of chlordiazepoxide and antianxiety effects. After a single oral dose of 25 mg, blood levels ranged from 0.26 to 1.63 μg/ml after 1½ to 2½ hr, with a mean of approximately 0.86 μg/ml. There appeared to be no correlation between plasma level and body weight.

Antianxiety effects, as determined by speech content analysis, were most evident among individuals with plasma levels of at least 0.7 μg/ml. These results are of interest, but the study of psychotropic drug blood levels in relation to clinical response is in a formative stage, and much more investigation is required.

Assays for chlordiazepoxide using polarography, colorimetry, and ultraviolet spectrophotometry have been described in the literature[24-26] and are useful in cases of overdosage or after large therapeutic doses. These methods are not adequate for low blood levels, and also do not distinguish chlordiazepoxide from its metabolites. Zingales[27] presented a specific GLC assay for chlordiazepoxide which is sensitive at low levels. Single oral doses of 5 mg in two volunteers produced blood levels of 0.18 μg/ml 2 hr later; after 10 mg, the level was 0.4 μg/ml. After chronic therapy with total daily doses of 75 to 150 mg, blood levels in patients were found to range from 3.2 to 6.9 μg/ml. The reliability of this GLC method has not yet been confirmed by other groups.

Autoradiographic studies have added to our knowledge of chlordiazepoxide pharmacokinetics.[28] When injected intravenously into mice, there is immediate uptake into the brain, heart, kidney, liver, and skeletal muscle. Initially, the brain radioactivity is more concentrated in the gray matter and thalamus, but within 10 min after injection the label is distributed evenly throughout the brain. There is no evidence of selective localization in limbic structures, postulated to be the site of antianxiety activity. Nor is there apparent correlation between brain distribution and sedative effects.[29] Within several hours the label becomes concentrated in excretory organs. A similar pattern is seen with diazepam and other benzodiazepines, as discussed below.

DIAZEPAM

Diazepam is lipid soluble and relatively water insoluble, and probably circulates strongly bound to serum albumin (95%) over a wide range of concentrations.[30] Parenteral administration of diazepam must utilize a nonaqueous solvent system, and the nature of the solvent may influence the bioavailability.[31] In the preparation supplied by Roche Laboratories (the composition of which is shown in Table 2-3), propylene glycol is a predominant constituent and can produce a variety of central depressant effects in animals (see Chapters 5, 7, and 12). Bioavailability after oral administration is also influenced by the formulation. One study showed that a diazepam suspension produced lower blood levels than tablets,[32] whereas another study showed no significant difference.[33] Between different tablet preparations which have been tested, however, there is no difference in bioavailability with either diazepam[32] or chlordiazepoxide.[34] Syrup preparations seem to be less well absorbed than suspensions,[35] although in one animal study absorption was enhanced by micronization of the drug.[36] In another study, rectal administra-

TABLE 2-3. *Solvent system for commercially available parenteral diazepam*

Propylene glycol	40%
Ethyl alcohol	10%
Sodium benzoate	5%
Benzyl alcohol	1.5%
Final diazepam concentration: 5 mg per ml	

tion of diazepam in suppository form produced higher overall blood levels than equivalent oral doses.[33] None of these studies is definitive, but they suggest that the question of the bioavailability of diazepam is one which cannot be neglected.

Autoradiographic studies on mice, monkeys, and cats have yielded few unexpected results.[37-42] Being lipid soluble, intravenous diazepam is rapidly taken up into fat and brain, as well as liver, kidneys, heart, and muscle. The distribution in brain within 1 hr of administration is uniform, showing no selective uptake by the limbic system. Six hr after the dose, radioactivity is concentrated in the gastrointestinal tract.

Diazepam in body fluids may be determined by polarography[43] or mass spectrometry and nuclear magnetic resonance,[44] but GLC has been the analytic mainstay. deSilva and associates[45] described the first GLC assay technique in 1964. In this report acid hydrolysis was performed prior to chromatography. deSilva and Puglisi[46] subsequently reported a method for GLC of intact diazepam using electron-capture detection. This method is adequately sensitive, and can quantitate diazepam and all of its metabolites in body fluids with no loss of specificity. Without electron capture, GLC of intact diazepam is inadequate except in cases of poisoning or overdosage.[47]

The metabolism of diazepam in man has been studied by a number of groups, and their results are in general agreement.[30,32,45,46,48-53] Diazepam is rapidly absorbed after oral administration. After a single oral dose of 10 to 15 mg, peak levels in the range of 0.2 to 0.3 μg/ml occur within 2 hr. There is wide variation between individuals.[2] Nearly all subjects show subjective signs of drowsiness in this range of plasma concentrations. Blood levels then fall, first rapidly, then slowly. The initial rapid disappearance, with a half-life of only a few hours, represents distribution, following which the drug is slowly biotransformed and excreted, with a half-life ranging between individuals from 20 to 50 hr. This biphasic elimination pattern is most marked after intravenous administration. A 10- to 20-mg dose produces a level at 4 min of about 1 μg/ml, coincident with profound clinical sedation and a short period of anterograde amnesia. Blood levels rapidly fall to about 0.25 μg/ml within an hour, accompanied by clinical "recovery." The rate of elimination then slows. Baird and Hailey[51] have noted a "resurgence" of blood levels at approximately 6 hr following the dose, at which time subjects again become drowsy. This phenomenon may be related either to

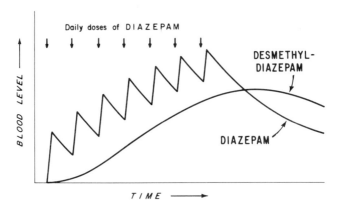

FIG. 2-4. Blood levels of diazepam and desmethyldiazepam during and after repeated daily administration of diazepam (see J Pharmaceut Sci 62:1789-1796, 1973).

mobilization of diazepam from lipid storage sites or to release of diazepam or its active metabolites from the enterohepatic circulation.

Repeated oral administration of diazepam in man leads to accumulation. If the drug is given daily in divided doses, blood levels gradually rise until a plateau is reached after 5 to 7 days of therapy. The usual plateau blood levels are in the range of 0.1 to 0.4 μg/ml, depending on the size and frequency of the doses. Pharmacologically active metabolites, temazepam and desmethyldiazepam, are detectable in the blood following a single dose.[51] After several days of therapy, blood levels of desmethyldiazepam, the major metabolite in man, begin to accumulate. At steady state (equilibrium), levels of desmethyldiazepam are close to, or may exceed, those of diazepam.[53] When therapy is stopped, levels of both drugs decline, but desmethyldiazepam, with an apparent half-life as long as 96 hr in some subjects, persists in the plasma longer than diazepam. The situation is pictured schematically in Fig. 2-4.

Radiolabeled diazepam studies in man[54] have shown that 65 to 75% of an oral dose is eventually excreted in the urine and 9 to 10% in the feces. Essentially all of the urinary products are conjugated metabolites—primarily glucuronides and, to a lesser extent, sulfates. Conjugates of oxazepam predominate over conjugates of desmethyldiazepam. Dogs metabolize diazepam much more rapidly than man.[55] The major blood metabolite also is desmethyldiazepam, but dogs excrete more radioactivity in the feces (31 to 36%). Nearly all urinary activity is accounted for by oxazepam conjugates. The postulated scheme for diazepam metabolism in man and dog is shown in Fig. 2-5.

Species differences in drug-metabolizing capacities are of considerable interest to investigators. In mice, both the intact animal and *in vitro* extracts of hepatic tissue readily form all diazepam metabolites.[2,56-61] Levels of diazepam in blood and brain rapidly rise and fall when the drug is administered, but anticonvulsant effects may persist long after diazepam has become undetectable in brain tissue. Since oxazepam is conjugated and excreted relatively slowly in mice, the demethylated metabolites (desmethyldiazepam and oxazepam) are thought to be responsible for the persistent anticonvulsant effect.[56,62] These two metabolites accumulate in tissues, including brain. In rats, metabolic capacities are reversed. This species metabolizes diazepam slowly, forming small amounts of desmethyldiazepam and no temazepam or oxazepam.[60,61] When administered desmethyldiazepam, the intact rat forms no oxazepam; when temazepam is given, small amounts of oxazepam are formed. Yet, the rat excretes oxazepam more rapidly than the mouse when this drug is administered, so that whatever small amounts may be formed are rapidly eliminated. In the rat, intact diazepam accumulates in the brain and probably is responsible for anticonvulsant effects. The metabolizing deficiencies of the rat liver are less profound *in vitro* than *in vivo*.[57,59,63]

Still another situation exists in the guinea pig. This species rapidly forms desmethyldiazepam from diazepam, but produces oxazepam from desmethyldiazepam only slowly. No temazepam is formed after administration of diazepam, but if temazepam is given exogenously, oxazepam is formed rapidly. Oxazepam, however produced or administered, is conjugated and excreted slowly.[61,64-66] A single study in rabbits yielded limited results, but this species appears at least to be able to N-demethylate. There is evidence also of *para*-hydroxylation of the 5-phenyl ring.[67]

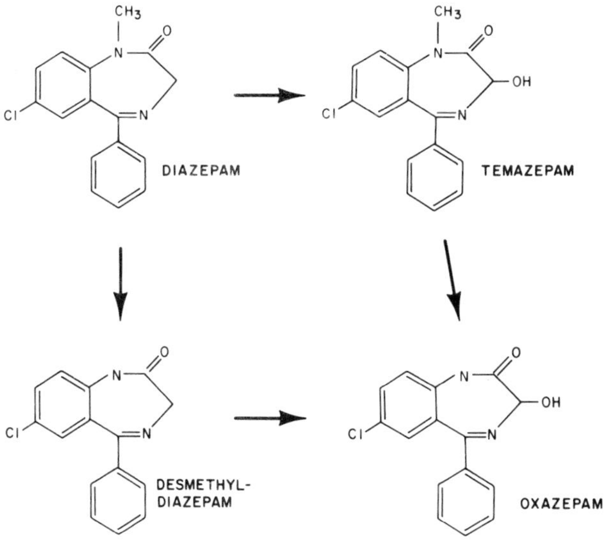

FIG. 2-5. Metabolic transformations of diazepam.

OXAZEPAM AND LORAZEPAM

Oxazepam itself is water insoluble, but has been prepared as a conjugate of succinic acid, the sodium salt of which is water soluble. Oxazepam hemisuccinate (Wy 4426) has pharmacologic activity similar or identical to free oxazepam,[68] but its activity is influenced by stereostructure.[69,70] When given parenterally, the *dextro*isomer is more potent than the *levo* in all screening tests except the reduction of spontaneous motor activity where the relationship is reversed, and in lethal effects in which the isomers are approximately equivalent. After oral administration, the differences are far less pronounced. Oxazepam hemisuccinate probably becomes active after deconjugation and release of free oxazepam, with the ease of deconjugation differing between isomers.

Assays for oxazepam may be performed by polarography,[71] spectroscopy,[72] and most recently by GLC of the hydrolyzed derivative.[73-75] In man a single oral dose of 45 mg produces maximal blood levels of free oxazepam in the range of 1.1 μg/ml between 1 and 4 hr after administration. The serum half-life of oxazepam ranges from 3 to 21 hr in different individuals; in one study the mean half-life was 4 hr[73] and in another the mean was 15 hr.[74] Oxazepam glucuronide, the major metabolite, rapidly appears in the plasma. Eighty percent of the total dose is excreted in the urine after 72

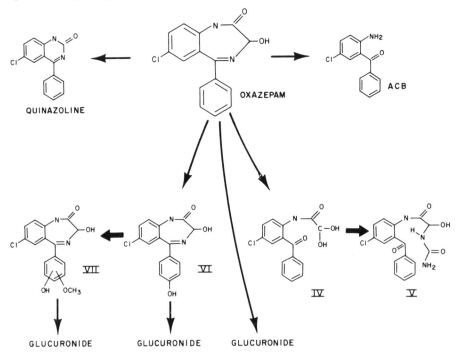

FIG. 2-6. Metabolic transformations of oxazepam.

hr; 10% or less appears in the feces. In dogs and rats, fecal elimination is greater than in humans.[76,77]

Unlike diazepam, repeated administration of oxazepam to humans produces little accumulation. One implication of this fact is that diazepam could be given in decreasing doses over time, while oxazepam might require steady dosing. A second is that oxazepam might be more appropriate for parenteral anticonvulsant therapy, inasmuch as cumulative sedation from repeated dosage would not occur. At the present time, however, a parenteral preparation of oxazepam is not available.

Numerous oxazepam metabolites have been identified in various species.[77] In man, dog, and swine, oxazepam glucuronide is by far the major metabolite. The rat excretes primarily the 5-parahydroxyphenyl analogue of oxazepam (VI), both free and conjugated. Figure 2-6 shows some of the identified metabolites of oxazepam.

Lorazepam, the 5-orthochlorophenyl analogue of oxazepam, has a high milligram potency. After a 7.5-mg oral dose in man, free lorazepam concentrations barely exceed 0.05 μg/ml despite profound sedative effects; levels fall slowly over 48 hr.[78] Lorazepam glucuronide is detectable in the blood within a few hours after administration of free lorazepam, and reaches maximum levels of about 0.1 μg/ml 4 to 12 hr after the dose. Sixty-five percent of the dose is recoverable in the urine after 3 days, with lorazepam glucuronide the major urinary constituent in man, dog, pig, and cat.[79] Rats excrete a number of hydroxylated and acetylated derivatives in addition to lorazepam glucuronide.

NITRAZEPAM

Nitrazepam (NTZ) can be qualitatively identified by TLC.[80] Quantitative assays using colorimetry[81] or infrared spectrophotometry[82] have also been described, which are adequate when high levels of the drug are present in body fluids. GLC analysis of the intact drug has been used by some groups, with column temperatures and carrier gas flow rates higher than those used in chromatography of other benzodiazepines. The sensitivity and reliability of GLC may be considerably improved by acid hydrolysis prior to analysis, but, again, some specificity is lost.[83] The hydrolysis product of nitrazepam is 2-amino-5-nitrobenzophenone (ANB). The two major metabolites, formed by reduction and acetylation in the 7-position, both yield 2,5-diaminobenzophenone (DAB) on hydrolysis. The internal standard is 2-amino-5-nitro-2´-chlorobenzophenone (ANCB), the hydrolysis product of clonazepam. GLC has not yet been used for extensive pharmacokinetic analysis of nitrazepam, and most of our knowledge of the metabolism and distribution of this drug has been reported by groups using spectrophotometric assays. Unfortunately, the assay utilizing the Bratton-Marshall reaction[81,84] does not appear to be sufficiently sensitive. Sawada and Shinohara[84] estimated the

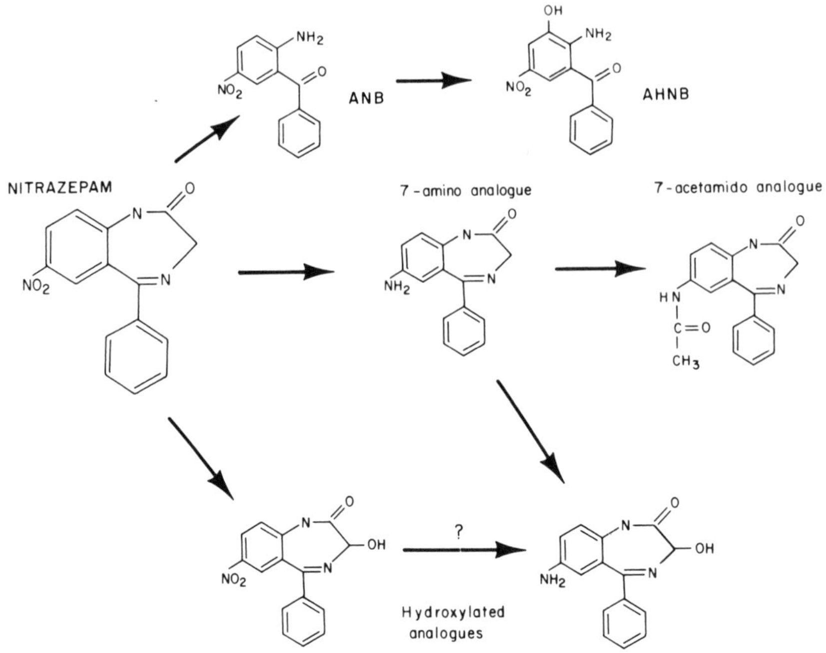

FIG. 2-7. Metabolic transformations of nitrazepam.

plasma half-life of nitrazepam in man to be about 7 hr. Subsequent studies by Reider and associates, using a more reliable fluorometric method, have suggested that this figure is an underestimate.[85-87]

The absorption of nitrazepam following oral administration is variable, ranging between individuals from 53 to 94% of the total dose. In most subjects, 10 mg taken orally produces maximum blood levels of 0.08 to 0.10 μg/ml 2 hr after ingestion. Nitrazepam is 87% protein bound. The half-life of unchanged nitrazepam is 25 hr after oral administration and 21 hr when the drug is given intravenously. Repeated administration results in some degree of accumulation. A daily dose of 5 mg produces a steady-state blood level of approximately 0.04 μg/ml after 4 days of continuous therapy. Both the 7-amino and the 7-acetamido derivatives (Fig. 2-7) also accumulate in the plasma, but both of these metabolites are essentially inactive.

The disposition of nitrazepam is dependent upon the route of administration. When given orally, 65 to 71% of the dose eventually appears in the urine, and 14 to 20% in the feces. After intravenous dosage, 93% is recovered in the urine and 2 to 13% in the feces. In both cases, the unchanged 7-acetamido derivative is the major metabolite, accounting for up to 68% of urinary radioactivity. The 7-amino metabolite (free and conjugated) is quantitatively more important after intravanenous than after oral administration (free only). The two benzophenone metabolities—2-amino-5-nitro-benzophenone (ANB) and 2-amino-3-hydroxy-5-nitrobenzophenone (AHNB)

—on the other hand, are more important when nitrazepam is given orally. Both these metabolites appear predominantly as glucuronides. The hydroxylated analogues are relatively minor metabolites, and only traces of free and conjugated nitrazepam can be detected.

Rats, mice, and rabbits metabolize nitrazepam more rapidly than do humans.[84,88–90] Both rats and mice can reduce the 7-nitro group to form the 7-amino derivative, but rats form the 7-acetamido analogue with more ease than mice.

FLURAZEPAM

Flurazepam is metabolized and excreted so rapidly by humans that within several hours of a very large dose (90 mg), plasma levels of the intact drug became barely detectable by spectrophotofluorometric assay (less than 0.01 μg/ml).[91,92] More than 50% of the total dose appears in the urine in 24 hr, with eventual urinary excretion accounting for 80% or more of the total dose.[93] Eight to nine percent appears in the feces. Dogs excrete the drug even more rapidly.[93] Intravenous flurazepam (2 mg/kg) disappears from the plasma with half-lives of 11 min and 1.4 hr in the two phases

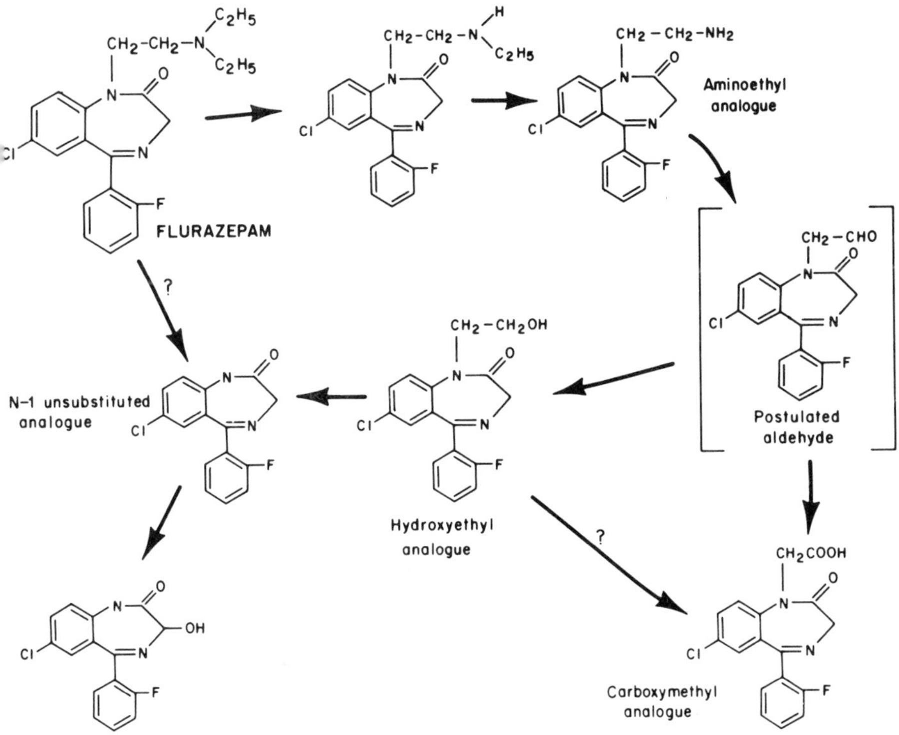

FIG. 2-8. Metabolic transformations of flurazepam.

of the elimination curve. As much as 90% of the total dose may be excreted in 2 days, with the fecal route of elimination predominating.[93]

Metabolism proceeds by stepwise dealkylation of the 1-diethylaminoethyl side chain, followed by oxidation of the amino group to an alcohol or carboxyl (Fig. 2-8). The aldehyde intermediate is postulated. In man the major urinary metabolite is the 1-hydroxyethyl analogue in conjugated form; in dog, the 1-carboxymethyl derivative predominates. Other metabolites are present in smaller or trace amounts. After oral flurazepam in man (90 mg), the 1-hydroxyethyl and 1-unsubstituted analogues are present in plasma in higher concentrations than the parent drug, but even these levels do not exceed 0.1 μg/ml.

MEDAZEPAM

GLC has been adapted for sensitive and specific assays of medazepam in blood and urine.[46] An oral dose of 50 mg in man results in a brief blood level peak of about 1 μg/ml 1 to 2 hr after the dose. Levels rapidly fall to about 0.1 μg/ml in 2 to 3 hr, then slowly decline to 0.03 μg/ml over 24 hr. Diazepam is detectable in blood shortly after a single oral dose of medazepam, together with traces of desmethyldiazepam.[46] After several single daily doses of 50 mg, medazepam does not accumulate in the plasma to any significant degree since each dose is rapidly metabolized and eliminated. Its metabolites (diazepam, desmethyldiazepam, and desmethylmedazepam) do, however, show a tendency to accumulate. In man, 55 to 63% of a dose is eventually recoverable in the urine, with 7 to 22% appearing in the feces.[94] Of the identifiable metabolites, oxazepam glucuronide predominates, with slightly smaller amounts of free and conjugated desmethylmedazepam (DMMDZ) also present. The glucuronides of temazepam and of 2-amino-3-hydroxy-5-chlorobenzophenone (AHCB) are also present in significant quantities.[94] In the dog, urinary and fecal contributions to total excretion are about equal. Conjugates of oxazepam and of 2-amino-3-hydroxy-5-chlorobenzophenone are the major urinary metabolites. Dogs produce only small amounts of desmethyldiazepam and diazepam *in vitro* as well as *in vivo*.[95]

Figure 2-9 shows the postulated metabolic pathways for medazepam. With the exception of the bracketed 1-desmethyl-2-hydroxy analogue, all of the indicated metabolites have been identified in one species or another, either from the intact organism or from an *in vitro* system. Several 5-parahydroxyphenyl metabolites formed by the rat are not shown.

In autoradiographic studies, medazepam behaves similarly to other benzodiazepines.[41,96] The drug is rather evenly distributed initially, with highest concentrations in the brain, liver, kidneys, and adipose tissue. At 6 hr, most of the radioactivity is in the kidneys and the gastrointestinal tract.

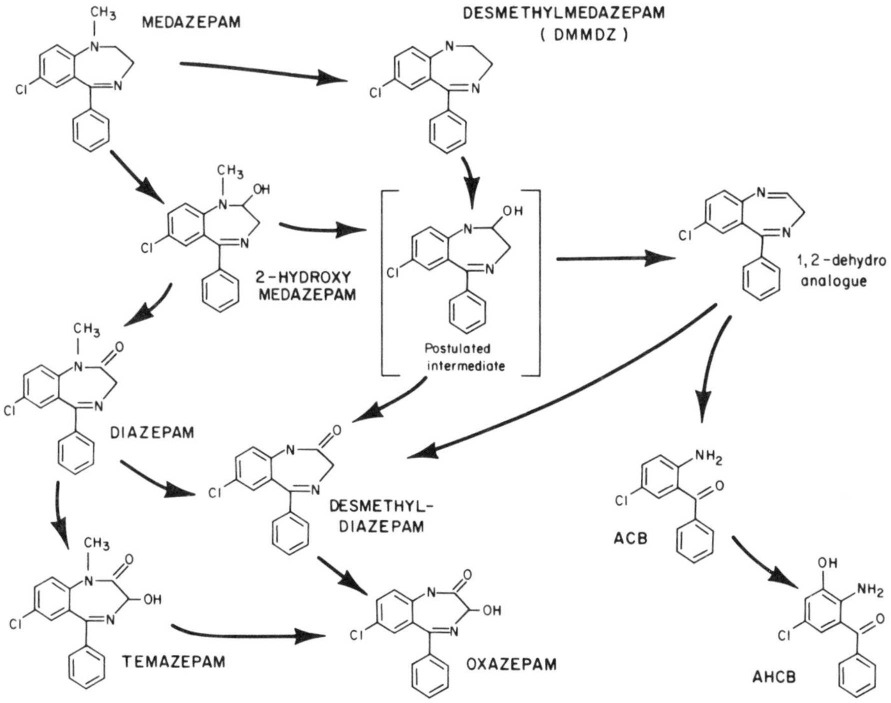

FIG. 2-9. Metabolic transformations of medazepam.

PRAZEPAM

Prazepam (PRZ) is slowly absorbed and slowly metabolized.[97] After an oral dose in man (25 mg), blood levels rise very gradually over 4 to 6 hr. In general, benzodiazepines circulate enterohepatically, but the slow absorption of prazepam in addition suggests some sort of "hang-up" in the gastrointestinal tract, perhaps due to binding by mucosal cells.

The pharmacokinetics of prazepam have been studied by radioactive tracer investigations. The half-life of total radioactivity in human blood was found to be 43 to 57 hr in four of five subjects in one study,[98] and approximately 78 hr in another.[99] Most of the radioactivity in plasma was located in unconjugated compounds, which were eliminated more slowly than the conjugated metabolites. Fourteen percent of the total dose appears in the urine after 24 hr and 22% in 48 hr. Fecal excretion is 7% in 48 hr. Nearly all the urinary radioactivity is found in glucuronide metabolites, primarily the glucuronides of oxazepam and 3-hydroxyprazepam. Small amounts of unchanged desmethyldiazepam can also be identified. Metabolic pathways of prazepam are shown in Fig. 2-10.

In the dog, prazepam is excreted into the urine even more slowly than in man,[100,101] with only 9% of the total dose appearing after 3 days. Oxazepam

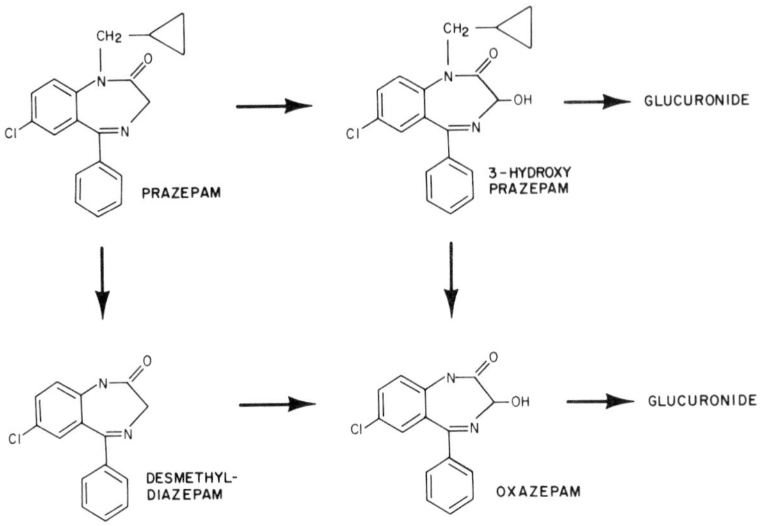

FIG. 2-10. Metabolic transformations of prazepam.

glucuronide makes up nearly 75% of urinary radioactivity, with free oxazepam and 3-hydroxyprazepam glucuronide also contributing substantially. The 5-parahydroxyphenyl derivatives of desmethyldiazepam and oxazepam are detectable in dog urine as well as traces of free prazepam and desmethyldiazepam. Eighty to 95% of total radioactivity appears in the feces, almost all of which is unchanged prazepam, indicating that intestinal binding and/or enterohepatic circulation of prazepam is prominent in dogs.

These results suggest that N-dealkylation of prazepam to form desmethyldiazepam is achieved with difficulty in the intact animal. Metabolism proceeds instead to 3-hydroxylation, followed either by conjugation with glucuronide and excretion or by N-dealkylation to form oxazepam. N-Dealkylation therefore occurs more easily after 3-hydroxylation than before. *In vitro* studies with liver homogenates from a number of species (man, dog, rat, mouse) at first glance would seem to contradict this.[102] The results are the same in all species: after incubation with prazepam, desmethyldiazepam and oxazepam are detected in the system, but 3-hydroxyprazepam is absent. In fact, these results are consistent with the *in vivo* findings. Prazepam is readily 3-hydroxylated, but since glucuronidation does not occur *in vitro*, 3-hydroxyprazepam is completely transformed to oxazepam. Desmethyldiazepam is formed slowly, but accumulates, since 3-hydroxylation of prazepam occurs more readily than 3-hydroxylation of desmethyldiazepam.

OTHER BENZODIAZEPINES

The pharmacokinetics of several other benzodiazepines have been studied. A GLC assay based on the hydrolysis product of bromazepam (2-amino-5-bromobenzoylpyridine) has been described by deSilva and Kaplan.[103] In two of three subjects, the plasma half-life of bromazepam was 18 to 19 hr; in the third, the half-life was 64 hr. Blood levels after a 15-mg oral dose reached a maximum in the range of 0.3 to 0.4 μg/ml. Sawada[104] identified the glucuronide conjugate of 2-amino-5-bromobenzoylpyridine as a urinary metabolite of bromazepam in the rabbit and the dog.

Oxazolam[105,106] is a benzodiazepine with a 4,5-heterocyclic ring appended to ring B (Fig. 2-11). The half-life in man is estimated at 4½ hr. Eighty percent of a dose is recovered in the urine after 48 hr, with the predominant metabolite being the glucuronide conjugate of 2-amino-3-hydroxy-5-chlorobenzophenone. A similar drug, ketazolam, is currently under investigation.[5]

At present there are no published data available on the pharmacokinetics of chlorazepate (Fig. 1-4). The manufacturer indicates that the drug is rapidly biotransformed to desmethyldiazepam. If this is the case, then long-acting pharmacologic effects could be expected.

INFLUENCE OF OTHER DRUGS ON BENZODIAZEPINE METABOLISM

Only a few examples exist of alterations in benzodiazepine metabolism in man by other drugs. Leevy[107] noted that chlordiazepoxide elimination was greatly delayed in an alcoholic patient with advanced cirrhosis. Presumably, this impairment was the result of liver disease rather than alcohol itself. In general, alcoholics without severe liver disease require larger doses of benzodiazepines to achieve sedation than do normals. Ethanol is known to stimulate hepatic microsomal enzymes,[108] but it is not clear whether alcohol has acted as an enzyme inducer in such patients, or whether their anxiety and agitation is so severe as to require more medication. Viala and associates[52] noted, in a few epileptic children receiving long-term diazepam therapy, that desmethyldiazepam blood levels exceeded diazepam concentrations when phenobarbital was administered concurrently. Without phenobarbital, diazepam levels exceeded those of desmethyldiazepam. This observation suggests that formation of desmethyldiazepam might be enhanced by phenobarbital-induced enzyme stimulation. Much more study is needed, how-

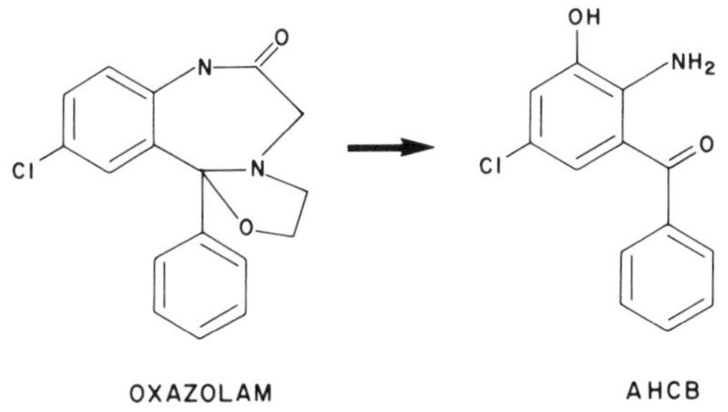

OXAZOLAM   AHCB

FIG. 2-11. Metabolic transformation of oxazolam.

ever, to elucidate the effects of phenobarbital and alcohol on benzodiazepine metabolism.

Other investigations involve animal systems, both *in vitro* and *in vivo*. The effects of phenobarbital, a powerful enzyme inducer, are uniform: this drug enhances the formation of benzodiazepine metabolites from the parent drugs.[17,63,102,109–111] Other agents which stimulate benzodiazepine metabolism include DDT,[112] lynestrol,[113] and spironolactone.[114] Meyers and associates[115] noted that after long-term nortriptyline therapy, the acute toxicity of chlordiazepoxide in animals was greater than without treatment. An interesting explanation for this phenomenon is impairment of drug metabolism by nortriptyline, documented by Vesell et al[116] in humans. The enzyme-inducing properties of the benzodiazepines themselves will be considered in Chapter 12.

COMMENT

A great deal is known about the metabolism of 1,4-benzodiazepines, but much remains to be learned. As time passes, less expensive, less tedious analytic techniques such as radioimmunoassay may become available to more investigators, allowing many important questions to be answered.

The benzodiazepines seem to be suitable for oral administration. Significant amounts are absorbed from the gastrointestinal tract, and, with the exception of prazepam, absorption is rapid. The degree to which gastric acidity or the concurrent administration of other drugs influences absorption has not been studied. Nor is it known if the benzodiazepines themselves influence the rate of gastric emptying.

Biotransformation of the benzodiazepines is extensive, but some derivatives are metabolized and excreted slowly. Animal studies suggest that the drugs have an affinity for the gastrointestinal tract, and it may be that the slow removal of certain benzodiazepines from the body is related more to binding in the gastrointestinal tract or enterohepatic circulation, with prolonged delayed release, rather than sluggish metabolism. Such a mechanism, if applicable, must apply whether the drug is given parenterally or orally, since elimination proceeds at approximately the same rate regardless of the route of administration.

The metabolites of chlordiazepoxide and diazepam are pharmacologically active, whereas those of nitrazepam and oxazepam are inactive. When either the parent drug or an active metabolite thereof has an elimination half-life which exceeds the interval between doses, cumulative clinical effects may be anticipated. This is well documented for diazepam and its biotransformation product desmethyldiazepam. Chlordiazepoxide has not been studied, but in theory it should produce cumulative sedation owing to the slow excretion of desmethylchlordiazepoxide and demoxepam. Clinical experience appears to be consistent with this prediction. The half-life of nitrazepam

TABLE 2-4. *Summary of pharmacokinetic and metabolic data in humans*

Drug	Half-life (hr)	Blood metabolites	% excreted in urine	Major urinary metabolites
Chlordiazepoxide	7-28	Desmethylchlordiazepoxide Demoxepam	60-64	Demoxepam Conjugated oxazepam Opened lactam
Diazepam	{ 1-6 (1st phase) 20-50 (2nd phase) }	{ Desmethyldiazepam (major) Temazepam (minor) }	60-75	Conjugated oxazepam Conjugated desmethyldiazepam
Oxazepam	3-21	Oxazepam glucuronide	80[a]	Oxazepam glucuronide
Lorazepam		Lorazepam glucuronide	65	Lorazepam glucuronide
Nitrazepam	18-28	7-Amino derivative 7-Acetamido derivative	65-93	Free 7-acetamido derivative Conjugated ANB and AHNB Free and conjugated 7-amino derivatives
Flurazepam		1-Hydroxyethyl derivative 1-Unsubstituted derivative	80	Conjugated 1-hydroxyethyl derivative
Medazepam		Diazepam Desmethyldiazepam Desmethylmedazepam	55-63	Oxazepam glucuronide Conjugated desmethylmedazepam Free desmethylmedazepam Conjugated temazepam Conjugated AHCB
Prazepam		3-Hydroxyprazepam glucuronide[b] Oxazepam glucuronide[b]	22[c]	3-Hydroxyprazepam glucuronide Oxazepam glucuronide

[a] after 72 hr
[b] probable metabolites
[c] after 48 hr

is about 1 day, and some degree of accumulation does occur; its metabolites, however, are inactive. Oxazepam is more rapidly excreted and has inactive biotransformation products.

This analysis suggests that in many clinical situations multiple daily doses of chlordiazepoxide or diazepam are not necessary for adequate antianxiety effects. A larger dose may be taken in the evening, enhancing sleep at bedtime and producing residual antianxiety effects during the next day. A smaller supplemental dose may be taken during the daytime. At present, there are no studies which investigate the relation of dosage schedules to antianxiety effects.

The data also suggest that major differences between various benzodiazepines may in large part be pharmacokinetic rather than neuropharmacologic. Benzodiazepines such as flurazepam which are rapidly biotransformed to inactive metabolites are suitable as hypnotics, since the effective dose is largely eliminated overnight, leaving minimal residual sedation during the next day. Adequate doses of chlordiazepoxide and diazepam clearly will produce sleep, but sedation can persist well into the following day and, after repeated administration, cumulative effects will occur. It has been claimed that oxazepam produces drowsiness less frequently than chlordiazepoxide and diazepam; if true, this probably is due to more rapid elimination and lack of accumulation rather than to an intrinsically more favorable toxic-to-therapeutic ratio. Oxazepam would appear to be useful as a hypnotic, but it is seldom administered for this purpose.

Understanding of many of the other properties and uses of the benzodiazepines is dependent upon knowledge of their pharmacokinetics. Pertinent data applicable to humans, where available, are summarized in Table 2-4.

REFERENCES

1. Garattini S, Mussini E, Marcucci F, Guaitani A: Metabolic studies on benzodiazepines in various animal species. In, *The Benzodiazepines.* Edited by S Garattini, E Mussini, LO Randall. New York, Raven Press, 1973, p. 75-97
2. Schwartz MA: Pathways of metabolism of the benzodiazepines. In, *The Benzodiazepines.* Edited by S Garattini, E Mussini, LO Randall. New York, Raven Press, 1973, p. 53-74
3. Scott CG, Bommer P: The liquid chromatography of some benzodiazepines. J Chrom Sci 8:446-448, 1970
4. Senkowski BZ, Levin MS, Urbigkit JR, Wollish EG: Polarography of some benzodiazepines. Anal Chem 36:1991-1994, 1964
5. Weber DJ: High pressure liquid chromatography of benzodiazepines: analysis of ketazolam. J Pharmaceut Sci 61:1797-1800, 1972
6. Jacobsen E, Jacobsen TV: Electrochemical reduction of chlordiazepoxide at mercury electrodes. Anal Chim Acta 55:293-301, 1971
7. Sadee W, van der Kleijn E: Thermolysis of 1,4-benzodiazepines during gas chromatography and mass spectroscopy. J Pharmaceut Sci 60:135-137, 1971

8. Marcucci F, Fanelli R, Mussini E: A method for gas chromatographic determination of benzodiazepines. J Chrom 37:318-320, 1968

9. Forgione A, Martelli P, Marcucci F, Fanelli R, Mussini E, Jommi GC: Gas-liquid chromatography and mass spectrometry of various benzodiazepines. J Chrom 59:163-168, 1971

10. Garattini S, Marcucci F, Mussini E: Gas chromatographic analysis of benzodiazepines. In, *Gas Chromatography in Biology and Medicine*. Edited by R Porter. London, JA Churchill Ltd, 1969, pp 161-172

11. van der Kleijn E, Beelen GC, Frederick MA: Determination of tranquillizers by GLC in biological fluids. Clin Chim Acta 34:345-356, 1971

12. van der Kleijn E: Protein binding and lipophilic nature of ataractics of the meprobamate- and diazepine-group. Arch Int Pharmacodyn 179:225-250, 1969

13. Smyth D, Pennington GW, Jackson N: Identification reactions of chlordiazepoxide ("Librium") and the product of acid hydrolysis 2-amino-4-chlorobenzophenone. Arch Int Pharmacodyn 145:147-153, 1963

14. Smyth D, Pennington GW: The detection and excretion of chlordiazepoxide ("Librium") in human plasma and urine. Arch Int Pharmacodyn 145:154-165, 1963

15. Koechlin BA, D'Arconte L: Determination of chlordiazepoxide (Librium) and of a metabolite of lactam character in plasma of humans, dogs, and rats by a specific spectrofluorometric micro method. Anal Biochem 5:195-207, 1963

16. Koechlin BA, Schwartz MA, Krol G, Oberhansli W: The metabolic fate of C[14]-labeled chlordiazepoxide in man, in the dog, and in the rat. J Pharmacol Exp Ther 148:399-411, 1965

17. Schwartz MA, Postma E: Metabolic N-demethylation of chlordiazepoxide. J Pharmaceut Sci 55:1358-1362, 1966

18. Schwartz MA, Postma E, Gaut Z: Biological half-life of chlordiazepoxide and its metabolite, demoxepam, in man. J Pharmaceut Sci 60:1500-1503, 1971

19. Schwartz MA, Postma E: Metabolites of demoxepam, a chlordiazepoxide metabolite, in man. J Pharmaceut Sci 61:123-125, 1972

20. Kimmel HB, Walkenstein SS: Oxazepam excretion by chlordiazepoxide-^{14}C-dosed dogs. J Pharmaceut Sci 56:538-539, 1967

21. Schwartz MA, Postma E, Kolis SJ: Metabolism of demoxepam, a chlordiazepoxide metabolite, in the dog. J Pharmaceut Sci 60:438-444, 1971

22. Kaplan SA, Lewis M, Schwartz MA, Postma E, Cotler S, Abruzzo CW, Lee TL, Weinfeld RE: Pharmacokinetic model for chlordiazepoxide • HCl in the dog. J Pharmaceut Sci 59:1569-1574, 1970

23. Gottschalk LA, Kaplan SA: Chlordiazepoxide plasma levels and clinical responses. Compr Psychiat 13:519-527, 1972

24. Cimbura G, Gupta RC: Polarographic determination of chlordiazepoxide and diazepam in toxicological analyses. J Forensic Sci 10:282-293, 1965

25. Frings CS, Cohen PS: Rapid colorimetric method for the quantitative determination of Librium (chlordiazepoxide hydrochloride) in serum. Amer J Clin Pathol 56:216-219, 1971

26. Jatlow P: Ultraviolet spectrophotometric measurement of chlordiazepoxide in plasma. Clin Chem 18:516-518, 1972

27. Zingales IA: Determination of chlordiazepoxide plasma concentrations by electron capture gas-liquid chromatography. J Chrom 61:237-252, 1971

28. Placidi GF, Cassano GB: Distribution and metabolism of ^{14}C-labelled-chlordiazepoxide in mice. Int J Neuropharmacol 7:383-389, 1968

29. Cassano GB, Gliozzi E, Ghetti B: The relationship between dynamic features of the brain distribution of C[14]-chlordiazepoxide and motor behaviour changes in mice. In, *The Present Status of Psychotropic Drugs. Pharmacological and Clinical Aspects*. Edited by A Cerletti, FJ Bové. Amsterdam, Excerpta Medica Foundation, 1969, pp 342-346

30. van der Kleijn E, van Rossum JM, Muskens ETJM, Rijntjes NVM: Pharmacokinetics of diazepam in dogs, mice, and humans. Acta Pharmacol Toxicol 29(supp 3):109-127, 1971

31. Carstensen JT, Su KSE, Maddrell P, Johnson JB, Newmark HN: Thermodynamic and kinetic aspects of parenteral benzodiazepines. Bull Parenteral Drug Assoc 25:193-202, 1971

32. Berlin A, Siwers B, Agurell S, Hiort A, Sjoqvist F, Strom S: Determination of bioavailability of diazepam in various formulations from steady state plasma concentration data. Clin Pharmacol Ther 13:733-744, 1972

33. Schwartz DE, Vecchi M, Ronco A, Kaiser K: Blood levels after administration of 7-chloro-1,3-dihydro-1-methyl-5-phenyl-2H-1,4-benzodiazepine-2-one (diazepam) in various forms. Arzneim-Forsch 16:1109-1110, 1966

34. Foldes EG, Campbell KN, Wohlman A: Comparative blood level study of different brands of chlordiazepoxide hydrochloride and their coadministration with chymotrypsin. Int J Clin Pharmacol 3:338-343, 1970

35. Munzel K: The desorption of medicinal substances from adsorbents in oral pharmaceutical suspensions. Acta Pharmacol Toxicol 29 (supp 3):81-87, 1971

36. Bernareggi V, Bugada G, Levi G: Absorption and pharmacological activities of a new diazepam preparation. Arzneim-Forsch 20:1250-1252, 1970

37. van der Kleijn E: Kinetics of distribution and metabolism of diazepam and chlordiazepoxide in mice. Arch Int Pharmacodyn 178:193-215, 1969

38. van der Kleijn E: Kinetics of distribution and metabolism of diazepam in animals and humans. Arch Int Pharmacodyn 182:433-436, 1969

39. van der Kleijn E, Wijffels CCG: Whole-body distribution of diazepam in newborn rhesus monkeys. Arch Int Pharmacodyn 192:255-264, 1971

40. Idanpaan-Heikkila JE, Taska RJ, Allen HA, Schoolar JC: Autoradiographic study of the fate of diazepam-C^{14} in the monkey brain. Arch Int Pharmacodyn 194:68-77, 1971

41. van der Kleijn E, Guelen PJM, Beelen TCM, Rijntjes NVM, Zuidgeest TLB: Kinetics of general and regional brain distribution of closely related 7-chloro-1,4-benzodiazepines. In, The Benzodiazepines. Edited by S Garattini, E Mussini, LO Randall. New York, Raven Press, 1973, pp 145-164

42. Morselli PL, Cassano GB, Placidi GF, Muscettola GB, Rizzo M: Kinetics of the distribution of ^{14}C-diazepam and its metabolites in various areas of cat brain. In, The Benzodiazepines. Edited by S Garattini, E Mussini, LO Randall. New York, Raven Press, 1973, pp 129-143

43. Berry DJ: The cathode ray polarographic determination of diazepam, 7-chloro-1,3-dihydro-1-methyl-5-phenyl-2H-1,4-benzodiazepine-2-one, in human plasma. Clin Chim Acta 32:235-241, 1971

44. Schwartz MA, Bommer P, Vane FM: Diazepam metabolites in the rat: characterization by high-resolution mass spectrometry and nuclear magnetic resonance. Arch Biochem Biophys 121:508-516, 1967

45. deSilva JAF, Schwartz MA, Stefanovic V, Kaplan J, D'Arconte L: Determination of diazepam (Valium) in blood by gas liquid chromatography. Anal Chem 36:2099-2105, 1964

46. deSilva JAF, Puglisi CV: Determination of medazepam (Nobrium), diazepam (Valium) and their major biotransformation products in blood and urine by electron capture gas-liquid chromatography. Anal Chem 42:1725-1736, 1970

47. Foster LB, Frings CS: Determination of diazepam (Valium) concentrations in serum by gas-liquid chromatography. Clin Chem 16:177-179, 1970

48. van der Kleijn E: Pharmacokinetics of distribution and metabolism of ataractic drugs and an evaluation of the site of antianxiety action. Ann NY Acad Sci 179:115-125, 1971

49. Garattini S: Metabolism of diazepam in animals and man. In, *The Present Status of Psychotropic Drugs. Pharmacological and Clinical Aspects.* Edited by A Cerletti, FJ Bové. Amsterdam, Excerpta Medica Foundation, 1969, pp 84-89

50. deSilva JAF, Koechlin BA, Bader G: Blood level distribution patterns of diazepam and its major metabolite in man. J Pharmaceut Sci 55:692-702, 1966

51. Baird ES, Hailey DM: Delayed recovery from a sedative: correlation of the plasma levels of diazepam with clinical effects after oral and intravenous administration. Brit J Anaesth 44:803-808, 1972

52. Viala A, Cano JP, Dravet C, Tassinari CA, Roger J: Blood levels of diazepam (Valium) and N-desmethyl diazepam in the epileptic child. Psychiat Neurol Neurochirur 74:153-158, 1971

53. Zingales IA: Diazepam metabolism during chronic medication. Unbound fraction in plasma, erythrocytes, and urine. J Chrom 75:55-78, 1973

54. Schwartz MA, Koechlin BA, Postma E, Palmer S, Krol G: Metabolism of diazepam in rat, dog, and man. J Pharmacol Exp Ther 149:423-435, 1965

55. Ruelius HW, Lee JM, Alburn HE: Metabolism of diazepam in dogs: transformation to oxazepam. Arch Biochem Biophys 111:376-380, 1965

56. Marcucci F, Mussini E, Fanelli R, Garattini S: Species differences in diazepam metabolism—I. Metabolism of diazepam metabolites. Biochem Pharmacol 19:1847-1851, 1970

57. Kvetina J, Marcucci F, Fanelli R: Metabolism of diazepam in isolated perfused liver of rat and mouse. J Pharm Pharmacol 20:807-808, 1968

58. Marcucci F, Fanelli R, Frova M, Morselli PL: Levels of diazepam in adipose tissue of rats, mice, and man. Eur J Pharmacol 4:464-466, 1968

59. Marcucci F, Fanelli R, Mussini E, Garattini S: The metabolism of diazepam by liver microsomal enzymes of rats and mice. Eur J Pharmacol 7:307-313, 1969

60. Marcucci F, Fanelli R, Mussini E, Garattini S: Further studies on species difference in diazepam metabolism. Eur J Pharmacol 9:253-256, 1970

61. Bertagni P, Marcucci F, Mussini E, Garattini S: Biliary excretion of conjugated hydroxyl benzodiazepines after administration of several benzodiazepines to rats, guinea pigs, and mice. J Pharmaceut Sci 61:965-966, 1972

62. Marcucci F, Guaitani A, Kvetina J, Mussini E, Garattini S: Species differences in diazepam metabolism and anticonvulsant effect. Eur J Pharmacol 4:467-470, 1968

63. Schwartz MA, Postma E: Metabolism of diazepam *in vitro.* Biochem Pharmacol 17:2443-2449, 1968

64. Marcucci F, Guaitani A, Fanelli R, Mussini E, Garattini S: Metabolism and anticonvulsant activity of diazepam in guinea pigs. Biochem Pharmacol 20:1711-1713, 1971

65. Mussini E, Marcucci F, Fanelli R, Garattini S: Metabolism of diazepam metabolites in guinea pigs. Chemico-Biol Interactions 5:73-76, 1972

66. Mussini E, Marcucci F, Fanelli R, Garattini S: Metabolism of diazepam and its metabolites by guinea pig liver microsomes. Biochem Pharmacol 20:2529-2531, 1971

67. Jommi G, Mannito P, Silanos MA: Metabolism of diazepam in rabbits. Arch Biochem Biophys 108:334-340; 562-568, 1964

68. Babbini M, DeMarchi F, Montanaro N, Strocchi P, Torrielli MV: Chemistry and CNS-pharmacological properties of two hydrosoluble benzodiazepine derivatives. Arzneim-Forsch 19:1931-1936, 1969

69. Mussini E, Marcucci F, Fanelli R, Guaitani A, Garattini S: Analytical and pharmacokinetic studies on the optic isomers of oxazepam succinate half-ester. Biochem Pharmacol 21:127-129, 1972

70. deAngelis L, Predominato M, Vertua R: Stereostructure-activity relationships for oxazepam hemisuccinate. Effects on central nervous system. Arzneim-Forsch 22:1328-1333, 1972

71. Fazzari FR, Riggleman OH: Polarographic determination of oxazepam. J Pharmaceut Sci 58:1530-1531, 1969

72. Salim EF, Deuble JL, Papariello G: Qualitative and quantitative tests for oxazepam. J Pharmaceut Sci 57:311-313, 1968

73. Knowles JA, Ruelius HW: Absorption and excretion of 7-chloro-1,3-dihydro-3-hydroxy-5-phenyl-2H-1,4-benzodiazepin-2-one (oxazepam) in humans. Determination of the drug by gas-liquid chromatography with electron capture detection. Arzneim-Forsch 22:687-692, 1972

74. Vessman J, Alexanderson B, Sjoqvist F, Strindberg B, Sundwall A: Comparative pharmacokinetics of oxazepam and nortriptyline after single oral doses in man. In, *The Benzodiazepines*. Edited by S Garattini, E Mussini, LO Randall. New York, Raven Press, 1973, pp 139-147

75. Vessman J, Freij G, Stromberg S: Determination of oxazepam in serum and urine by electron capture gas chromatography. Acta Pharm Suecica 9:447-456, 1972

76. Walkenstein SS, Wiser R, Gudmundsen CH, Kimmel HB, Corradino RA: Absorption, metabolism, and excretion of oxazepam and its succinate half-ester. J Pharmaceut Sci 53:1181-1186, 1964

77. Sisenwine SF, Tio CO, Shrader SR, Ruelius HW: The biotransformation of oxazepam (7-chloro-1,3-dihydro-3-hydroxy-5-phenyl-2H-1,4-benzodiazepin-2-one) in man, miniature swine, and rat. Arzneim-Forsch 22:682-687, 1972

78. Knowles JA, Comer WH, Ruelius HW: Disposition of 7-chloro-5-(o-chlorophenyl)-1,3-dihydro-3-hydroxy-2H-1,4-benzodiazepin-2-one (lorazepam) in humans. Arzneim-Forsch 21:1055-1059, 1971

79. Schillings RT, Shrader SR, Ruelius HW: Urinary metabolites of 7-chloro-5-(o-chlorophenyl)-1,3-dihydro-3-hydroxy-2H-1,4-benzodiazepin-2-one (lorazepam) in humans and four animal species. Arzneim-Forsch 21:1059-1065, 1971

80. Sawada H, Shinohara K: Detection and identification of nitrazepam and related compounds by thin-layer chromatography. Arch Toxikol 27:71-78, 1970

81. Sawada H, Shinohara K: Colorimetric determination of nitrazepam. J Hygenic Chem 16:318-321, 1970

82. Tompsett SL: Nitrazepam (Mogadon) in blood serum and urine and Librium in urine. J Clin Path 21:366-371, 1968

83. Beharrell GP, Hailey DM, McLaurin MK: Determination of nitrazepam (Mogadon) in plasma by electron capture gas-liquid chromatography. J Chrom 70:45-52, 1972

84. Sawada H, Shinohara K: On the urinary excretion of nitrazepam and its metabolites. Arch Toxikol 28:214-221, 1971

85. Rieder J: A fluorimetric method for determining nitrazepam and the sum of its main metabolites in plasma and urine. Arzneim-Forsch 23:207-212, 1973

86. Rieder J: Plasma levels and derived pharmacokinetic characteristics of unchanged nitrazepam in man. Arzneim-Forsch 23:212-218, 1973

87. Rieder J, Wendt G: Pharmacokinetics and metabolism of the hypnotic nitrazepam. In, *The Benzodiazepines*. Edited by S Garattini, E Mussini, LO Randall. New York, Raven Press, 1973, pp 99-127

88. Bartosek I, Mussini E, Garattini S: Reduction of nitrazepam by rat liver. Biochem Pharmacol 18:2263-2264, 1969

89. Bartosek I, Kvetina J, Guaitani A, Garattini S: Comparative study of nitrazepam metabolism in perfused isolated liver of laboratory animals. Eur J Pharmacol 11:378-382, 1970

90. Bartosek I, Mussini E, Saronio C, Garattini S: Studies on nitrazepam metabolism *in vitro*. Eur J Pharmacol 11:249-253, 1970

91. Schwartz MA, Vane FM, Postma E: Urinary metabolites of 7-chloro-1-(2-diethylaminoethyl)-5-(2-fluorophenyl)-1,3-dihydro-2H-1,4-benzodiazepin-2-one dihydrochloride. J Med Chem 11:770-774, 1968

92. deSilva JAF, Strojny N: Determination of flurazepam and its major biotransformation products in blood and urine by spectrophotofluorometry and spectrophotometry. J Pharmaceut Sci 60:1303-1314, 1971

93. Schwartz MA, Postma E: Metabolism of flurazepam, a benzodiazepine, in man and dog. J Pharmaceut Sci 59:1800-1806, 1970

94. Schwartz MA, Carbone JJ: Metabolism of ^{14}C-medazepam hydrochloride in dog, rat, and man. Biochem Pharmacol 19:343-361, 1970

95. Schwartz MA, Kolis SJ: Pathways of medazepam metabolism in the dog and rat. J Pharmacol Exp Ther 180:180-188, 1972

96. Rentsch G: Distribution of ^{14}C-labelled madazepam in the mouse as examined by whole body autoradiography. Naunyn-Schmied Arch Pharmakol 266:434, 1970

97. DiCarlo FJ, Viau J-P, Epps JE, Haynes LJ: Biotransformation of prazepam in man. Ann NY Acad Sci 179:487-492, 1971

98. Vesell ES, Passananti GT, Viau J-P, Epps JE, DiCarlo FJ: Effects of chronic prazepam administration on drug metabolism in man and rat. Pharmacology 7:197-206, 1972

99. DiCarlo FJ, Viau J-P, Epps JE, Haynes LJ: Prazepam metabolism by man. Clin Pharmacol Ther 11:890-897, 1970

100. DiCarlo FJ, Crew MC, Melgar MD, Haynes LJ: Prazepam metabolism by dogs. J Pharmaceut Sci 58:960-962, 1969

101. DiCarlo FJ, Viau J-P: Prazepam metabolites in dog urine. J Pharmaceut Sci 59:322-325, 1970

102. Viau J-P, Epps JE, DiCarlo FJ: Prazepam metabolism *in vitro*. Biochem Pharmacol 21:563-569, 1972

103. deSilva JAF, Kaplan J: Determination of 7-bromo-1,3-dihydro-5-(2-pyridyl)-2H-1,4-benzodiazepin-2-one (Ro 5-3350) in blood by gas-liquid chromatography. J Pharmaceut Sci 55:1278-1283, 1966

104. Sawada H: An urinary metabolite of bromazepam. Experientia 28:393, 1972

105. Shindo H, Nakajima E, Yasumura A, Murata H, Hiraoka T, Sasahara K: Studies on the metabolism of oxazolam. I. Distribution and excretion studies. Chem Pharm Bull 19:61-70, 1971

106. Yasumura A, Murata H, Hattori K, Matsuda K: Studies on the metabolism of oxazolam. II. Isolation and identification of the metabolites of oxazolam in rats. Chem Pharm Bull 19:1929-1936, 1971

107. Leevy CM: Cirrhosis in alcoholics. Med Clin NA 52:1445-1455, 1968

108. Misra PS, Lefevre A, Ishii H, Rubin E, Lieber CS: Increase of ethanol, meprobamate, and pentobarbital metabolism after chronic ethanol administration in man and rats. Amer J Med 51:346-351, 1971

109. Manzo L, Berte F, DeBernardi M: Oxazepam glucuronidation "in vitro" in some maternal and fetal tissues of the rat. Effects of pretreatment with oxazepam and phenobarbital. Estratto Boll Chim Farm 108:19-24, 1969

110. Berte F, Manzo L, DeBernardi M, Benzi G: Ability of the placenta to metabolize oxazepam and aminopyrine before and after drug stimulation. Arch Int Pharmacodyn 182:182-185, 1969

111. Marcucci F, Fanelli R, Mussini E, Garattini S: Effect of phenobarbital on the *in vitro* metabolism of diazepam in several animal species. Biochem Pharmacol 19:1771-1776, 1970

112. Datta PR, Nelson MJ: Enhanced metabolism of methyprylon, meprobamate, and chlordiazepoxide hydrochloride after chronic feeding of a low dietary level of DDT to male and female rats. Toxicol Appl Pharmacol 13:346-352, 1968

113. Blackham A, Spencer PSJ: Response of female mice to anticonvulsants after pretreatment with sex steroids. J Pharm Pharmacol 22:304-305, 1970

114. Haataja M, Nieminen L, Kangas L, Mottonen M, Bjondahl K: Effect of spironolactone on pentobarbital anaesthesia, diazepam metabolism, and toxicity of spironolactone and furosemide. Ann Med Exp Biol Fenn 50:57-60, 1972

115. Meyers DB, Kanyuck DO, Anderson RC: Effect of chronic nortriptyline pretreatment on the acute toxicity of various medicinal agents in rats. J Pharmaceut Sci 55:1317-1318, 1966

116. Vesell ES, Passananti T, Greene FE: Impairment of drug metabolism in man by allopurinol and nortriptyline. New Eng J Med 283:1484-1488, 1970

Chapter 3
Behavioral Pharmacology

Numerous reputable investigators have devoted painstaking efforts to the study of drug-induced changes in animal behavior. In many studies the design is straightforward and the results are readily understood. Others involve highly complex designs with multiple contingencies and results which may be obscure to the nonbehavioral scientist. Interpretation of results in terms of human behavior is complicated by dosage relationships. Laboratory animals tolerate large quantities of sedative and tranquilizing drugs: the smaller the animal, the larger the amount necessary to produce behavioral effects. Doses of 50 mg/kg of chlordiazepoxide may produce no effects whatsoever in mice; in humans, this dose would cause obtundation and coma.

The benzodiazepines and propanediols have been collectively classified as *minor tranquilizers, anxiolytics,* or *antianxiety agents,* in part because of the similarity of their animal psychopharmacology. The principal behavioral effects of minor tranquilizers can be summarized as follows:[1-6]

1. Reduction of hostile and aggressive behavior, both spontaneous and evoked.
2. Attenuation of the behavioral consequences of frustration, fear, and punishment, including
   a. restoration of behavior suppressed by punishment or lack of reward, and
   b. reduction of behavior motivated by punishment.

The second property, also termed the "disinhibition" effect, is the most consistently observed behavioral sequel of minor tranquilizer treatment. When aggression and hostility are inhibited by fear or anxiety, minor tranquilizers can produce an apparently "paradoxical" increase in aggresion. This situation will be discussed subsequently.

Barbiturates and other central depressant drugs also can produce antiaggressive and disinhibitory effects in certain animal models. What distinguishes the minor tranquilizers from barbiturates is their ability to produce these behavioral changes at doses distinctly below those which are "neurotoxic." Unfortunately, much confusion and apparent inconsistency results from the lack of a uniform definition of neurotoxicity. Endpoints for neurologic impairment range between studies from reduction in locomotor activity to ataxia and incoordination to narcosis and coma. In a given study, the difference between disinhibitory and neurotoxic doses will obviously depend upon the author's choice of endpoint. Regardless of the criteria for neurologic impairment, however, benzodiazepines and propanediols are generally characterized by larger toxic-to-effective dose ratios than barbiturates, ethanol, or other central depressants. The *major tranquilizers* or *neuroleptics* (phenothiazines, thioxanthenes, and butyrophenones) stand in distinct contrast to the minor tranquilizers and barbiturates. Major tranquilizers do not produce disinhibition at any dose. These drugs weaken all forms of response, regardless of the role of punishment, and reduce psychomotor and locomotor activity.

Clinical psychopharmacologists have long been plagued by the influence of "nonspecific" factors upon the results of drug trials in neurotic patients. Numerous factors unrelated to the pharmacology of the drug being tested may alter the response to drug and/or placebo, and may either exaggerate or negate overall drug-placebo differences. Some clinical aspects of this problem are discussed in Chapter 4.

In animal investigations, analogous nonspecific effects have received less attention. Most studies utilize animals with fixed, "stable" baseline response rates. Incentive strengths and intensities of aversive stimuli likewise are usually fixed. Although the influences of drug dosage variation are almost always studied in detail, the effects of alterations in baseline response rate and stimulus strength upon drug-induced behavioral change usually are not. Several research groups have demonstrated that benzodiazepines, meprobamate, or barbiturates may facilitate avoidance responses in animals with low baseline response rate, and impair avoidance in those with high rates.[7-9] Wuttke and Kelleher[10] showed that benzodiazepines selectively facilitated punished behavior in pigeons with higher response rates, but facilitated *all* examined behavior in low-responding pigeons. Others have similarly shown drug effects upon approach-and-avoidance behavior to be dependent upon the relative intensities and frequencies of the stimuli.[11,11a,12] The failure of most investigators to deal with these influences constitutes a major weakness in the field of experimental psychopharmacology as a whole.

APPETITE AND SENSATION

Hunger and pain are two of the most important unconditioned stimuli exploited in the experimental analysis of behavior. Starved animals want food; shocked animals dislike the pain associated with the shock. Since most drug studies investigate the interaction of these two drives, it obviously is crucial to know if drugs alter the intensity of the primary drives themselves as well as the effect of their interaction. Unfortunately, the appetite-stimulating, appetite-depressing, and analgesic properties of the benzodiazepines are not well understood.

Appetite stimulation by chlordiazepoxide was demonstrated in early pharmacologic screening (see Chapter 1), but in other studies this effect has not been so obvious. MacDonald et al.,[13] using high doses of chlordiazepoxide in rats (50 to 150 mg/kg per day), showed body weight to be increased after 5 days of treatment but reduced after 4 weeks of treatment when compared with controls. Since sedative effects were minimal, "chronic fatigue" did not appear to account for the results. Clark[14] demonstrated reduced food consumption in animals treated with chlordiazepoxide, but only at doses which reduced locomotor activity. Matsuda[15] found no change in food consumption either in normal rats or in those with hypothalamic lesions. Poschel[16] showed that five different benzodiazepines increased food consumption in nonstarved rats presented with an unfamiliar food; in seemingly comparable doses, phenobarbital had a lesser effect, whereas all other psychotropic drugs tested, including meprobamate, had no effect. Intake of an unpleasant food may also be enhanced in a food-deprived animal.[17] The influence of benzodiazepines on food consumption and body weight is undoubtedly complex, involving not only appetite and hunger, but also the nature of the foodstuff, its ease of availability, and the circumstances under which it is presented. Studies utilizing food consumption as a dependent variable must therefore control for the possibility of drug-induced alteration in appetite, particularly if comparative claims are made to other classes of drugs. Unfortunately, this usually has not been the case.

Analgesic effects may likewise confound studies using pain as an aversive stimulus. Tests of analgesia produced by benzodiazepines alone, however, have been negative,[18-20] except in high doses when the escape from pain is impaired by muscular relaxation and neurotoxicity.[21,22] In two studies in which chlordiazepoxide alone did not produce analgesia, the analgesic effects of morphine and acetaminophen were potentiated.[20,23] Leslie,[24] however, found that chlordiazepoxide did not potentiate oxotremorine analgesia in mice, while Weis[25] showed that chlordiazepoxide antagonized morphine analgesia. It appears that the effects of benzodiazepines on the sensation of pain *per se* are secondary to nonspecific sedation at high doses. There is a suggestion that other analgesics may be potentiated; this has been noted in humans as well (see Chapters 7 and 10).

SPONTANEOUS ACTIVITY

The "inverted U" model has been used to describe the effect of benzodiazepines and other minor tranquilizers on spontaneous motor activity and responses not altered by punishment. At low doses, no effects are seen, and responding remains at the baseline rate; at high doses, neuromuscular toxicity ensues and response rates are at baseline or below.[26-29] Intermediate doses tend to increase responding,[26-34] giving the "inverted U" shape to the dose-response curve. Exceptions are numerous. In some studies, activity is unaltered until neurotoxic doses are reached.[35–41] Dosage ranges are highly variable even within the same species, and depend upon many of the "nonspecific" parameters discussed previously. In rats given chlordiazepoxide, the effective parenteral dose range usually falls between 5 and 30 mg/kg, with greater than 40 mg/kg being toxic. Some authors have reported maximum effects at 2.5 to 3.75 mg/kg with 5.0 being toxic;[26] others report maximum effects at 30 to 60 mg/kg.[42] The effective doses for diazepam and nitrazepam are about five to 10 times smaller than those for chlordiazepoxide. Rats and mice in general approach a new environment with caution and tend to choose a familiar environment when given a choice between that and one which is novel. Several authors have reported increases in "exploratory" behavior produced by benzodiazepines, manifested by increased activity in unfamiliar surroundings,[27] or by increased preference for a novel setting over a familiar one.[26,29,42,43] Drug effects are most obvious in those animals who are least familiar with the setting.[29,30,43a]

Amphetamine-induced activity and hypermotility are similarly affected by benzodiazepines. Low doses of chlordiazepoxide (0.5 mg/kg) have no effect on amphetamine-induced behavior,[44] whereas amphetamine effects are potentiated by chlordiazepoxide in the dose range of 1 to 50 mg/kg.[41,45–47] At very high doses (100 mg/kg), amphetamine effects are antagonized.[41,43,48] The interaction between amphetamine and barbiturates shows a similar dose-dependent variation in animals.[41] Many commercially available anorectic drug preparations contain combinations of amphetamines and barbiturates, based upon the idea that the sedative agent modifies some of the unwanted amphetamine-induced stimulation. Interestingly, the amphetamine-barbiturate ratio in some of these preparations is the same ratio which produces maximum behavioral stimulation in animal studies.[41]

The benzodiazepines also may modify behavioral changes induced by organic brain lesions. In rats made hypermotile by removal of the olfactory bulb[49] or by lesions in the septal region of the brain,[50] chlordiazepoxide in doses of 10 to 20 mg/kg reduces hypermotility. Olds and associates[51–55] have extensively studied the behavior of rats with electrodes implanted in the hypothalamic pleasure center. High rates of self-stimulation rapidly become established in such animals. The benzodiazepines enhance self-stimulation with an "inverted U" type of dose dependence. Phenobarbital and meprobamate produce similar enhancement;[56] diphenylhydantoin does not.[53–56] This suggests that the anticonvulsant effects of these drugs do not explain their enhancement of self-stimulation. It may be that under non-drug conditions self-stimulation is modulated by inhibitory effects, perhaps elicited at the site of stimulation. Antianxiety drugs may remove the inhibitory influences, causing an increase in self-stimulation rate.

AGGRESSIVE BEHAVIOR

A number of studies have confirmed the findings of early investigators that the benzodiazepines reduce aggression and fighting behavior in animals. In some species such behavior occurs spontaneously. Subneurotoxic doses of benzodiazepines can reduce spontaneous aggression and fighting in mice,[57-61] monkeys,[62,63] baboons,[64,65] mink,[66] and cats.[67,68] Aggression may also be induced in animals by a variety of methods. Such experimental models of aggression include the septal rat,[30,69-71] the shocked mouse,[30,72] animals with brain stimulation through implanted electrodes,[73-75] the mouse administered D,L-DOPA,[76] and mice reared in isolation and grouped at maturity.[68,77-81] The benzodiazepines have shown antiaggressive properties in all of the above models.

Other studies using the same models of spontaneous and induced aggression have yielded contradictory results. Many authors have found that the benzodiazepines reduce aggression only at neurotoxic doses.[71,82-86] Others have found that benzodiazepines actually potentiate hostility and fighting. Cole and Wolf[77] showed that chlordiazepoxide (30 to 54 mg/kg) increased fighting time among mice of a spontaneously aggressive strain. Guaitini and associates[87] noted an increase in traumatic skin lesions among grouped male mice fed diazepam, oxazepam, or desmethyldiazepam over a 6-month period. Fox et al.[88-90] studied the effects of benzodiazepines (chlordiazepoxide, diazepam, nitrazepam, flurazepam) added to the food supply of mice reared in isolation, then subsequently grouped. Mortality from fighting among drugged mice was two to six times greater than among the nondrugged control group.

The net effect of the benzodiazepine tranquilizers on aggressive behavior in animals undoubtedly depends upon many interrelated factors, including the animal species and sex, drug dosage and route of administration, the social environment, and the manner in which aggressive behavior is induced.[91,92] Given one set of circumstances, the benzodiazepines can enhance aggression; in other situations, the drugs have taming effects. The type of aggression under study seems to be of great importance. Studying two animal species (mice and cats), Hoffmeister and Wuttke[68] found that chlordiazepoxide was a potent inhibitor of "defensive-aggressive" behavior (hostility induced by intrusion or provocation). "Attack-aggression," on the other hand, was almost completely resistant to chlordiazepoxide effects. Behavior in some aggressive animals appears to be motivated in part by fear or anxiety. Valzelli, for example, has noted that spontaneous activity and exploratory behavior of aggressive mice was less than that of normals.[60,93] Administration of benzodiazepines to the aggressive animals enhanced activity and exploration, whereas no effect was seen in nonaggressive mice. Anxiolytic drugs are most likely to enhance hostility by disinhibition when the animal's aggression is "bound" by anxiety. The applicability of this model to human behavior remains uncertain.

PUNISHED BEHAVIOR

The restoration of behavior suppressed by punishment is one of the most predictable effects of minor tranquilizers. A typical experiment is designed as follows. Food-deprived rats are taught to press a lever for a food reward on a schedule of intermittent reinforcement such as a 2-min variable interval (VI 2 min). A conditioned stimulus (CS), either light or noise, is then presented, at which time the reinforcement schedule changes to reward each response (continuous reinforcement, CRF) and also to deliver a painful shock from the floor of the cage. As the reinforcement schedule is alternated between VI 2 min and CRF with response-contingent shock, the animals learn to stop responding during the CS-CRF period, despite availability of reward for each response; in other words, their behavior has been suppressed by the threat of shock, signaled by the CS. Responses in the absence of CS continue unchanged.

Administration of benzodiazepines to trained rats approximately 1 hr before an experimental session changes the pattern of behavior. Response rates during the CS period are invariably increased over control levels. Unpunished responses during VI 2 min are generally unchanged. This restoration of punished behavior has been demonstrated in numerous studies using an experimental design identical or similar to the one described above.[11a,94–106] All benzodiazepines tested have shown similar properties. For chlordiazepoxide, the effective dose range is usually between 5 and 25 mg/kg; doses greater than 30 mg/kg usually are neurotoxic, reducing both punished and unpunished response rates because of motor impairment. In some studies using high doses of benzodiazepines, neuromuscular toxicity is noted after the first few administrations of the drug.[103–106] On repeated administration, evidence of oversedation seems to disappear as "tolerance" develops, and the disinhibition of punished behavior becomes fully manifest.

Meprobamate and certain barbiturates show disinhibitory effects similar to the benzodiazepines. For the barbiturates, differences between fear-attenuating and toxic doses may be small and difficult to demonstrate.[99] The major tranquilizers show quite different properties, producing suppression of both punished and unpunished behavior.[11a]

Operant responses for a food reward may be suppressed by an aversive stimulus (shock), even if the shock is not contingent upon response. This phenomenon, termed "conditioned suppression" or "conditioned emotional response," is also altered by the benzodiazepines. Rats trained to associate a conditioned stimulus with shock, not contingent upon ongoing responses, will show reduced response rates when the CS is presented. Pretreatment with benzodiazepines produces "disinhibition," and response rates during the CS return toward baseline.[107-114] The release of conditioned suppression has been interpreted as another aspect of the fear-attenuating or disinhibitory properties of the benzodiazepines.

AVOIDANCE BEHAVIOR

Behavior *motivated* by punishment (*active* avoidance), as well as that *suppressed* by punishment (*passive* avoidance), may be influenced by minor tranquilizers. Rats are easily taught that the appearance of a conditioned stimulus means they will soon be shocked, unless they avoid the shock by climbing a pole, jumping a hurdle, or entering a chamber. Treatment with benzodiazepines prior to testing reduces the active avoidance responses evoked by presentation of the CS in trained rats. Some authors claim that active avoidance inhibition is not due to fear attenuation, but rather to nonspecific sedation and neuromuscular impairment.[115-118] Others provide good evidence that the benzodiazepines produce suppression of active avoidance at doses well below those which produce significant central nervous system depression.[119-127] It appears that disinhibition of passive avoidance occurs at somewhat lower doses than suppression of active avoidance. Again, the barbiturates and meprobamate have similar properties, but the differential between effective and toxic doses is, in general, much smaller.

FRUSTRATION

Frustrating situations have adverse behavioral consequences in animals, producing hesitation, fixation, and reduced response rates. Benzodiazepines attenuate the behavioral consequences of frustration.

These situations may be created experimentally in a number of ways. "Incentive shift" is a common one, in which the reward associated with a given operant pattern is suddenly reduced or made more difficult to obtain. Reducing the dextrose concentration in a liquid nourishment or reducing the quantity of food in a "goal box" will be followed by diminished liquid consumption and a delay in reaching the goal box, respectively, in undrugged trained rats. Administration of chlordizepoxide, however, will restore response rates close to "pre-shift" levels.[128,129] The effect is not produced by appetite stimulation, since no change in response rate occurs in control animals not subjected to incentive shift. "Progressive-ratio" reinforcement schedules also create frustration. Starved pigeons can be taught to peck a key for food. The number of responses necessary for a reward is increased by consecutive multiples of an arbitrary integer—eight, for example. With this design, eight responses are required for the first reward, 16 for the second, 24 for the third, and so on. The pigeon soon reaches a "breaking point" when it stops responding. Both chlordiazepoxide (20 mg/kg) and phenobarbital

(40 mg/kg) significantly delay the breaking point phenomenon.[130] The "time-out" maneuver is another inducer of frustration. Rats rewarded on a fixed ratio-25 schedule, paired with a CS, learn to stop responding or respond less when the CS disappears and no rewards are given. After chlordiazepoxide, the incentive-shift inhibitory effect is attenuated, and unrewarded response rates during the "time-out" period approach those maintained by the fixed-ratio schedule without drugs.[131,132]

Animals presented with insoluble problems develop prolonged decision times and hesitation. They may also develop "fixations," making an identical choice each time they are forced to make a decision, inasmuch as a "correct" decision cannot be made. Established fixations are not easily broken even when an insoluble problem is made soluble. If a soluble problem is complicated by rewarding the incorrect response or failing to reward the correct one, behavior is disrupted and response rates fall. The experiments upon which these observations are based are complex. Most involve a jumping platform opposite two doors with lights above each. Unlocked doors are "correct," and have food behind them; locked doors are "incorrect." Rats are placed on the platform and forced to jump to one of the two windows, based upon some combination of light on, light off, left, or right. Rats making "correct" responses get the food behind the door; those responding incorrectly bounce off the locked window and fall into a net. Learning to make the correct choice can be made either possible or impossible for the rat.

In several studies using designs such as these, the benzodiazepines have been shown to attenuate the behavioral consequences of the insoluble problem.[133–140] Hesitancy and decision times are reduced, and the development of fixations is prevented. The disruptive effect of incorrect reinforcement is also attenuated. Fixations once developed are more easily abandoned when the problem becomes soluble. These effects are thought to be consistent with a drug-induced reduction in the consequences of negative incentives. An analogy in human terms is an individual's willingness to keep trying despite a feeling of "hitting one's head against a wall" or of "talking to deaf ears."

LEARNING AND MEMORY

The previous sections have considered the effect of benzodiazepines upon patterns of behavior established in undrugged animals. The question of the influence of these drugs upon the learning process itself is at least as important, and far more difficult to answer.

Geller and associates studied "stupid" animals who were unable to learn a discrimination task after 6 months of training.[141] Administration of chlordiazepoxide to these animals produced a fall in the frequency of incorrect discriminative responses, suggesting a drug-induced enhancement of learning. This, in general, has not been the experience of others. Chisholm and Moore[142] and Kamano and Arp[143] found the acquisition of conditioned avoidance unaffected by chlordiazepoxide. Others have demonstrated the learning process to be impaired by benzodiazepines in a dose-dependent manner.[113,114,122,144-148] Sansone and associates[149] demonstrated that acquisition of conditioned avoidance in mice was facilitated by low doses of chlordiazepoxide (5 mg/kg) and retarded by higher doses (15 mg/kg). Steiner et al[150] showed that chlordiazepoxide (10 mg/kg) produced variable effects on learned avoidance in rats depending upon the task. Shuttle avoidance was facilitated, but pole-climbing avoidance was impaired. Extinction of learned behavior also is variably affected, being enhanced in some studies[143] and impaired in others.[147,150-153]

Several other observations have further compounded the confusion. It appears that minor tranquilizers may in themselves serve as discriminative stimuli.[154-156] Animals faced with a choice situation can be taught to make one choice when drugged and another while undrugged. Overton, among others, described this situation as "dissociated" or "state-dependent" learning in which behavior acquired under drug or non-drug conditions is manifested during later testing only under the same drug or non-drug condition that exisited during training.[157] Other investigators have confirmed that chlordiazepoxide may produce dissociated learning.[153,158,159] Workers at Wyeth Laboratories, studying shock-induced suppression of water drinking, in addition have demonstrated that "asymmetrical dissociation" may occur with oxazepam and lorazepam.[104,160,161] Behavior acquired in the drug state is later manifested when tested in the drug state but not if tested with the animal undrugged. But behavior acquired under undrugged conditions is manifested under subsequent testing of both drugged and undrugged animals. A further fascinating observation is that regardless of the testing condition, oxazepam- or lorazepam-treated animals show *exaggerated* responses when later tested, with much longer drinking latencies than animals trained and tested under non-drug conditions. The authors conclude with a clinical interpretation that lorazepam and oxazepam may enhance the retrieval of unpleasant memories. It may be that the drugs produce a disinhibition of mechanisms suppressing these memories.

No simple generalization can be made regarding the effects of benzodiazepines on learning. The drugs do seem to influence the acquisition of conditioned behavior in some circumstances, depending upon the nature of the response and of the reinforcement or punishment. The subsequent expression of conditioning may depend on the drug state during testing.

COMMENT

In animals, the most consistent effect of the benzodiazepines is disinhibition—attenuation of the behavioral consequences of fear, conflict, and frustration. Enhancement of appetite, increased responding at low rates, potentiation of amphetamine hyperactivity, increased exploratory behavior, decreased fixation, enhanced self-stimulation, "paradoxical" hostility, and enhanced retrieval of unpleasant memories are other observed drug effects which may be explained in part if not entirely by the underlying mechanism of disinhibition—the release of behavior that is suppressed by punishment or by lack of reward. For the clinician, animal studies can at best suggest avenues of investigation. The antianxiety effects of these drugs have been exhaustively studied in humans (Chapter 4). Yet there has been relatively little investigation in humans of the influence of the benzodiazepines upon discrete dysfunctional syndromes postulated to be induced by fear, conflict, or anxiety (e.g., impotence, phobias, conversion symptoms, obsessive-compulsive behavior, etc.). Although the prediction of clinical effects on the basis of animal studies should be undertaken only with great caution, the minor tranquilizers could in fact be of considerable value in the treatment of such syndromes.

REFERENCES

1. Cook L, Kelleher RT: Effects of drugs on behavior. Ann Rev Pharmacol 3:205-222, 1963
2. Margules DL, Stein L: Neuroleptics vs. tranquilizers: evidence from animal behavior studies of mode and site of action. In, *Neuro-Psycho-Pharmacology*. Edited by H Brill. Amsterdam, Excerpta Medica Foundation, 1966, pp 108-120
3. Zbinden G, Randall LO: Pharmacology of benzodiazepines: laboratory and clinical correlations. Adv Pharmacol 5:213-291, 1967
4. Barry H, Buckley JP: Drug effects on animal performance and the stress syndrome. J Pharmaceut Sci 55:1159-1183, 1966
5. Cook L, Catania AC: Effects of drugs on avoidance and escape behavior. Fed Proc 23:818-835, 1964
6. Valzelli L: Drugs and aggressiveness. Adv Pharmacol 5:79-108, 1967
7. Bignami G, deAcetis L, Gatti GL: Facilitation and impairment of avoidance responding by phenobarbital sodium, chlordiazepoxide, and diazepam—the role of performance base lines. J Pharmacol Exp Ther 176:725-732, 1971
8. Gatti GL, Bignami G: Effects of chlordiazepoxide, diazepam, phenobarbital, meprobamate, and phenytoin on continuous lever-pressing avoidance with or without warning stimulus. In, *The Present Status of Psychotropic Drugs. Pharmacological and Clinical Aspects*. Edited by A Cerletti, FJ Bové. Amsterdam, Excerpta Medica Foundation, 1969, pp 255-256
9. Takaori S, Yada Y, Mori G: Effects of psychotropic agents on Sidman avoidance response in good- and poor-performed rats. Jap J Pharmacol 19:587-596, 1969
10. Wuttke W, Kelleher RT: Effects of some benzodiazepines on punished and unpunished behavior in the pigeon. J Pharmacol Exp Ther 172:397-405, 1970
11. King AR: The significance of drive level as a determinant of drug effects on approach and avoidance behavior in the rat. In, *The Present Status of Psychotropic Drugs. Pharmacological and Clinical Aspects*. Edited by A Cerletti, FJ Bové. Amsterdam, Excerpta Medica Foundation, 1969, pp 260-262
11a. Cook L, Davidson AB: Effects of behaviorally active drugs in a conflict-punishment procedure in rats. In, *The Benzodiazepines*. Edited by S Garattini, E Mussini, LO Randall. New York, Raven Press, 1973, pp 327-345

12. Bernstein BM, Cancro LP: The effect of two temporal variables of avoidance conditioning on drug-behavior interaction. Psychopharmacologia 3:105-113, 1962
13. McDonald DG, Stern JA, Hahn WW: Behavioral, dietary, and autonomic effects of chlordiazepoxide in the rat. Dis Nerv Syst 24:95-103, 1963
14. Clark R: A rapid method for testing antiappetite drugs in mice. Toxicol Appl Pharmacol 15:212-215, 1969
15. Matsuda Y: Effects of some centrally acting drugs on food intake of normal and hypothalamus-lesioned rats. Jap J Pharmacol 16:276-286, 1966
16. Poschel BPH: A simple and specific screen for benzodiazepine-like drugs. Psychopharmacologia 19:193-198, 1971
17. Falk JL, Burnidge GK: Fluid intake and punishment-attenuating drugs. Physiol Behav 5:199-202, 1970
18. Collins RJ, Weeks JR, MacGregor DW: An attempt to demonstrate ceiling efficacy of analgesics in rats. Arch Int Pharmacodyn 147:76-82, 1964
19. Weller CP, Ibrahim I, Sulman FG: Analgesic profile of tranquilizers in multiple screening tests in mice. Arch Int Pharmacodyn 176:176-192, 1968
20. Gupta SK, Gaitonde BB: Analgesic activity of a new quinoline derivative RO-4-1778. Indian J Physiol Pharmacol 7:27-32, 1964
21. Palosi E, Szporny L: New, simple method for the investigation of sedatives. Psychopharmacologia 12:44-49, 1967
22. Silvestrini B, Quadri E: Investigations on the specificity of the so-called analgesic activity of non-narcotic drugs. Eur J Pharmacol 12:231-235, 1970
23. Grotto M, Sulman FG: Interaction of analgesic effects of psychopharmaca. Arch Int Pharmacodyn 170:257-263, 1967
24. Leslie GB: The effect of anti-parkinsonian drugs on oxotremorine-induced analgesia in mice. J Pharm Pharmacol 21:248-250, 1969
25. Weis J: Morphine antagonistic effect of chlordiazepoxide (Librium®). Experientia 25:381, 1969
26. Hughes RN: Chlordiazepoxide modified exploration in the rat. Psychopharmacologia 24:462-469, 1972
27. Marriott AS, Smith EF: An analysis of drug effects in mice exposed to a simple novel environment. Psychopharmacologia 24:397-406, 1972
28. Ahtee L, Shillito E: The effect of benzodiazepines and atropine on exploratory behavior and motor activity of mice. Brit J Pharmacol 40:361-371, 1970
29. Marriott AS, Spencer PSJ: Effects of centrally acting drugs on exploratory behavior in rats. Brit J Pharmacol Chemother 25:432-441, 1965
30. Christmas AJ, Maxwell DR: A comparison of the effects of some benzodiazepines and other drugs on aggressive and exploratory behavior in mice and rats. Neuropharmacology 9:17-29, 1970
31. Richelle M, Xhenseval B, Fontaine O, Thone L: Action of chlordiazepoxide on two types of temporal conditioning in rats. Int J Neuropharmacol 1:381-391, 1962
32. Richelle M: Combined action of diazepam and d-amphetamine on fixed-interval performance in cats. J Exp Anal Behav 21:989-998, 1969
33. Hanson HM, Witoslawski JJ, Campbell EH: Drug effects in squirrel monkeys trained on a multiple schedule with a punishment contingency. J Exp Anal Behav 10:565-569, 1967
34. Longoni A, Mandelli V, Pessotti I: Variable interval in rats treated with temazepam, diazepam, oxazepam, and chlordiazepoxide. Pharmacol Res Comm 3:165-173, 1971
35. Cole J, Dearnaley DP: A technique for measuring exploratory activity in rats: some effects of chlorpromazine and chlordiazepoxide. Arzneim-Forsch 21:1359-1362, 1971
36. Gray WD, Osterberg AC, Rauh CE: Neuropharmacological actions of mephenoxalone. Arch Int Pharmacodyn 134:198-215, 1961

37. Shillito EE: A method for recording the effects of drugs on the activity of small animals over long periods of time. Brit J Pharmacol Chemother 26:248-255, 1966

38. Bignami G, Gatti GL: Analysis of drug effects on multiple fixed ratio 33-fixed interval 5 min in pigeons. Psychopharmacologia 15:310-332, 1969

39. Schneider CW, Chenoweth MB: Effects of hallucinogenic and other drugs on the nest-building behavior of mice. Nature (London) 225:1262-1263, 1970

40. Douglas RJ, Scott DW: The differential effects of nitrazepam on certain inhibitory and exploratory behavior. Psychonom Sci 26:164-166, 1972

41. Rushton R, Steinberg H, Tomkiewicz M: Effects of chlordiazepoxide alone and in combination with amphetamine on animal and human behavior. In, *The Benzodiazepines*. Edited by S Garattini, E Mussini, LO Randall. New York, Raven Press, 1973, pp 355-366

42. Morrison CF, Stephenson JA: Drug effects on a measure of unconditioned avoidance in the rat. Psychopharmacologia 18:133-143, 1970

43. Morrison CF, Stephenson JA: Drug effects on unconditioned light-avoidance in the rat. Psychopharmacologia 24:456-461, 1972

43a. Nolan NA, Parkes MW: The effect of benzodiazepines on the behavior of mice on a hole board. Psychopharmacologia 29:277-288, 1973

44. Herman ZS: Influence of some psychotropic and adrenergic blocking agents upon amphetamine stereotyped behavior in white rats. Psychopharmacologia 11:136-142, 1967

45. Sethy VH, Naik PY, Sheth UK: Effect of d-amphetamine sulphate in combination with CNS depressants on spontaneous motor activity of mice. Psychopharmacologia 18:19-25, 1970

46. Babbini M, Montanaro N, Strocchi P, Gaiardi M: Enhancement of amphetamine-induced stereotyped behavior by benzodiazepines. Eur J Pharmacol 13:330-340, 1971

47. Rushton R, Steinberg H: Combined effects of chlordiazepoxide and dexamphetamine on activity of rats in an unfamiliar environment. Nature (London) 211:1312-1313, 1966

48. Borella LE, Paquette R, Herr F: The effect of some CNS depressants on the hypermotility and anorexia induced by amphetamine in rats. Canad J Physiol Pharmacol 47:841-847, 1969

49. Kumadaki N, Hitomi M, Kumada S: Effect of psychotherapeutic drugs on hypermotility of rats in which the olfactory bulb was removed. Jap J Pharmacol 17:659-667, 1967

50. Stark P, Henderson JK: Differentiation of classes of neurosedatives using rats with septal lesions. Int J Neuropharmacol 5:385-389, 1966

51. Olds ME: Alterations by centrally acting drugs of the suppression of self-stimulation behavior in the rat by tetrabenazine, physostigmine, chlorpromazine, and pentobarbital. Psychopharmacologia 25:299-314, 1972

52. Olds ME: Facilitatory action of diazepam and chlordiazepoxide on hypothalamic reward behavior. J Comp Physiol Psychol 62:136-140, 1966

53. Domino EF, Olds ME: Effects of d-amphetamine, scopolamine, chlordiazepoxide, and diphenylhydantoin on self-stimulation behavior and brain acetylcholine. Psychopharmacologia 23:1-16, 1972

54. Olds ME: Comparative effects of amphetamine, scopolamine, chlordiazepoxide, and diphenylhydantoin on operant and extinction behavior with brain stimulation and food reward. Neuropharmacology 5:519-532, 1970

55. Olds ME: Comparative effects of amphetamine, scopolamine, and chlordiazepoxide on self-stimulation behavior. Rev Canad Biol 31(supp):25-47, 1972

56. Weinreich D, Clark LD: Anticonvulsant drugs and self-stimulation in rats. Arch Int Pharmacodyn 185:269-273, 1970

57. Boissier J-R, Grasset S, Simon P: Effect of some psychotropic drugs on mice from a spontaneously aggressive strain. J Pharm Pharmacol 20:972-973, 1968

58. Kostowski W: A note on the effects of some psychotropic drugs on the aggressive behavior in the ant, *Formica rufa*. J Pharm Pharmacol 18:747-749, 1966

59. Macko E, Wilfon G, Greene L, Bender AD, Tedeschi RE: Pharmacological properties of the isopropyl ester of o-sulfamoyl-benzoic acid. Arch Int Pharmacodyn 168:220-234, 1967

60. Valzelli L: Further aspects of the exploratory behavior in aggressive mice. Psychopharmacologia 19:91-94, 1971

61. Shibata S, Sasakawa S, Fujita Y: The central depressant profile of carbamate ester of glycerol ether: 3-(1,2,3,4-tetrahydro-7-naphthyloxy)-2-hydroxypropyl carbamate. Toxicol Appl Pharmacol 11:591-602, 1967

62. Scheckel CL, Boff E: Effects of drugs on aggressive behavior in monkeys. In, *Neuro-Psycho-Pharmacology*. Edited by H Brill. Amsterdam, Excerpta Medica Foundation, 1966, pp 789-795

63. Delgado JMR: Antiaggressive effects of chlordiazepoxide. In, *The Benzodiazepines*. Edited by S Garattini, E Mussini, LO Randall. New York, Raven Press, 1973, pp 419-432

64. Beattie IA, Berry PA, Lister RE: Methods for detecting anti-anxiety activity using baboons (*Papio cynocephalus*). Brit J Pharmacol 38:460P-461P, 1970

65. Lister RE, Beattie IA, Berry PA: Effects of drugs on the social behavior of baboons. In, *Advances in Neuro-Psychopharmacology*. Edited by O Vinar, Z Votava, PB Bradley. Amsterdam, North-Holland Publishing Co., 1971, pp 299-303

66. Bauen A, Possanza GJ: The mink as a psychopharmacological model. Arch Int Pharmacodyn 186:133-136, 1970

67. Langfeldt T, Ursin H: Differential action of diazepam on flight and defense behavior in the cat. Psychopharmacologia 19:61-66, 1971

68. Hoffmeister F, Wuttke W: On the actions of psychotropic drugs on the attack- and aggressive-defensive behavior of mice and cats. In, *Aggressive Behavior*. Edited by S Garattini, EB Sigg. New York, Wiley-Interscience, 1969, pp 273-280

69. Usher DR, Ling GM, MacConaill M: Some endocrine and behavioral effects of chlordiazepoxide in septal-lesioned rats. Int J Clin Pharmacol 1:191-196, 1968

70. Malick JB, Sofia RD, Goldberg ME: A comparative study of the effects of selected psychoactive agents upon three lesion-induced models of aggression in the rat. Arch Int Pharmacodyn 181:459-465, 1969

71. Sofia RD: Effects of centrally active drugs on four models of experimentally-induced aggression in rodents. Life Sci 8(part I):705-716, 1969

72. Irwin S, Kinohi R, Van Sloten M, Workman MP: Drug effects on distress-evoked behavior in mice: methodology and drug class comparisons. Psychopharmacologia 20:172-185, 1971

73. Panksepp J: Drugs and stimulus-bound attack. Physiol Behav 6:317-320, 1971

74. Baxter BL: The effect of chlordiazepoxide on the hissing response elicited via hypothalamic stimulation. Life Sci 3:531-537, 1964

75. Malick JB: Effects of selected drugs on stimulus-bound emotional behavior elicited by hypothalamic stimulation in the cat. Arch Int Pharmacodyn 186:137-141, 1970

76. Yen HCY, Katz MH, Krop S: Effects of various drugs on 3,4-dihydroxyphenylalanine (DL-DOPA)-induced excitation (aggressive behavior) in mice. Toxicol Appl Pharmacol 17:597-604, 1970

77. Cole HF, Wolf HH: Laboratory evaluation of aggressive behavior in the grasshopper mouse *(Onychomys)*. J Pharmaceut Sci 59:969-971, 1970

78. Scriabine A, Blake M: Evaluation of centrally acting drugs in mice with fighting behavior induced by isolation. Psychopharmacologia 3:224-226, 1962

79. Valzelli L, Giacalone E, Garattini S: Pharmacological control of aggressive behavior in mice. Eur J Pharmacol 2:144-146, 1967

80. LeDouarec JC, Broussy L: Dissociation of the aggressive behavior in mice produced by certain drugs. In, *Aggressive Behavior*. Edited by S Garattini, EB Sigg. New York, Wiley-Interscience, 1969, pp 281-295

81. Davanzo JP: Observations related to drug-induced alterations in aggressive behavior. In,

Aggressive Behavior. Edited by S Garattini, EB Sigg. New York, Wiley-Interscience, 1969, pp 263-272

82. Valzelli L, Bernasconi S: Differential activity of some psychotropic drugs as a function of emotional level in animals. Psychopharmacologia 20:91-96, 1971

83. Goldberg ME: Pharmacologic activity of a new class of agents which selectively inhibit aggressive behavior in rats. Arch Int Pharmacodyn 186:287-297, 1970

84. Horovitz ZP, Furguiele AR, Brannick LJ, Burke JC, Craver BN: A new chemical structure with specific depressant effects on the amygdala and on the hyper-irritability of the 'septal rat.' Nature (London) 200:369-370, 1963

85. Horovitz ZP, Ragozzino PW, Leaf RC: Selective block of rat mouse-killing by antidepressants. Life Sci 4:1909-1912, 1965

86. Horovitz ZP, Piala JJ, High JP, Burke JC, Leaf RC: Effects of drugs on the mouse-killing (muricide) test and its relationship to amygdaloid function. Int J Neuropharmacol 5:405-411, 1966

87. Guaitani A, Marcucci F, Garattini S: Increased aggression and toxicity in grouped male mice treated with tranquilizing benzodiazepines. Psychopharmacologia 19:241-245, 1971

88. Fox KA, Webster JC, Guerriero FJ: Increased aggression among grouped male mice fed nitrazepam and flurazepam. Pharmacol Res Comm 4:157-162, 1972

89. Fox KA, Tuckosh JR, Wilcox AH: Increased aggression among grouped male mice fed chlordiazepoxide. Eur J Pharmacol 11:119-121, 1970

90. Fox KA, Snyder RL: Effects of sustained low doses of diazepam on aggression and mortality in grouped male mice. J Comp Physiol Psychol 69:663-666, 1969

91. Valzelli L, Ghezzi D, Bernasconi S: Benzodiazepine activity on some aspects of behavior. Totus Homo 3:73-79, 1971

92. Valzelli L: Activity of benzodiazepines on aggressive behavior in rats and mice. In, *The Benzodiazepines.* Edited by S Garattini, E Mussini, LO Randall. New York, Raven Press, 1973, pp 405-417

93. Valzelli L: The exploratory behavior in normal and aggressive mice. Psychopharmacologia 15:232-235, 1969

94. Geller I, Kulak JT, Seifter J: The effects of chlordiazepoxide and chlorpromazine on a punishment discrimination. Psychopharmacologia 3:374-385, 1962

94a. Longoni A, Mandelli V, Pessotti I: Study of antianxiety effects of drugs in the rat, with a multiple punishment and reward schedule. In, *The Benzodiazepines.* Edited by S Garattini, E Mussini, LO Randall. New York, Raven Press, 1973, pp 347-354

94b. Miczek KA: Effects of scopolamine, amphetamine, and chlordiazepoxide on punishment. Psychopharmacologia 28:373-389, 1973

95. Geller I: Relative potencies of benzodiazepines as measured by their effects on conflict behavior. Arch Int Pharmacodyn 149:243-247, 1964

96. Goldberg ME, Ciofalo VB: Effect of diphenylhydantoin sodium and chlordiazepoxide alone and in combination on punishment behavior. Psychopharmacologia 14:233-239, 1969

97. Morrison CF: The effect of nicotine on punished behavior. Psychopharmacologia 14:221-232, 1969

98. Bremner FJ, Cobb HW, Hahn WC: The effect of chlordiazepoxide on the behavior of rats in a conflict situation. Psychopharmacologia 17:275-282, 1970

99. Blum K: Effects of chlordiazepoxide and pentobarbital on conflict behavior in rats. Psychopharmacologia 17:391-398, 1970

100. Vogel JR, Beer B, Clody DE: A simple and reliable conflict procedure for testing anti-anxiety agents. Psychopharmacologia 21:1-7, 1971

101. Aron C, Simon P, Larousse C, Boissier J-R: Evaluation of a rapid technique for detecting minor tranquilizers. Neuropharmacology 10:459-469, 1971

102. Cannizzaro G, Nigito S, Provenzano PM, Vitikova T: Relationship between inhibitory factors and behavior after treatment with medazepam. Arzneim-Forsch 22:772-776, 1972

103. Cannizzaro G, Nigito S, Provenzano PM, Vitikova T: Modification of depressant and disinhibitory action of flurazepam during short term treatment in the rat. Psychopharmacologia 26:173-184, 1972

104. Stein L, Berger BD: Psychopharmacology of 7-chloro-5-(o-chlorophenyl)-1,3-dihydro-3-hydroxy-2H-1,4-benzodiazepin-2-one (lorazepam) in squirrel monkey and rat. Arzneim-Forsch 21:1073-1078, 1971

105. Margules DL, Stein L: Increase of "antianxiety" activity and tolerance of behavioral depression during chronic administration of oxazepam. Psychopharmacologia 13:74-80, 1968

106. Matsuki K, Iwamoto T: Development of tolerance to tranquillizers in the rat. Jap J Pharmacol 16:191-197, 1966

107. Maser JD, Hammond LJ: Disruption of a temporal discrimination by the minor tranquilizer, oxazepam. Psychopharmacologia 25:69-76, 1972

108. Tenen SS: Recovery time as a measure of CER strength: effects of benzodiazepines, amobarbital, chlorpromazine, and amphetamine. Psychopharmacologia 12:1-17, 1967

109. Bainbridge JG: The effect of psychotropic drugs on food reinforced behavior and on food consumption. Psychopharmacologia 12:204-213, 1968

110. Boissier J-R, Simon P, Aron C: A new method for rapid screening of minor tranquillizers in mice. Eur J Pharmacol 4:145-151, 1968

111. Lauener H: Conditioned suppression in rats and the effect of pharmacological agents thereon. Psychopharmacologia 4:311-325, 1963

112. Ross N, Monti JM: Effects of haloperidol, trifluperidol, nitrazepam, and chlordiazepoxide upon conditioned midbrain behavioral responses. Psychopharmacologia 22:31-44, 1971

113. Cicala GA, Hartley DL: Drugs and the learning and performance of fear. J Comp Physiol Psychol 64:175-178, 1967

114. Chisholm DC, Couch JV, Moore JW: Chlordiazepoxide and aversive conditioning: effects of acquisition and performance on the conditioned nictating membrane response in the rabbit. Psychonom Sci 23:203-204, 1971

115. Delini-Stula A: Drug-induced suppression of conditioned hyperthermic and conditioned avoidance behavior response in rats. Psychopharmacologia 20:153-159, 1971

116. Molinengo L, Gamalero SR: Behavioral action and tranquillizing effect of reserpine, diazepam, and hydroxyzine. Arch Int Pharmacodyn 180:217-231, 1969

117. Morpurgo C: Drug-induced modifications of discriminated avoidance behavior in rats. Psychopharmacologia 8:91-99, 1965

118. Dinsmoor JA, Bonbright JC, Lilie DR: A controlled comparison of drug effects on escape from conditioned aversive stimulation ("anxiety") and from continuous shock. Psychopharmacologia 22:323-332, 1971

119. Chittal SM, Sheth UK: Effect of drugs on conditioned avoidance response in rats. Arch Int Pharmacodyn 114:471-480, 1963

120. Oishi H, Iwahara S, Yang K-M, Yogi A: Effects of chlordiazepoxide on passive avoidance responses in rats. Psychopharmacologia 23:373-385, 1972

121. Fuller JL: Strain differences in the effects of chlorpromazine and chlordiazepoxide upon active and passive avoidance in mice. Psychopharmacologia 16:261-271, 1970

122. Chisholm DC, Moore JW: Effects of chlordiazepoxide on the acquisition of shuttle avoidance in the rabbit. Psychonom Sci 19:21-22, 1970

123. Sansone M, Marino A: Benzodiazepines on avoidance conditioning in guinea pigs. Pharmacol Res Comm 1:122-126, 1969

124. Hughes FW, Rountree CB, Forney RB: Suppression of learned avoidance and discriminative responses in the rat by chlordiazepoxide (Librium) and ethanol-chlordiazepoxide combinations. J Genetic Psychol 103:139-145, 1963

125. Heise GA, McConnell H: Differences between chlordiazepoxide-type and chlorpromazine-type action in "trace" avoidance. In, *Proceedings of the Third World Congress of Psychia-*

try, Vol. II. Montreal, University of Toronto and McGill University Press, 1961, pp 917-921

126. Cole HF, Wolf HH: The effects of some psychotropic drugs on conditioned avoidance and aggressive behaviors. Psychopharmacologia 8:389-396, 1966

127. Heise GA, Boff E: Continuous avoidance as a base-line for measuring behavioral effects of drugs. Psychopharmacologia 3:264-282, 1962

128. Rosen AJ, Tessel RE: Chlorpromazine, chlordiazepoxide, and incentive-shift performance in the rat. J Comp Physiol Psychol 72:257-262, 1970

129. Vogel JR, Principi K: Effects of chlordiazepoxide on depressed performance after reward reduction. Psychopharmacologia 21:8-12, 1971

130. Thompson DM: Enhancement of progressive-ratio performance by chlordiazepoxide and phenobarbital. J Exp Anal Behav 17:287-292, 1972

131. Wedeking PW: Stimulating effects of chlordiazepoxide in rats on a food reinforced FR schedule. Psychonom Sci 12:31-32, 1968

132. Wedeking PW: Disinhibition effect of chlordiazepoxide. Psychonom Sci 15:232-233, 1969

133. Liberson WT, Kafka A, Schwartz E, Gagnon V: Effects of chlordiazepoxide (Librium) on fixated behavior in rats. Int J Neuropharmacol 2:67-78, 1963

134. Feldman RS: The prevention of fixations with chlordiazepoxide. J Neuropsychiat 3:254-259, 1962

135. Feldman RS: Further studies on assay and testing of fixation-preventing psychotropic drugs. Psychopharmacologia 6:130-142, 1964

136. Lewis EM, Feldman RS: The depressive effect of chlordiazepoxide on a negative incentive. Psychopharmacologia 6:143-150, 1964

137. Feldman RS: The mechanism of fixation prevention and "dissociation" learning with chlordiazepoxide. Psychopharmacologia 12:384-399, 1968

138. Bremner FJ, Cobb HD, Nagy TJ: Comparison of the effect of two minor tranquilizers on escape behavior. Psychonom Sci 17:159-160, 1969

139. Yen HCY, Krop S, Mendez HC, Katz MH: Effects of some psychoactive drugs on experimental 'neurotic' (conflict induced) behavior in cats. Pharmacology 3:32-40, 1970

140. Soubrie P, Schoonhoed L, Simon P, Boissier J-R: Conflict behavior in a heated-floor maze: effects of oxazepam. Psychopharmacologia 26:317-320, 1972

141. Geller I, Hartmann R, Blum K: Effects of nicotine, nicotine monomethiodide, lobeline, chlordiazepoxide, meprobamate, and caffeine on a discrimination task in laboratory rats. Psychopharmacologia 20:355-365, 1971

142. Chisholm DC, Moore JW: Effects of chlordiazepoxide on discriminative fear conditioning and shuttle avoidance performance in the rabbit. Psychopharmacologia 18:162-171, 1970

143. Kamano DK, Arp DJ: Effects of chlordiazepoxide (Librium) on the acquisition and extinction of avoidance responses. Psychopharmacologia 6:112-119, 1964

144. Cicala GA, Hartley DL: The effects of chlordiazepoxide on the acquisition and performance of a conditioned escape response in rats. Psychol Rec 15:435-440, 1965

145. Stolerman IP: A method for studying the influences of drugs on learning for food rewards in rats. Psychopharmacologia 19:398-406, 1971

146. Scobie SR, Garske G: Chlordiazepoxide and conditioned suppression. Psychopharmacologia 16:272-280, 1970

147. Tessel RE, Lash S: Effects of chlordiazepoxide on the acquisition and extinction of a running response. Proc Amer Psychol Assoc 3:149-150, 1968

148. Thompson DM: Repeated acquisition as a behavioral base line for studying drug effects. J Pharmacol Exp Ther 184:506-514, 1973

149. Sansone M, Renzi P, Amposta B: Effects of chlorpromazine and chlordiazepoxide on discriminated lever-press avoidance behavior and intertrial responding in mice. Psychopharmacologia 27:313-318, 1972

150. Steiner SS, Fitzgerald HL, Taber RI: Effect of chlordiazepoxide (CDP) on acquisition

and extinction of shuttle box and pole-climbing avoidance. Pharmacologist 9:200, 1967

151. Taber RI, Latranvi MB, Steiner SS: Prevention of extinction of an active avoidance response by "anti-anxiety" agents. Pharmacologist 9:200, 1967

152. Kumar R: Extinction of fear II: effects of chlordiazepoxide and chlorpromazine on fear and exploratory behavior in rats. Psychopharmacologia 19:297-312, 1971

153. Sachs E, Weingarten M, Klein NW: Effects of chlordiazepoxide on the acquisition of avoidance learning and its transfer to the normal state and other drug conditions. Psychopharmacologia 9:17-30, 1966

154. Overton DA: State-dependent learning produced by depressant and atropine-like drugs. Psychopharmacologia 10:6-31, 1966

155. Berger BD: Conditioning of food aversions by injections of psychoactive drugs. J Comp Physiol Psychol 81:21-26, 1972

156. Brown A, Feldman RS, Moore JW: Conditional discrimination learning based upon chlordiazepoxide. J Comp Physiol Psychol 66:211-215, 1968

157. Overton DA: Dissociated learning in drug states (state dependent learning). In, *Psychopharmacology: A Review of Progress 1957-1967*. Edited by DH Efron. Washington, DC, USPHS publication #1836, 1968, pp 918-930

158. Iwahara S, Matsushita K: Effect of drug-state changes upon black-white discrimination learning in rats. Psychopharmacologia 19:347-358, 1971

159. Henriksson BG, Jarbe T: Effects of diazepam on conditioned avoidance learning in rats and its transfer to normal state conditions. Psychopharmacologia 20:186-190, 1971

160. Berger BD, Stein L: Asymmetrical dissociation of learning between scopolamine and Wy 4036, a new benzodiazepine tranquilizer. Psychopharmacologia 14:351-358, 1969

161. Stein L, Berger BD: Paradoxical fear-increasing effects of tranquilizers: evidence of repression of memory in the rat. Science 166:253-256, 1969

Chapter 4
The Treatment of Emotional Disorders

This chapter will consider the efficacy of the benzodiazepines in the clinical treatment of emotional disorders.

The ethical and financial implications of this problem are staggering in view of epidemiologic studies of the extent of psychotropic drug use. Most psychotropic drug users are outpatients; only a few are hospitalized. In 1967, psychotropic drugs accounted for 17% of the 1.1 billion prescriptions written in the United States.[1,2] Two-thirds were refills while one-third were new prescriptions. Minor tranquilizers or antianxiety agents, predominantly benzodiazepines, accounted for 20.4 million or nearly 30% of new psychotropic drug prescriptions. General practitioners wrote the majority (75%) of these prescriptions; only 5% were written by psychiatrists. Several surveys have suggested that 5 to 15% of all adult Americans take antianxiety agents in a year's time.[3-5] Among patients receiving psychiatric outpatient care, the figure exceeds 30%. The benzodiazepines not only predominate among antianxiety agents, but also comprise a substantial proportion of total psychotropic drug prescriptions and of all drug prescriptions taken together. Chlordiazepoxide and diazepam invariably are at or near the top of lists of drugs most frequently used by outpatients.[6,7] An estimated 42 million dollars was spent on prescriptions for these two drugs in 1968 in the United States. In Great Britain, 12.7 million prescriptions for benzodiazepines were written in 1968.[8] Surveys performed in Australia yield similar findings.[9]

The benzodiazepines likewise are frequently administered to hospitalized patients, both psychiatric[10,11] and medical.[12,13] The Boston Collaborative Drug Surveillance Program[14] monitors drug use among hospitalized medical patients in nine hospitals located in the United States, Canada, Israel, and New Zealand. Of 13,349 patients monitored from 1966 to 1972, 2,086 (15.6%) received chlordiazepoxide and 2,623 (18.9%) received diazepam during one or more admissions.

The use of the benzodiazepines is becoming more widespread with each year that passes. No less than one in 10 adult Americans may be expected to ingest one of these drugs in a year's time. In this setting, a critical survey of what the benzodiazepines do, and how well they do it, is of considerable importance.

WHO TAKES MINOR TRANQUILIZERS?

General practitioners and internists will attest that the most common disease they treat is non-disease or "dys-ease." Gynecologists and gastroenterologists might agree. Anxious neurotic patients with no demonstrable organic disease fill the waiting rooms of physicians and clinics in all parts of the world. Most doctors have been schooled to evaluate, diagnose, and treat objective pathology. Confronted with patient after patient whose diseases do not show up in physical findings, lab tests, or X-rays, they often feel plagued and frustrated, and may respond curtly as if the patient's symptoms were not real. Yet patients seek this medical care because something is wrong. Nearly all turn first to their internist or family physician for help, and, in fact, do not require formal psychiatric intervention. What they do need is the busy physician's least available commodity, *time*—time to work toward delineating and resolving the conflicts and stresses in their lives. Such clarifications, carried out by an understanding physician who does not become anxious at hearing the patient's story, may be a sufficient intervention, obviating the need for the prescription of psychotropic drugs. For the practitioner who is unable or unwilling to provide this time-consuming support, the prescription pad alone often becomes the automatic answer. Minor tranquilizers are most often prescribed by nonpsychiatrists for their anxious neurotic patients. Although this is an appropriate target population, iatrogenic drug overuse is always a potential problem.

Anxiety must be understood as a ubiquitous term. In contrast to actual fear, anxiety reactions may occur in the absence of an observable threat, or the resultant anxiety may seem disproportionate to or incongruous with the objective reality.[15] Anxiety may be intimately linked to depression and other dysphoric affects. Occasionally, anxiety may be acute, free-floating, and culminate in panic.

Anxiety states may be communicated through many terms and symptoms, and the understanding clinician must listen with an ear that is tuned to recognize the multiple clusterings which may be expressed by the patient (Table 4-1). Some individuals are overtly anxious but have no specific somatic complaints. "I'm nervous all the time," or, "Little things bother me," are common complaints. Others, in addition to overt anxiety, have somatic symptoms: headaches, fatigue, dizziness, palpitations, breathlessness, chest pain, diarrhea. A few have physical symptoms only. It is not uncommon for patients to make statements such as, "It's not that I'm anxious, it's just that I'm nervous," or "I don't know what it is, I just feel these times when I get breathless, my heart seems to pound, and I feel all keyed up." The clinician should rule out organic disease (hypoglycemia, pheochromocytoma, thyrotoxicosis, pulmonary emboli, etc.) as causes of the patient's symptoms. When the emotional etiology of these complaints is established and the presence of anxiety recognized, the clinician can then proceed to consider what pharmacotherapy has to offer.

Inasmuch as most of the benzodiazepines are classified as antianxiety agents, one would expect these drugs to be of greatest value in the treatment of anxiety. This simplistic concept, however, does not consider the important distinction between syndrome and disease. Because our understanding of emotional disorder is relatively primitive, we have aggregated certain patterns of psychopathology into broad categories of disease—neurosis, psychosis, personality disorder, depression. Whether these arbitrary categories have correspondingly distinct biochemical or physiological bases is largely unknown. Psychotropic drugs interact with the patient and his symptoms, not with our disease categories. Anxiety—the symptom—may be prominent in many diseases. The benzodiazepines accordingly have been used in numerous disease states other than "anxiety neurosis," with varying degrees of success. With some justification one might predict that the value of the benzodiazepines in emotional disorders might depend on the importance and severity of anxiety and agitation in the patient's complex of symptomatology.

TABLE 4-1. *Common subjective descriptors of anxiety experiences*

Anxious
Apprehensive
Avoiding fright
Breathless
Choking sensations
Danger
Dizzy
Fear
Feeling of dread
Flushing
Giddy
Head pounding
Heart racing
Keyed up
Muscle tension
Nervous
Overconcerned
Palpitations
Panic
Phobic
Restless
Scared for no reason
Shaky
Sweating
Tense
Threatened
Tightness in chest
Tired easily
Tremulous
Urge to urinate
Worried

UNCONTROLLED TRIALS

The uncontrolled trial is one of the most straightforward approaches to drug evaluation. The pharmacologic agent is administered to the subject, and the investigator observes the target effects. Numerous limitations are inherent in this approach, the most important of which is the failure to assess the contribution of "placebo" effects in psychotropic drug research. It is well known that target symptoms may appear or disappear either spontaneously, in response to the aura of investigation, in response to the expectation of change, or because of investigator bias. Uncontrolled trials can suggest whether further controlled study is indicated, but, when taken alone as conclusive, drug studies without properly controlled design frequently confuse the issue of efficacy.

Chapter 1 discusses uncontrolled trials of chlordiazepoxide appearing in 1960. Appendix 3 lists studies of the benzodiazepines in psychiatric disorders appearing during or after 1961 (references cited in this paragraph and the following one are given in Appendix 3). Trials in patients with acute and chronic alcoholism have not been included, since they are discussed in Chapter 11. There are nearly 100 studies, all with inadequate or no controls, involving thousands of patients. The results are given in Table 4-2. Of some 1,500 patients with psychoneurotic anxiety, depression, agitation, or behavior problems treated with chlordiazepoxide, the overall improvement rate was 74%. In nearly 250 psychotic patients, 69% improved on chlordiazepoxide. Details of response to therapy among the psychotic patients are not always available, but in most cases there was improvement of anxiety and agitation rather than amelioration of the thought disorder or other psychotic manifestations. Three studies (Sargant, 1962; Sargant and Dally, 1962; Kearney, 1964) describe the use of chlordiazepoxide combined with monoamine oxidase inhibitors in the treatment of anxiety or depression. Settel (1963) and Matlin (1963) used chlordiazepoxide with or without amphetamines to treat obesity. Ayd (1962) was the least enthusiastic of investigators, pointing out the substantial frequency of oversedation from chlordiazepoxide at daily doses

TABLE 4-2. *Summary of uncontrolled clinical trials**

	Psychoneurotics		Psychotics	
Drug	Total patients studied	% improved	Total patients studied	% improved
Chlordiazepoxide	1,500	74	250	69
Diazepam	2,500	73	300	64
Oxazepam	1,000	78	—	—
Medazepam	314	68	—	—

*See Appendix 3 for complete bibliography.

of more than 50 mg. He also noted the occurrence of paradoxical excitement, garrulity, rage, and mania early in the course of treatment, as well as appetite stimulation and weight gain in some patients. Other investigators also noted increased agitation and hostility, and at least three mentioned weight gain associated with treatment.

Among nearly 2,500 psychoneurotic individuals treated with diazepam, the improvement rate was 73%. Darling (1963) thought that chlordiazepoxide and diazepam were interchangeable at equipotent doses. Of some 300 psychotic patients, 64% improved on diazepam. Feldman (1962) emphasized that diazepam has little or no effect upon psychotic thinking and may encourage the development of hostility. Others (Galambos, 1964a; Barsa and Saunders, 1964; Hollister et al., 1963) noted deterioration of some psychotic patients on diazepam. Irvine and Schaechter (1969), on the other hand, successfully treated 25 schizophrenics with refractory hallucinations using oral diazepam. Galambos (1964b, 1965) found that diazepam improved disturbed behavior in mentally retarded, institutionalized adults. Kalina (1964) used diazepam in male prison inmates with personality disorders. Paradoxical agitation was rarely reported by investigators in trials with diazepam, and weight gain was not reported at all.

Studies involving oxazepam, medazepam, lorazepam, and chlorazepate are fewer in number. This may reflect the more recent availability of the drugs, as well as an increasing tendency for controlled trials to be performed early in the course of drug evaluation. The improvement rates with oxazepam and medazepam are close to those reported with chlordiazepoxide and diazepam. Seventy-eight percent of 1,000 oxazepam-treated neurotic patients improved; with medazepam the figure is 68% of 300. Isolated trials with a number of other benzodiazepines are included in Appendix 3.

THE CONTROLLED CLINICAL TRIAL: DELIVERANCE OR DECEPTION?

The obvious necessity for dealing with placebo reactivity and investigator bias in psychotropic drug evaluation has led to the concept of the double-blind trial, now accepted as an essential parameter of design in any reliable drug assessment.[16-21] Yet, the double-blind approach has hardly solved all the methodological problems of psychotropic drug research. Numerous valid criticisms of the concept of the controlled trial have been raised.[22-27] Many can be answered or adjusted for, although others cannot. A summary of points of debate is given in Table 4-3. The objection to the crossover trial is a valid one, from both a pharmacologic and a psychiatric point of view. Many antianxiety agents, particularly benzodiazepines, are slowly excreted from the human body; significant amounts of the parent drug and pharmacologically active metabolites may be detectable for days after drug therapy is discontinued (see Chapter 2). Patients in whom the testing sequence

TABLE 4-3. *Criticisms of the double-blind: Claims and counter-claims*

Claim	Counter-claim
Administering a placebo to a symptomatic patient is unethical.	a) The treatment of millions of patients with a drug whose efficacy is not established is hardly ethical.
	b) Depriving a neurotic patient of active medication during a drug study is not akin to withholding penicillin from a patient with pneumococcal pneumonia.
	c) An active medication may be used instead of placebo as a reference substance.
Drug-placebo differences may be demonstrable only with large sample sizes (50 or more patients per treatment group).	For clinically useful agents which differ markedly from placebo, significant differences may appear in trials with 10—15 patients.
Controlled trials are performed in a rigid, sterile, investigative setting; results therefore are not applicable to the setting of the usual doctor-patient relationship.	Valid psychopharmacological research may be performed within ongoing private practices and clinics, with no disruption of the therapeutic relationship.
Studies using fixed drug dosage are unrealisitic, since most patients on psychotropic drugs require trial-and-error titration of dosage.	Optional dosage adjustment is easily incorporated into the design of a controlled trial.
The onset of action of the drug may not occur within the duration of the trial.	Effects of antianxiety agents, when they occur, are almost always seen within 7 days of therapy. Most drug trials last at least this long.
Overall results of studies on large numbers of patients do not predict whether the drug will be of benefit to an individual patient.	Nothing can unequivocally predict an individual's response to a drug. Physicians deal with probabilities, most reliably provided from experience with large numbers of patients.
Effects of the first drug administered on a crossover trial may influence the post-crossover response.	A drug-free "washout" period at the time of crossover may be interpolated between drug exposures.
"Double-blind" is seldom realistically valid. Both patient and investigator can distinguish between active and inactive medications.	None.

is "drug $\rightarrow$ placebo" may be pharmacologically influenced by the active drug even when receiving placebo, tending to negate drug-placebo differences. Interposition of a "washout" period of several days, during which no medications are ingested, between test-drug exposures may solve the pharmacologic aspect of this problem, but a more fundamental psychiatric one remains. Numerous studies have demonstrated that the relative responses to drugs and placebo, and thus drug-drug or drug-placebo differences, may be profoundly influenced by the sequence of administration in a crossover trial. The crossover design is being utilized by fewer investigators as time passes. The second major weakness of the double-blind trial is that it often is unachievable in reality.[27] Both patient and physician can accurately differentiate active drug from inactive placebo on the basis of pharmacologic effects and side effects.[28] The problem is no less serious in trials comparing two active drugs. Studies on antipsychotic and antidepressant agents may use "active" placebos (such as atropine and/or phenobarbital) having side effects similar to the drug being tested. In studies of antianxiety agents versus placebo, however, there is no reliable method of dealing with this potential source of non-blindness in the double-blind design. This is a weakness which must be recognized and with which investigators must live.

Another set of problems which plagues psychotropic drug research on a much broader scale includes the "nonspecific" factors in drug therapy: characteristics of patient, physician, treatment setting, and disease which influence the response to drug and placebo, and hence alter the potential drug-placebo difference. Numerous reviews discuss the subject in great detail.[29-38] Table 4-4 summarizes important non-drug factors and their influence on drug trials in anxious neurotics. The "strength" of these various factors differs from study to study. In some cases, different investigators have found the same nonspecific factor to influence results in different directions. In a series of drug trials involving the benzodiazepines, Rickels and associates[45,47,48] demonstrated that in patients with high pretreatment anxiety levels, the placebo response was minimal, thus exaggerating the drug-placebo differences in this group. In those with less severe illnesses, the drug-placebo difference was less marked. In a study of meprobamate, Uhlenhuth and co-workers[40] found the reverse: the most anxious patients responded best to placebo. These two groups of investigators have also reported opposite influences of sex, race, and duration of illness (Table 4-4).

Computerized multivariate data analysis has enhanced the possibilities for discovery of nonspecific factors in drug therapy. Undoubtedly, many more of these factors will be described as time passes and as drug studies become more sophisticated and involve larger sample sizes. One possible sequel of this increased sophistication is that generalizations about drug efficacy—whether the drug is "effective" or "ineffective"—will be made with increasing reservation and limitation. We now realize that in a well-designed but simple and straightforward study, a positive result could be due either to strong drug effects which overwhelm the nonspecific factors or to a fortuitous combination of non-drug factors which exaggerate the drug-placebo difference. Likewise, a negative result could be due to an ineffective drug or to a wrong choice of "set." Judgments of drug efficacy may come to be stringently

TABLE 4-4. Nonspecific factors in antianxiety drug studies

Ref.	Author(s)	Factor	Effect
39	Uhlenhuth et al., 1968	Age	Old patients respond more to drug than placebo. Young patients respond as much or more on placebo than on drug.*
40	Uhlenhuth et al., 1972		
40	Uhlenhuth et al., 1972	Sex	Females improve more on both drug and placebo than males.*
41	Rickels et al., 1971a		Males improve more on drug than females, but the same on placebo.**
39	Uhlenhuth et al., 1968	Race	Negroes improve more on both drug and placebo than whites.*
40	Uhlenhuth et al., 1972		
41	Rickels et al., 1971a		Whites improve more on drug and less on placebo than Negroes.**
39	Uhlenhuth et al., 1968	Body weight	Heavy patients improve slightly more on drug and less on placebo than light patients.*
39	Uhlenhuth et al., 1968	Marital status	Married or widowed patients respond more to drug and less to placebo than single, separated, or divorced patients.*
40	Uhlenhuth et al., 1972	Education	Response to drug and placebo is greater in those with more education.**
41	Rickels et al., 1971a		
42	Lewis et al., 1961		
43	Hesbacher et al., 1970a	Social class	Clinic patients drop out of therapy and fail to take medications more often than private patients.
44	Hesbacher et al., 1970b		Private patients respond more to drugs and less to placebo than clinic patients.**
45	Rickels et al., 1970a		
46	Rickels et al., 1970d		
42	Lewis et al., 1961		Patients with higher annual income respond more to drugs.***
47	Rickels and Downing, 1967	Severity of illness	Patients with more severe anxiety respond slightly more to drug and much less to placebo than those with mild illness.**
45	Rickels et al., 1970a		
48	Rickels et al., 1970b		
46	Rickels et al., 1970d		
49	Gardos et al., 1968		Normal volunteers with high characterological anxiety scores respond more to drug than to placebo; those with low anxiety scores respond little to either.**
50	DiMascio et al., 1969		
51	Barrett and DiMascio, 1966		
52	DiMascio and Barrett, 1965		
53	Salzman et al., 1969		

Ref.	Source	Category	Finding
40	Uhlenhuth et al., 1972		Patients with more severe anxiety respond much more to placebo and slightly more to drug than those with mild illness.*
54	Rickels et al., 1966	Duration of illness	Superiority of drug over placebo is greatest in those with long illness.**
41	Rickels et al., 1971a		
40	Uhlenhuth et al., 1972		Superiority of drug over placebo is not evident in those with long illness.*
54	Rickels et al., 1966	Prior drug therapy	Better response to drug is found in those with previous improvement on drug therapy. Poor response to placebo is found in those who took many drugs previously.**
55	Uhlenhuth et al., 1959	Physician attitude	Drug-placebo differences greatest in patients with physicians perceived as "warm" and having an enthusiastic attitude toward pharmacotherapy.***
56	Uhlenhuth et al., 1966		
39	Uhlenhuth et al., 1968		
41	Rickels et al., 1971a		
57	Rickels et al., 1971b		
58	Lipman et al., 1969		
59	McNair et al., 1970a	Patient attitude	Low-acquiescent patients respond more to drug than to placebo.**
60	McNair et al., 1970b		
61	McNair et al., 1966		
62	Rickels and Downing, 1966		Compliant patients improve more on drugs than noncompliant.* **
63	Rickels and Anderson, 1967		Patients who complete the drug trial improve more than patients who drop out.
64	Lipman et al., 1971	Life events	Patients experiencing positive life event during trial respond better to drug and placebo than those reporting negative events. Patients treated with drug report positive events more often than those on placebo.***
65	Lipman et al., 1965		
66	Uhlenhuth et al., 1965	Pattern of pill-taking	Greater placebo response is found with more placebo pills taken.***
67	Rickels et al., 1970c		
68	Hussain and Ahad, 1970		Slightly greater response to drug is found when drug is packaged as capsule rather than tablet.**
69	Hussain, 1972		Slightly greater response to drug is found when drug is packaged as green tablet rather than yellow or red tablet.**
70	Schapira et al., 1970		

*Demonstrated in studies involving propanediols (meprobamate or tybamate).
**Demonstrated in studies involving benzodiazepines.

qualified according to the parameters of measurement, the magnitude and variability of differences, and the details of patient population characteristics and the treatment setting.

MEASURING ANXIETY

The quantitation of human behavior is one of the most primitive fields of medical science. Life appears to be relatively easy for the renal physiologist. He administers a diuretic which alters the renal excretion of salt and water—easily measured parameters. Few would dispute the reliability of his results, since they could be verified by other scientists who, if they wished, could exactly replicate the design and measurements. For the psychopharmacologist studying antianxiety drug effects, life is much more complicated. A single satisfactory method for measuring the elusive parameter of anxiety has not been devised. Moreover, drug effects at times are so variable and unpredictable that an investigator across the street doing the same study a week later may derive totally different results.

Available approaches to the quantitation of anxiety in humans are so numerous as to suggest that none are totally adequate. Anxiety may be inferred and measured from projective tests. It may appear in overt behavior such as pacing, foot-tapping, or shakiness. It can also be ascertained from patient self-reports or from reports by observers—family, health care personnel, or physicians. Results of projective tests and patient self-ratings do not necessarily correlate well.[71] Two major strategies of measurement involve the estimation of *global* and *target symptom* change (Table 4-5). Global estimates are the easiest to perform and are probably of the most clinical significance, but they are the least specific. Patient, physician, nurse, and even family or friends may perform global ratings of drug effects by specifying their impression of whether the patient was or was not improved, and perhaps the degree of improvement. Target symptom ratings are more specific but less reliable.[72] Patient and physician can estimate drug effects on symptoms and symptom groups, such as anxiety, tension, depression, somatic complaints, insomnia, etc. These may be determined by simple verbal interview or checklist, or by more elaborate psychological testing. In crossover trials, patients may be asked to specify a drug preference. Many investigators devise their own rating system appropriate for their testing design. A number of rating scales have been standardized and used by different investigators in different studies. Some of the more popular rating scales are listed in Table 4-5. Many of these allow quantitation of target symptoms and also provide some type of overall score or global rating.

Complicated, highly specific rating systems enhance sophistication but make interpretation of results more difficult. When strong drug-placebo differences are evident in all measures, there is no problem, but frequently the different measures conflict. Physician ratings, for example, may reveal drug-

TABLE 4-5. *Approaches to quantitation in antianxiety drug studies*

Physician Global Rating
Patient Global Self-Rating
Physician Rating Scales
    Brief Psychiatric Rating Scale (BPRS)
    Hamilton Anxiety Rating Scale
    Hamilton Depression Rating Scale
    Physician Questionnaire (Rickels)
    Verdun Target Symptom Rating Scale
    Wittenborn Psychiatric Rating Scale
Patient Self-Rating Scales
    Clyde Mood Scale
    Maudsley (Eysenck) Personality Inventory
    Institute for Personality and Ability Testing (IPAT) Anxiety Forms
    Minnesota Multiphasic Personality Inventory (MMPI)
    Patient Symptom Checklist (SCL-35, SCL-90, NIMH Self-Rating Scale)
    Scheier-Cattell Anxiety Battery (SCAB)
    Taylor Manifest Anxiety Scale (TMAS)
    Zung Self-Rating Anxiety Scale
    Zung Self-Rating Depression Scale

---

placebo differences, while concomitant patient self-reports yield no distinction between active drug and the control substance. Equally perplexing are situations in which global and target symptom ratings conflict. A drug trial, for example, may show more overall global improvement on active drug, but no significant drug-placebo difference in important target symptoms such as anxiety. To make a single "yes or no" statement as to drug efficacy in some situations may boil down to the clinician's or investigator's judgment of the relative value of various modes of evaluation.

REVIEW OF CONTROLLED TRIALS

No single study can unequivocally determine whether the benzodiazepines are effective psychotropic drugs, but an overview of many controlled studies may begin to provide an answer. The following section presents a review of such studies published in the English language. The emotional disorders considered herein are "primary" rather than "secondary"—studies on patients with anxiety or depression associated with disease in specific organ systems (cardiovascular, dermatologic, gynecologic, gastrointestinal) are reviewed in Chapter 7. Also excluded are studies involving patients whose major manifestations of anxiety are somatic (hyperkinetic heart syndromes, functional gastrointestinal disorders, excema, asthma, etc.). The use of the benzodiazepines in the treatment of acute and chronic alcoholism is the subject of Chapter 11.

All of the studies reviewed give a global estimate of relative efficacy

TABLE 4-6. *The treatment of anxious-neurotic patients: Benzodiazepines versus placebo*

		Superiority of drug over placebo			
(Ref.)	Strong	(Ref.)	Weak	(Ref.)	None
CHLORDIAZEPOXIDE					
(73)	Azima et al., 1962[x]	(88)	Chien et al., 1963[f]	(97)	Claghorn, 1973
(74)	Chesrow et al., 1965[j]	(89)	Gore and McComisky, 1961[x]	(98)	Kingstone et al., 1969
(75)	Daneman, 1964	(90)	Grosser and Ryan, 1965[x]	(99)	Maggs and Neville, 1964[x]
(76)	Dunlop and Weisberg, 1968	(64)	Lipman et al., 1971[h]	(100)	Oliver, 1968[x,w]
(77)	Hanysova et al., 1966[x,w]	(91)	McNair et al., 1965[h]	(101)	Orvin, 1967[x]
(78)	Jenner et al., 1961a[x]	(54)	Rickels et al., 1966[n]	(102)	Schwartzberg and Van de Castle, 1961[x]
(79)	Kelly et al., 1969	(46)	Rickels et al., 1970d	(103)	Scrignar et al., 1967
(80)	Lader and Wing, 1965[x]	(92)	Rickels et al., 1971[g]	(104)	Tobin et al., 1964[x]
(81)	Leedy, 1970[x]	(57)	Rickels et al., 1971b[h]		
(82)	Lipman et al., 1966	(93)	Rickels et al., 1972a[h]		
(83)	Moriarty and Mebane, 1962	(94)	Rickels et al., 1972b		
(84)	Rickels et al., 1965	(95)	Silver et al., 1969[n]		
(85)	Rickels and Clyde, 1967	(96)	Silverstone et al., 1972		
(45)	Rickels et al., 1970a	(66)	Uhlenhuth et al., 1965[n]		
(41)	Rickels et al., 1971a				
(86)	Rickels and Hesbacher, 1973				
(87)	Shah et al., 1962				
DIAZEPAM					
(105)	Bonn et al., 1971	(114)	Arfwidsson et al., 1971[h]	(123)	Bonn, 1972
(106)	Brandsma, 1967	(115)	deLemos et al., 1965p[,j]	(124)	Gundlach et al., 1966
(107)	Cromwell, 1963[x]	(116)	Itoh et al., 1971[h]	(125)	Nesselhof et al., 1965[n]
(75)	Daneman, 1964	(117)	Kearnie and Bonime, 1966[x]		
(108)	Eaves et al., 1973	(118)	McLaughlin et al., 1965[n,x]		
(77)	Hanysova et al., 1966[x,w]	(119)	McLeod et al., 1970[x,w,n]		
(109)	Hare, 1963[x]	(120)	McLeod, 1972[x,w,n]		
(44)	Hesbacher et al., 1970b[g]	(61)	McNair et al., 1966[g]		

(110) Kellner et al., 1968[x]
(111) Okasha and Sadek, 1973
(112) VenkobaRao, 1964b
(113) Zapella and Wodinsky, 1967

OXAZEPAM
(126) Beber, 1965[j]
(127) Canning, 1966
(74) Chesrow et al., 1965[j]
(128) Csillag, 1967[x]
(129) LeGassicke and Harry, 1971[x]
(130) LeGassicke and McPherson, 1965[x]
(131) Sanders, 1965[j]

OTHER BENZODIAZEPINES
(134) Cassano et al., 1968 (NTZ)
(135) Charalampous et al., 1973 (CZP)
(136) Dull et al., 1970[x] (MDZ)
(76) Dunlop and Weisberg, 1968 (PRZ)
(108) Eaves et al., 1973 (LRZ)
(137) Haider, 1971a (LRZ)
(138) Krakowski, 1967 (MDZ)
(111) Okasha and Sadek, 1973 (LRZ)
(121) Ricca, 1972 (CZP)
(139) Sarteschi et al., 1972 (TMZ)

(59) McNair et al., 1970a[g]
(121) Ricca, 1972
(122) VenkobaRao, 1964a[n]

(132) Janecek et al., 1966
(133) McPherson and LeGassicke, 1965[n,x]
(101) Orvin, 1967[x]

(116) Itoh et al., 1971[h] (MDZ)
(98) Kingstone et al., 1969 (PRZ)
(95) Silver et al., 1969[n] (PRZ)
(96) Silverstone et al., 1972 (MDZ)

(125) Nesselhof et al., 1965
(104) Tobin et al., 1964[x]

(119) McLeod et al., 1970[x,w,n] (BMZ)
(84) Rickels et al., 1965 (NTZ)

f: sample size not specified
g: nonspecific factors prominent
x: crossover trial
h: drug-placebo differences present early in trial then diminish

n: less than 12 patients per treatment per group
w: less than 1 week of drug exposure
p: placebo reactors excluded from study
j: geriatric patients with behavioral problems

among the drugs tested. Target symptom ratings are included in many of the trials. When the two measures do not agree, the global rating is considered the more important. We have performed appropriate statistical tests in cases where they have not been done by the authors. Each study has been categorized into those which demonstrate the benzodiazepine to have strong, weak, or no superiority over the comparison drug. Judgments of "weak" are made on the basis of dubious design, small sample sizes, borderline statistical significance, inconsistent ratings, or strong influence of nonspecific factors.

ANXIOUS NEUROTIC PATIENTS

Benzodiazepines versus Placebo

Table 4-6 summarizes controlled trials involving benzodiazepines and placebo in the treatment of anxious neurotics. For each drug there is substantial documentation of clinical superiority over placebo, with studies showing strong drug-placebo differences outnumbering those which show no difference. In many of the studies showing only a "weak" difference, the problem is one of small sample sizes. If the placebo-treated patients in these studies are collected and pooled (approximately 750), one finds that 28% had a "satisfactory" response to the inert medication—a surprisingly low placebo response rate. If drug effects were similarly classified either as "satisfactory" or "unsatisfactory," then the drug must theoretically produce improvement in 70 to 80% or more of patients to reach statistical significance in a trial involving 12 patients in each treatment group and a 30% placebo improvement rate. With a higher placebo response—not at all uncommon—then an even higher drug response rate (90%) is needed to demonstrate statistical significance in a sample of this size. Some studies do not report the number of patients showing particular degrees of improvement on each treatment regimen, but instead compare the mean change scores observed in each treatment group. These two approaches do not always yield the same results in terms of statistical significance. Similarly, two treatment means can differ significantly in a statistical sense, but the size of the difference may not be clinically meaningful. Unfortunately, few if any studies present both parametric and nonparametric analyses.

Another important phenomenon is that of drug "washout." In a number of studies, significant drug-placebo differences are present early in the trial, but then diminish or disappear as the study continues for several weeks or months. The cyclic or intermittent nature of symptomatology in patients with situational ("state") anxiety probably explains this observation. A substantial proportion of patients who are symptomatic at the beginning of a drug trial will experience spontaneous remission or improvement within 1 to 3 months, thus diminishing the apparent drug effect. Patients with characterological ("trait") anxiety may have more continuous symptomatology, but such individuals often respond poorly to drugs. The "washout" effect lends credence to the contention of some authors that antianxiety drugs are most useful and efficacious when administered on an intermittent or "p.r.n." basis rather than continuously.

Benzodiazepines versus Barbiturates, Propanediols, and Hydroxyzine

The superiority of benzodiazepines over inert placebo seems reasonably well established. At least as important is the question of whether benzodiazepines are the antianxiety agents of choice when a drug of this type is clinically indicated. Several other drugs, marketed earlier than the benzodiazepines, are available as anxiolytics. These include various barbiturates (phenobarbital, amobarbital, butabarbital), meprobamate, hydroxyzine, and others. Studies comparing benzodiazepines to older anxiolytics in the treatment of anxious neurotics are reviewed in Table 4-7. The superiority over barbiturates appears striking, but nearly all studies showing a strong benzodiazepine-barbiturate difference are crossover trials in which the patient's drug preference is a major parameter of quantitation. In non-crossover trials using more sophisticated quantitative techniques, the differences are somewhat less striking. Dosages compared are the commonly prescribed ones. Unfortunately, there has been no systematic study of multiple-dosage levels which would clarify the range of dosages for which one treatment is superior to another. A small number of trials involve direct comparison of benzodiazepines with meprobamate or tybamate. In general, these demonstrate a weak superiority in favor of the benzodiazepines. Comparison with hydroxyzine is made in three trials and with trichloroethyl phosphate in one. In none of the studies cited in Table 4-7 is the comparison drug more effective than the benzodiazepines.

Considering efficacy alone, the benzodiazepines appear to be superior to the barbiturates and meprobamate on the basis of this review. With respect to the danger of overdosage and the possibility of abuse, the benzodiazepines have a marked increment of safety, as discussed in Chapter 12. The barbiturates and meprobamate, especially in their generic forms, are much less expensive than the benzodiazepines. We conclude that the benzodiazepine tranquilizers are the antianxiety agents of choice considering the spectrum of currently available drugs. When drug cost is an overwhelming problem, a trial of a barbiturate or meprobamate could be considered.

Which Benzodiazepine is Best?

When new benzodiazepine derivatives become available, their efficacy is usually compared in comparative trials with older derivatives. Table 4-8 summarizes the results of these trials. There is no evidence that any one of

TABLE 4-7. *The treatment of anxious neurotic patients: Benzodiazepines versus older antianxiety agents*

Superiority of benzodiazepines over comparison drug:

(Ref.)	Strong	(Ref.)	Weak	(Ref.)	None
VS. BARBITURATE					
(140)	Capstick et al., 1965[x] (DZ)	(89)	Gore and McComisky, 1961[x] (CDX)	(80)	Lader and Wing, 1965[x] (CDX)
(141)	Daneman, 1969[x] (MDZ)	(148)	GPRG, 1965[x,y] (CDX)	(45)	Rickels et al., 1970a (CDX)
(142)	Dickel et al., 1962[x] (CDX)	(44)	Hesbacher et al., 1970b[g] (DZ)	(150)	Stotsky and Borzone, 1972 (CDX)
(136)	Dull et al., 1970[x] (MDZ)	(149)	Sterlin et al., 1972b (CDX)	(113)	Zapella and Wodinsky, 1967 (DZ)
(143)	Jenner et al., 1961b[x] (CDX)				
(144)	Jenner and Kerry, 1967[x] (DZ, CDX)				
(145)	Kerry and McDermott, 1968[x] (DZ)				
(146)	Kerry and McDermott, 1971[x] (MDZ)				
(147)	McDowall et al., 1966[x] (DZ)				
VS. MEPROBAMATE OR TYBAMATE					
		(151)	DeSilverio et al., 1969 (OXZ)	(142)	Dickel et al., 1962 (CDX)
		(64)	Lipman et al., 1967[h] (CDX)	(152)	Goldstein, 1967[j] (CDX)
		(118)	McLaughlin et al., 1965[n,x] (DZ)	(102)	Schwartzberg and Van de Castle, 1961 (CDX)
		(57)	Rickels et al., 1971b[h] (CDX)		
		(149)	Sterlin et al., 1972b (CDX)		
VS. HYDROXYZINE					
(110)	Kellner et al., 1968[x] (DZ)	(149)	Sterlin et al., 1972b (CDX)	(46)	Rickels et al., 1970d (CDX)
VS. TRICHLORETHYL PHOSPHATE					
(153)	GPRG, 1969[x] (CDX)				

x: crossover trial
y: no differences seen after one week: strong differences after 4 weeks
n: less than 12 patients per treatment group

g: nonspecific factors prominent
j: geriatric patients with behavioral problems
h: drug differences present early in trial, then diminish

the benzodiazepines is of consistently greater efficacy than any other. Occasionally evaluation is confounded by nonequivalence of dosage. Kerry and Jenner[164] compared 30 mg/day of diazepam and of chlordiazepoxide in a crossover study. Diazepam proved superior by patient preference, but the incidence of drowsiness was much higher with diazepam. The differences

TABLE 4-8. *The treatment of anxious-neurotic patients: Comparisons between benzodiazepines*

Ref.	Author(s)	Result of efficacy comparison
154	Bojanovsky and Chloupkova, 1964 [x,w]	CDX (90 mg/day) = CDX (30 mg/day)
74	Chesrow et al., 1965[j]	OXZ better than CDX
155	Coates, 1972	LRZ = DZ
75	Daneman, 1964	DZ better than CDX
156	DeBuck, 1973[x]	LRZ = DZ
151	DeSilverio et al., 1969	OXZ (100 mg/day) slightly better than OXZ (40-60 mg/day)
76	Dunlop and Weisberg, 1968	PRZ better than CDX
108	Eaves et al., 1973	LRZ (3-4.5 mg/day) better than LRZ (1.5 mg/day)
157	Gomez, 1972	LRZ slightly better than DZ
158	GPRG, 1967[x]	CDX better than OXZ
159	GPRG, 1971a	MDZ slightly better than CDX
160	Grozier, 1972	DZ = CDX
161	Haider, 1971b	LRZ = DZ
77	Hanysova et al., 1966[x,w]	DZ better than CDX
162	Holmberg and Livstedt, 1972[x]	CZP better than CDX
116	Itoh et al., 1971	MDZ = DZ
144	Jenner and Kerry, 1967[x]	DZ = CDX
164	Kerry and Jenner, 1962[x,d]	DZ better than CDX
165	Khorana et al., 1973	LRZ = DZ
98	Kingstone et al., 1969	PRZ slightly better than CDX
80	Lader and Wing, 1965[x]	CDX (45 mg/day) better than CDX (22.5 mg/day)
125	Nesselhof et al., 1965[n]	OXZ = DZ
166	Neville, 1967[x]	CDX (60 mg/day) slightly better than CDX (30 mg/day)
111	Okasha and Sadek, 1973	LRZ = DZ
101	Orvin, 1967[x]	OXZ better than CDX
121	Ricca, 1972	CZP = DZ
84	Rickels et al., 1965	NTZ = CDX
167	Sherliker, 1973[x]	LRZ better than DZ
95	Silver et al., 1969[n]	PRZ = CDX
96	Silverstone et al., 1972	MDZ = CDX
104	Tobin et al., 1964[x]	OXZ = CDX
168	Wiersum, 1972	CZP = DZ
169	Wig and Mohan, 1973[n]	LRZ = DZ

x: crossover trial   j: geriatric patients with behavioral problems
d: dosage of diazepam too high   n: less than 12 patients per treatment group
w: less than one week of drug exposure

in both therapeutic and adverse effects in this trial are probably attributable to the authors' failure to take account of the five- to 10-fold greater milligram potency of diazepam. It is also possible that nonequivalence of pharmacokinetic characteristics could confound comparisons between benzodiazepines despite administration of doses which are clinically equivalent in single-dose studies. Repeated administration of diazepam produces accumulation of both diazepam itself and its pharmacologically active metabolite desmethyldiazepam. Oxazepam, on the other hand, has a relatively short half-life and no active metabolites, so that cumulative effects are far less important (see Chapter 2). These factors could be of considerable significance when the clinical effects of diazepam and oxazepam are compared after 2 to 3 weeks of daily administration.

Lorazepam, medazepam, bromazepam, and prazepam are in the late stages of testing. Chlorazepate (Tranxene®) has recently been released for general use in the United States. Proof of the superiority of these drugs over chlordiazepoxide or diazepam is lacking. There is, however, some suggestion from the controlled trials that 3-hydroxy benzodiazepines derivatives (oxazepam and lorazepam) produce unwanted drowsiness and oversedation less frequently than benzodiazepines without the 3-hydroxy substitution. This was first noted in several early trials with oxazepam.[74,158] Recently lorazepam has been extensively evaluated in comparative trials with diazepam. In several of these studies,[111,161,165,169] drowsiness is noted less frequently with lorazepam than with diazepam; in others, however, oversedation is equally common with both drugs.[108,155–157,167] Both oxazepam and lorazepam are rapidly metabolized directly to inactive glucuronide conjugates (see Chapter 2). If these two drugs are in fact less "toxic" in clinical use, it probably is again attributable to lack of accumulation of drug and/or active metabolites after repeated use. An intrinsically more favorable toxic-to-therapeutic dosage ratio seems unlikely.

Benzodiazepines Versus Other Antianxiety Agents

Table 4-9 shows that only rarely do other antianxiety agents, regardless of how new or exotic, prove superior to the benzodiazepines. Doxepin has been marketed as an antidepressant with antianxiety properties. Yet only one study comparing this drug to a benzodiazepine in anxious neurotics shows doxepin to be superior. Doxepin often produces the anticholinergic side effects characteristic of the other tricyclic antidepressants. In most of the studies reviewed, doxepin-induced side effects are more frequent and troublesome than those associated with chlordiazepoxide or diazepam. Similarly, when major tranquilizers, tricyclic antidepressants, or tranquilizer-antidepressant combinations are administered to anxious neurotics, improvement is no greater than with benzodiazepine therapy. The hazards of major tranquilizers obviously are much greater. Clinical studies with other drugs (opipramol, oxypertine, benzoctamine, pimozide, propranolol) also demonstrate no superiority over the benzodiazepines. There appears to be little justification at the present time for undertaking antianxiety drug therapy with newer and usually more expensive agents when there is no evidence that they surpass the benzodiazepines in efficacy.

ANXIOUS DEPRESSION

Many neurotic patients are depressed as well as anxious. The benzodiazepines may be of value in patients with neurotic depression, particularly when anxiety or agitation is a prominent component.[211] A number of controlled trials have compared benzodiazepines with tricyclic antidepressants or with combinations of antidepressants and major tranquilizers. In two of these studies, the combination of amitriptyline and perphenazine was distinctly superior to chlordiazepoxide.[212,213] Three others showed the benzodiazepine and the antidepressant to be equivalent.[175,214,215] Verner[216] showed that imipramine produced much more overall improvement than chlordiazepoxide, but the two drugs were not significantly different with respect to the target symptom of anxiety. Beber[217] found overall equivalence of chlordiazepoxide and amitriptyline-perphenazine, but examination of target symptoms showed the minor tranquilizer to be superior against anxiety, whereas the antidepressant-neuroleptic combination produced more improvement in depression. Claghorn and Kellner[218] also found differential effects upon target symptoms despite global antidepressant-benzodiazepine equivalence. Rickels and associates[48] demonstrated that the relative contributions of tranquilizer and antidepressant to improvement in anxious-depressed neurotics depended on the relative severities of anxiety and depression in the patient's symptomatology. Rosenthal and Bowden[219] compared diazepam and thioridazine in patients with chronic anxiety and depression. There was no overall difference in efficacy between the drugs. Diazepam, however, produced more improvement in the target symptom of psychic anxiety; thioridazine proved more effective against feelings of guilt and worthlessness.

Drug combinations containing benzodiazepines and tricyclic antidepressants are being evaluated for the treatment of anxious depression.[220] In placebo-controlled studies, these preparations produce more improvement than placebo.[218,221-223] The most important question, however, is whether the addition of a minor tranquilizer to a tricyclic enhances the effect of the tricyclic antidepressant. In five studies, global improvement on the benzodiazepine-antidepressant combination was no better than that on the antidepressant alone.[218,223-226] One study showed the combination to be weakly superior,[227] and one demonstrated amitriptyline plus chlordiazepoxide to be superior to amitriptyline alone in hospitalized depressed patients.[228]

Kay and associates[229] compared diazepam and amitriptyline in hospitalized depressed patients undergoing electroconvulsive therapy. The clinical course

TABLE 4-9. *The treatment of anxious-neurotic patients: Benzodiazepines versus other antianxiety agents*

Benzodiazepine superior	No difference	Comparison drug superior
VS. DOXEPIN		
	(170) Ban et al., 1972	(186) Montgomery et al., 1970
	(171) Beaubein et al., 1970	
	(172) Bianchi and Phillips, 1972	
	(173) Fielding et al., 1969[x.w]	
	(174) Johnstone and Claghorn, 1968	
	(175) Jones et al., 1972	
	(176) Kingstone et al., 1970	
	(177) Krasner, 1971	
	(178) McLaughlin, 1969[p]	
	(179) Rickels et al., 1969	
	(180) Sim et al., 1971[a]	
	(181) Simeon et al., 1970[p]	
	(182) Smith, 1971	
	(149, 183-185) Sterlin et al., 1970, 1971, 1972a, 1972b	

VS. MAJOR TRANQUILIZER, TRICYCLIC ANTIDEPRESSANT, OR TRANQUILIZER-ANTIDEPRESSANT COMBINATION

Benzodiazepine superior	No difference	Comparison drug superior
(109) Hare, 1963[x]	(187) Carranza-Acevedo and Tovar-Acosta, 1972	(193) Donald, 1969[x]
(186a) Smith and Chassan, 1964	(97) Claghorn, 1973	(194) McKnight and Bodger, 1971
	(188) Goldstein et al., 1969	
	(189) Itoh et al., 1969[x]	
	(190) Lord and Kidd, 1973[x]	

(191) Myers, 1970
(192) Rickels et al., 1968
(92) Rickels et al., 1971c
(93) Rickels et al., 1972a
(139) Sarteschi et al., 1972
(103) Scrignar et al., 1967
(210) Yamamoto et al., 1973

VS. OPIPRAMOL, OXYPERTINE, BENZOCTAMINE, PIMOZIDE, OR PROPRANOLOL

(120) McLeod, 1972[x,w,n]

(114) Arfwidsson et al., 1971[h]
(195) Biddy et al., 1970
(196) Donald and McMillin, 1973
(197) Forrest and Maule, 1972[n]
(198) Goldstein and Weiner, 1970
(199) GPRG, 1971b
(200) GPRG, 1972
(201) Gringras and Beaumont, 1971
(90) Grosser and Ryan, 1965[x]
(202) Jepson and Beaumont, 1973
(203) Lo and Lo, 1973
(204) Murphy et al., 1970[h]
(205) Murphy, 1971
(206) Murphy and Donald, 1971
(94) Rickels et al., 1972b
(207) Sim et al., 1971b
(208) Wadzisz, 1972
(209) Wheatley, 1969

(105) Bonn et al., 1971
(123) Bonn, 1972

x: crossover trial
h: benzodiazepine superior to comparison drug early in trial, then differences diminish
w: less than one week of drug exposure
n: less than 12 patients per treatment group
p: placebo reactors excluded from study

of patients on amitriptyline was better than those on diazepam. In a study of newly hospitalized anxious-depressed patients, Hollister and colleagues[230] found diazepam superior to the major tranquilizer acetophenazine in individuals whose depression began late in life and was uncomplicated by alcoholism. Raskin[231] reports on an NIMH-sponsored collaborative study which compared diazepam, phenelzine, and placebo in newly admitted depressed individuals. The response to diazepam therapy depended upon the depression subtype. Patients with anxious depressions improved more on diazepam than on phenelzine or placebo; in those with hostile depressions, diazepam was inferior to the two other therapies. Some implications of these results will be discussed subsequently.

The benzodiazepines appear to have no specific antidepressant properties. In some patients with neurotic or endogenous depressions, the benzodiazepine tranquilizers may be of therapeutic value if anxiety or agitation is a significant component of the illness. When combined with tricyclic antidepressants, they neither enhance nor antagonize the primary action of the antidepressant. Individuals in whom tricyclic drugs cause tremulousness, excitement, or other manifestations of psychomotor stimulation can benefit from the addition of a benzodiazepine tranquilizer. However, drug combinations containing fixed doses of benzodiazepines and tricyclic antidepressants are probably not rational.

PSYCHOSES

Controlled trials have confirmed the impression that the benzodiazepines are of no particular benefit in the treatment of schizophrenic patients. Although anxiety and agitation may be improved in some cases,[232] the benzodiazepines have no effect on disordered thinking and other psychotic manifestations. In four studies, an overall drug-placebo difference was not detected.[73,112,124,233] In six comparisons with a major tranquilizer, four showed no superiority of a benzodiazepine over the neuroleptic.[234–237] Vilkin[238] found diazepam better than trifluoperazine in a crossover trial involving 45 borderline patients, although Hekimian and Friedhoff[239] showed chlorpromazine clearly superior to chlordiazepoxide in overtly psychotic patients. Sterlin and associates[240] added chlordiazepoxide to the ongoing antipsychotic medication of hospitalized chronic schizophrenics, but found no discernible improvement. The combined effects of haloperidol and lorazepam in hospitalized psychotic patients was investigated by Guz and co-workers.[241] The two drugs together produced slightly more clinical improvement than haloperidol plus placebo, but the differences did not reach statistical significance.

Two groups of investigators have demonstrated the futility of treating psychoses with benzodiazepines. Holden and associates[242] studied the effects of thioridazine, chlordiazepoxide, and placebo, given alone and in various combinations, on 22 male chronic schizophrenics in whom all previous medications were withdrawn for 1 month. Thioridazine and thioridazine plus chlordiazepoxide were clearly superior to placebo and to chlordiazepoxide alone. However, thioridazine plus chlordiazepoxide was no better than thioridazine alone, nor was chlordiazepoxide alone significantly different from placebo. All patients in whom deterioration was noted were in the chlordiazepoxide-treated group. Equally convincing results were reported in a series of publications from the Maryland Psychiatric Research Institute.[243–246] These investigators found that combined treatment with major tranquilizers and chlordiazepoxide produced no more benefit than did major tranquilizers alone. If anything, chlordiazepoxide produced a slight antagonism of some major tranquilizer effects.

THE PHARMACOLOGIC RELEASE OF HOSTILITY?

Chapter 3 reviews experimental evidence regarding benzodiazepine-induced reduction in spontaneous and experimentally produced aggression. Some animal studies show that benzodiazepines potentiate hostility and fighting. We speculated that this enhancement of hostility, when it occurs, could result from disinhibition of "anxiety-bound" hostility. Is there a counterpart to this phenomenon in human psychopharmacology? Clinical experience suggests an affirmative answer. Clinical reports from a variety of settings document occasional cases of increased rage or hostility in patients receiving chlordiazepoxide or diazepam. Feldman[247] described this phenomenon as follows: "...many of the patients receiving (diazepam) displayed a progressive development of dislikes or hates. The patients themselves deliberately used the term 'hate'. This hatefulness first involved nonsignificant figures in the patient's environment, progressed from there to the involvement of key figures such as aides, nurses and physicians, and went on to the involvement of important figures such as parents and spouses. The phenomenon was progressive and in some instances, culminated in overt acts of violence..."

We have previously described three cases drawn from our clinical experience.[248] The following additional case is quite typical:

A 39-year-old tree worker was placed on diazepam (20 mg) by his family physician following an accident at work in which he had injured his back. Three days after starting on this regimen, he began to be argumentative at home. He thought that this was related to being at home, so he returned to work on the fifth day on diazepam. At work he was also argumentative and got into a physical fight with a co-worker. Since this behavior seemed extreme for him (he hadn't had a fist fight since high school), his wife insisted that he seek psychiatric consultation. In the evaluation it became clear that this patient had a considerable amount of unexpressed resentment which he had previously contained by passive-aggressive behavior. Diazepam was discontinued immediately and the argumentativeness subsided in two days. He was referred for counselling to a neighborhood mental health clinic where he was supported and encouraged to examine and ventilate some of his long-standing resentments.

Dramatic cases such as these are not common. There is no possible way at present to estimate their frequency. Even acts of violence such as murder have been attributed to the use of chlordiazepoxide and diazepam,[248] but someone observing the individual patient has to connect the behavior to the drug. If the drug-induced behavior is rare, studies which analyze results by mean change scores might not reveal these cases, since reduction in hostility would probably be observed more commonly. Therefore, a study would have to include case-by-case evaluation, with an examination of those cases which did show increases. This approach would also require a rating system which has some specific focus on hostility and aggressive behavior, both before and after drug administration.

We know of no prospective clinical studies which have been designed to examine the association between changes in anxiety and hostility. However, one recent clinical trial in anxious outpatients provides some interesting results.[210] After 1 week on chlordiazepoxide (50 to 100 mg orally per day), 27 of 37 (73%) patients showed an improvement on the anxiety subscale of the Brief Psychiatric Rating Scale (BPRS). Of these 37 anxious patients, 24 also were rated at pretreatment as showing hostility. After 1 week, six were improved (25% of those with this target symptom). However, 14 patients showed *increased* hostility ratings. From the data presented it is not possible to determine whether these 14 are all from the 24 showing initial hostility or whether some may have initially shown no hostility at all. On none of the other measured dimensions of the BPRS did such a large number of chlordiazepoxide patients show a worsening.

This study[210] also contained a cohort receiving chlorpromazine. Of 29 with initial anxiety, 23 improved (79%) at one week. Nineteen of the chlorpromazine patients showed initial hostility and nine (47%) were improved at 1 week. Only seven chlorpromazine patients were considered more hostile at 1 week. Feldman,[249] using a similar rating approach, observed that chlordiazepoxide, diazepam, and oxazepam reduced hostility in only 7, 0, and 50% of patients, respectively. Are chlordiazepoxide and diazepam failing to reduce hostility or are they releasing or producing it?

At the Psychopharmacology Research Laboratory of the Massachusetts Mental Health Center (PRL-MMHC), a number of studies have been carried out with volunteer male subjects rather than with individuals with symptomatic emotional illness who seek medical help. Using the Taylor Manifest Anxiety Scale, a self-rating scale of characterological or trait anxiety, subjects are divided into "high-," "mid-," and "low-anxious" groups according to the number of points they score on the scale. Among subjects in the "high-anxious" group, more than half have had psychiatric treatment in the past. "Normal" and "asymptomatic" are, therefore, somewhat inappropriate adjectives for the "high-anxious" subjects. Administration of chlordiazepoxide, diazepam, and oxazepam for a period of 1 week produces an objective reduction in anxiety as measured before and after drug administration by the Scheier-Cattell Anxiety Battery in the "high-anxious" group.[49,52,250] In "low-anxious" subjects, the drugs produce no more change in anxiety than placebo, and in "mid-anxious" subjects, decrements in anxiety do not consistently reach statistical significance. Even after a single dose, these effects are evident.[251] When hostility is measured before and after 1 week of drug administration by the Buss-Durkee Hostility Inventory, chlordiazepoxide and diazepam produce an increase in hostility in the "high-anxious" subjects, while oxazepam does not.[49–52] MacDonald[252] found that single doses of diazepam (5 or 10 mg) produced an objective increase in hostility among female subjects judged to be "action-oriented."

Recent work at the PRL-MMHC has extended and replicated these observations.[253] Using male volunteers in three-person groups, chlordiazepoxide again was associated with significant increments in self-rated hostility as compared to placebo after 1 week. The hostility increments were most pronounced in the "high-" and "mid-anxious" subjects. These new studies permitted two new observational dimensions. Subjects could rate each other's hostility, and blind observers could rate interpersonal hostility among the subjects from videotaped recordings of group interactions. These group studies also included an experimental "frustration stimulus" at the end of the week. Following this stimulus, chlordiazepoxide subjects showed significantly greater increments in hostility than did placebo subjects when rated by each other and by the blind observers.

These studies provide objective documentation of the release of hostility induced by the chlordiazepoxide and diazepam concurrent with the reduction of anxiety. It is not clear why oxazepam failed to produce this effect in the PRL-MMHC investigations. This failure was observed in two independent replications. Feldman[249] also noted a dissociation of oxazepam from chlordiazepoxide and diazepam, reporting that oxazepam was more effective than the other two drugs in reducing hostility. Some animal studies, however, do demonstrate that oxazepam can cause increased aggression similar to other benzodiazepines.[254] It appears that the simple theory of disinhibition of anxiety-bound hostility is not entirely tenable. Pharmacokinetic differences between the drugs (see Chapter 2) may somehow contribute to differing effects upon hostility. Unlike chlordiazepoxide and diazepam, repeated administration of oxazepam does not lead to significant drug accumulation; its metabolites, moreover, are inactive.

Other clinical reports may also be related to these findings. The influence of depressive illness subtype upon the response to diazepam treatment has been discussed previously.[231] Diazepam was beneficial for anxious-depressed hospitalized patients; in those with depression associated with high levels of hostility, diazepam tended to produce no improvement or clinical deterioration. Bayliss and Gilbertson[255] compared chlordiazepoxide and placebo in a group of children with spastic musculature due to cerebral palsy. Chlordiazepoxide was of significant benefit in reducing spasticity, but increased aggression and agitation occurred in many of the children receiving the active drug. The effect of clonazepam upon refractory seizure disorders in children was reported by Bladin.[256] Adequate seizure control was achieved in most of the 27 children in the study. Ten patients, however, developed increased irritability and had episodes of irrational antisocial behavior and outbursts of aggressive temper. In two cases clonazepam had to be discontinued despite good control of seizures.

The frequency of such responses is unknown, but these studies do suggest that "paradoxical" increases in hostility can in some instances be an important factor in the overall clinical response to benzodiazepines.

DRUGS COMBINED WITH OTHER THERAPIES

A number of authors have observed that long-term psychotherapy is effectively complimented by concurrent treatment with benzodiazepine tranquilizers.[257–264] Both chlordiazepoxide and diazepam have been used for this purpose. Intravenous diazepam produces immediate antianxiety effects in high-anxious individuals.[265] Two reports describe the use of intravenous diazepam prior to psychotherapy.[266,267] In three controlled trials of drugs combined with interpersonal therapy, psychotherapy-plus-benzodiazepine groups did significantly better than those treated with psychotherapy plus placebo.[268–271] Bellak and Chassan,[272] in a multicrossover study of a single subject during psychotherapy, found that improvement was only slightly better during chlordiazepoxide periods than during placebo periods. Lorr and associates[273] conducted a 1-month trial on six groups of patients each receiving drug, placebo, or no medication, and psychotherapy or no psychotherapy. The drug-placebo differences were slight, as were the effects of psychotherapy. The greatest differences resulted from the medication (drug *or* placebo) versus no medication.

Measuring the interaction of psychotherapy and pharmacotherapy can be exceedingly complex. Rating scales for global and target symptom change used to measure drug effects may not be appropriate in the assessment of effects of psychotherapy. Moreover, the therapist himself is an important dependent variable. One therapist treating many patients is quite different from the situation in which many therapists each treat only a few patients. Despite these reservations, the studies cited above suggest that benzodiazepine treatment during psychotherapy can be a reasonable adjunct, particularly when it appears that excessive anxiety may interfere with the goals of psychotherapy, such as learning of new methods of handling conflict, increased tolerance for ambiguity or uncertainty, or increased capacity to bear certain dysphoric affects.

A possible role for benzodiazepines in phobic disorders is suggested in Chapter 3. Yeung[274] reported that intravenous diazepam facilitated desensitization. McCormick[275,276] described a technique whereby declining doses of intravenous diazepam are given over successive therapy sessions to facilitate desensitization. Marks and associates[277] reported that relief of phobias was enhanced by oral diazepam (0.1 mg/kg) given 4 hr prior to "flooding." Silverstone[278] compared diazepam, lorazepam, and placebo in a crossover study of six patients with phobias. Lorazepam produced more improvement than diazepam or placebo and caused fewer side effects than diazepam. Finally, Bryan[279] described the use of chlordiazepoxide as an aid to hypnosis.

Injection-site pain is known to occur with intravenous diazepam.[267] In some cases local phlebitis is a sequel (see Chapters 6, 7, and 12). The likelihood of phlebitis is greater if the same vein is used for repeated injections.[265,280] This may be an important limitation to the repeated use of intravenous diazepam for phobia desensitization.

EMOTIONAL DISORDERS IN CHILDREN AND ADOLESCENTS

One of the areas to which psychopharmacology has contributed relatively little to date is in the realm of emotional disorders in children. Much of the psychopathology observed in preadults can merge imperceptibly with organic disease, and the appropriate role of pharmacotherapy is often obscure. The benzodiazepines have been used at all points along the spectrum of disease, from mental retardation to psychopathic personality disorders to school phobias.[281–286] Gleser and associates[287] were able to show that a single dose of chlordiazepoxide reduced anxiety and overt hostility in teenaged juvenile delinquents. Lucas and Pasley[288] found that diazepam produced significant improvement in a small group of neurotic children and teenagers. In four other controlled trials involving children with behavior disorders and hyperkinetic syndromes, the benzodiazepines produced no improvement, and in some cases a trend toward deterioration was noted.[289–292]

The benzodiazepines have received trial in the treatment of enuresis.[293] Forsythe and associates[294] found that the addition of chloridiazepoxide to imipramine produced no additional antienuretic effect. Kline[295] reported a controlled trial of diazepam and placebo, in which diazepam given at bedtime was highly effective in the prevention of bedwetting. Wasz-Hockert[296] also reported significant results with 5 mg of nitrazepam given at bedtime. Electroencephalographic sleep studies have demonstrated that the benzodiazepines significantly reduce stage IV or "slow-wave" sleep time. This effect may account for the efficacy of several benzodiazepine derivatives in the treatment of enuresis (see Chapter 9).

COMMENT

Several authors have attempted overviews of the literature dealing with the efficacy of the benzodiazepines in emotional disorders.[297-299] These efforts have not yielded comprehensive surveys, and for this reason the practitioner has been exposed to widely differing opinions of the clinical usefulness of this group of drugs. Some reviews state that there are no important differences among benzodiazepines, meprobamate, and barbiturates in the treatment of anxiety.[300-302] Others are relatively noncommittal and tentative,[303-307] while some claim that the benzodiazepines are the safest and most effective of the available antianxiety agents.[308-311]

The present review supports the viewpoint we have stated in previous publications.[312,313] The benzodiazepine tranquilizers are currently the drugs of choice when antianxiety drug therapy is indicated. There is no substantial clinical basis upon which to choose among benzodiazepines. Substitution of meprobamate or a barbiturate reduces the dollar cost of drug therapy but also reduces safety and efficacy. On the basis of currently available data, there seldom appears to be justification for a preference for doxepin or major tranquilizers in neurotic anxiety. In patients with neurotic or endogenous depression, the benzodiazepines may be of value when anxiety is prominent in the complex of symptomatology. At present it is doubtful that the benzodiazepines have a role in the pharmacotherapy of psychoses or in the treatment of emotional disorders in children.

REFERENCES

1. Balter MB, Levine JO: The nature and extent of psychotropic drug usage in the United States. Psychopharmacol Bull 5:3-13 (Oct), 1969
2. Parry HJ: Use of psychotropic drugs by U.S. adults. Public Health Rep 83:799-810, 1968
3. Gottschalk LA, Bates DE, Fox RA, James JM: Psychoactive drug use. Patterns found in samples from a mental health clinic and a general medical clinic. Arch Gen Psychiat 25:395-397, 1971
4. Mellinger GD, Balter MB, Manheimer DI: Patterns of psychotherapeutic drug use among adults in San Francisco. Arch Gen Psychiat 25:385-394, 1971
5. Manheimer DI, Mellinger GD, Balter MB: Psychotherapeutic drugs. Use among adults in California. Calif Med 109:445-451, 1968
6. Friedman GD, Collen MF, Harris LE, VanBrunt EE, Davis LS: Experience in monitoring drug reactions in outpatients. The Kaiser-Permanente drug monitoring system. JAMA 217:567-572, 1971

7. Stolley PD, Becker MH, McEvilla JD, Lasagna L, Gainor M, Sloane LM: Drug prescribing and use in an American community. Ann Intern Med 76:537-540, 1972

8. Dunlop D: The use and abuse of psychotropic drugs. Proc Royal Soc Med 63:1279-1282, 1970

9. Rowe IL: Prescriptions of psychotropic drugs by general practitioners: 1. General. Med J Aust 1:589-593, 1973

10. Sheppard C, Collins L, Fiorentino D, Fracchia J, Merlis S: Polypharmacy in psychiatric treatment: I. Incidence at a state hospital. Curr Ther Res 11:765-774, 1969

11. Altman H, Evenson RC, Sletten IW, Cho DW: Patterns of psychotropic drug prescription in four midwestern state hospitals. Curr Ther Res 14:667-672, 1972

12. Palva IP, Sotaniemi E: Use of diazepam on medical wards. Scand J Clin Lab Invest 27(supp 116):81, 1971

13. Mayfield DG, Morrison D: The use of minor tranquilizers in a teaching hospital. Southern Med J 66:589-592, 1973

14. Miller RR: Drug surveillance utilizing epidemiologic methods: a report from the Boston Collaborative Drug Surveillance Program. Amer J Hosp Pharm 30:584-592, 1973

15. Lader M: The nature of anxiety. Brit J Psychiat 121:481-491, 1972

16. Lasagna L: The controlled clinical trial: theory and practice. J Chronic Dis 1:353-367, 1955

17. Ban TA: Methodological problems in the clinical evaluation of anxiolytic drugs. In, *Advances in Neuro-Psychopharmacology*. Edited by O Vinar, Z Votava, PB Bradley. Amsterdam, North-Holland Publishing Co., 1971, pp 211-224

18. Hollister LE: Methodological considerations in evaluating antianxiety agents. J Clin Pharmacol 10:12-18, 1970

19. Wittenborn JR: *The Clinical Psychopharmacology of Anxiety*. Springfield, Illinois, Charles C Thomas, 1966

20. Wittenborn JR: The design of clinical trials. In, *Principles and Problems in Establishing the Efficacy of Psychotropic Agents*. Edited by J Levine, BC Schiele, L Bouthilet. Washington, D.C., USPHS Publication #2138, 1971, pp 227-262

21. Downing RW, Rickels K, Wittenborn JR, Mattsson NB: Interpretation of data from investigations assessing the effectiveness of psychotropic agents. In, *Principles and Problems in Establishing the Efficacy of Psychotropic Agents*. Edited by J Levine, BC Schiele, L Bouthilet. Washington, D.C., USPHS Publication #2138, 1971, pp 321-369

22. Park LC, Imboden JB: Clinical and heuristic value of clinical drug research. J Nerv Ment Dis 151:322-340, 1970

23. Plutchik R, Platman SR, Fieve RR: Three alternatives to the double-blind. Arch Gen Psychiat 20:428-432, 1969

24. Rickels K, McLaughlin BE: Sample size in psychiatric drug research. Clin Pharmacol Ther 9:631-634, 1968

25. Hollister LE: Placebology: sense and nonsense. Curr Ther Res 2:477-483, 1960

26. Cromie BW: The feet of clay of the double-blind trial. Lancet 2:994-997, 1963

27. Barsa JA: The fallacy of the "double-blind." Amer J Psychiat 119:1174-1175, 1963

28. Rickels K, Lipman RS, Fisher S, Park LC, Uhlenhuth EH: Is a double-blind clinical trial really double-blind? A report of doctors' medication guesses. Psychopharmacologia 16:329-336, 1970

29. Overall JE, Hollister LE, Kimbell I, Shelton J: Extrinsic factors influencing responses to psychotherapeutic drugs. Arch Gen Psychiat 21:89-94, 1969

30. Rickels K (ed): *Non-Specific Factors in Drug Therapy*. Springfield, Illinois, Charles C Thomas, 1968

31. Uhlenhuth EH, Lipman RS, Chassan JB, Hines LR, McNair DM: Methodological issues in evaluating the effectiveness of agents for treating anxious patients. In, *Principles*

and Problems in Establishing the Efficacy of Psychotropic Agents. Edited by J Levine, BC Schiele, L Bouthilet. D.C., USPHS Publication # 2138, 1971, pp 137-161

32. Fisher S: Non-specific factors as determinants of behavioral response to drugs. In, *Clinical Handbook of Psychopharmacology.* Edited by A DiMascio, RI Shader. New York, Science House, 1970, pp 17-39

33. Honigfeld G: Non-specific factors in treatment. I. Review of placebo reactions and placebo reactors. Dis Nerv Syst 25:145-156, 1964

34. Honigfeld G: Non-specific factors in treatment. II. Review of social-psychological factors. Dis Nerv Syst 25:225-239, 1964

35. Shapiro AK: Iatroplacebogenics. Int Pharmacopsychiat 2:215-248, 1969

36. Downing RW, Rickels K: The prediction of placebo response in anxious and depressed outpatients. In, *Psychopharmacology and the Individual Patient.* Edited by JR Wittenborn, SC Goldberg, PRA May. New York, Raven Press, 1970, pp 160-188

37. Rickels K: Antineurotic agents: specific and non-specific effects. In, *Psychopharmacology: A Review of Progress 1957-1967.* Edited by DH Efron. Washington, D.C., USPHS Publication#1836, 1968, pp 231-247

38. Rickels K: Drug use in outpatient treatment. Amer J Psychiat 124 (Feb supp):20-31, 1968

39. Uhlenhuth EH, Lipman RS, Rickels K, Fisher S, Covi L: Predicting the relief of anxiety with meprobamate. Non-drug factors in the response of psychoneurotic outpatients. Arch Gen Psychiat 19:619-630, 1968

40. Uhlenhuth EH, Covi L, Rickels K, Lipman RS, Park LC: Predicting the relief of anxiety with meprobamate. Arch Gen Psychiat 26:85-91, 1972

41. Rickels K, Downing RW, Howard K: Predictors of chlordiazepoxide response in anxiety. Clin Pharmacol Ther 12:263-273, 1971a

42. Lewis NDC, Tobin JM, Boyle D, Caton J: Psychopharmacological research in an outpatient setting. In, *Proceedings of the Third World Congress of Psychiatry,* Vol. I. Toronto, University of Toronto and McGill University Press, 1961, pp 374-379

43. Hesbacher PT, Rickels K, Gordon PE, Gray B, Mecklenburg R, Weise CC, Vandervort WJ: Setting, patient, and doctor effects on drug response in neurotic patients. I. Differential attrition, dosage deviation, and side reaction responses to treatment. Psychopharmacologia 18:180-208, 1970a

44. Hesbacher PT, Rickels K, Hutchison J, Raab E, Sablosky L, Whalen EM, Phillips FJ: Setting, patient, and doctor effects on drug response in neurotic patients. II. Differential improvement. Psychopharmacologia 18:209-226, 1970b

45. Rickels K, Clark EL, Etezady MH, Sachs T, Sapra RK, Yee R: Butabarbital sodium and chlordiazepoxide in anxious neurotic outpatients: a collaborative controlled study. Clin Pharmacol Ther 11:538-550, 1970a

46. Rickels K, Gordon PE, Zamostien BB, Case W, Hutchison J, Chung H: Hydroxyzine and chlordiazepoxide in anxious neurotic outpatients: a collaborative controlled study. Compr Psychiat 11:457-474, 1970d

47. Rickels K, Downing RW: Drug- and placebo-treated neurotic outpatients. Arch Gen Psychiat 16:369-372, 1967.

48. Rickels K, Hesbacher P, Downing RW: Differential drug effects in neurotic depression. Dis Nerv Syst 31:468-475, 1970b

49. Gardos G, DiMascio A, Salzman C, Shader RI: Differential actions of chlordiazepoxide and oxazepam on hostility. Arch Gen Psychiat 18:757-760, 1968

50. DiMascio A, Gardos G, Harmatz J, Shader R: Tybamate: an examination of its actions in "high" and "low" anxious normals. Dis Nerv Syst 30:758-763, 1969

51. Barrett JE, DiMascio A: Comparative effects on anxiety of the "minor tranquilizers" in "high" and "low" anxious student volunteers. Dis Nerv Syst 27:483-486, 1966

52. DiMascio A, Barrett JE: Comparative effects of oxazepam in "high" and "low" anxious student volunteers. Psychosomatics 6:298-302, 1965

53. Salzman C, DiMascio A, Shader RI, Harmatz JS: Chlordiazepoxide, expectation, and hostility. Psychopharmacologia 14:38-45, 1969

54. Rickels K, Lipman R, Raab E: Previous medication, duration of illness, and placebo response. J Nerv Ment Dis 142:548-554, 1966

55. Uhlenhuth EH, Canter A, Neustadt JO, Payson HE: The symptomatic relief of anxiety with meprobamate, phenobarbital, and placebo. Amer J Psychiat 115:905-910, 1959

56. Uhlenhuth EH, Rickels K, Fisher S, Park LC, Lipman RS, Mock J: Drug, doctor's verbal attitude, and clinic setting in the symptomatic response to pharmacotherapy. Psychopharmacologia 9:392-418, 1966

57. Rickels K, Lipman RS, Park LC, Covi L, Uhlenhuth EH, Mock JE: Drug, doctor warmth, and clinic setting in the symptomatic response to minor tranquilizers. Psychopharmacologia 20:128-152, 1971b

58. Lipman RS, Uhlenhuth EH, Rickels K, Covi L: Medication attitudes and drug response. Dis Nerv Syst 30:454-459, 1969

59. McNair DM, Fisher S, Kahn RJ, Droppleman LF: Drug-personality interaction in intensive outpatient treatment. Arch Gen Psychiat 22:128-135, 1970a

60. McNair DM, Fisher S, Sussman C, Droppleman LF, Kahn RJ: Persistence of a drug-personality interaction in psychiatric outpatients. J Psychiat Res 7:299-305, 1970b

61. McNair DM, Kahn RJ, Droppleman LF, Fisher S: Compatibility, acquiescence, and drug effects. In, *Neuro-Psycho-Pharmacology.* Edited by H Brill. Amsterdam, Excerpta Medica Foundation, 1966, pp 536-542

62. Rickels K, Downing R: Compliance and improvement in drug-treated and placebo-treated neurotic outpatients. Arch Gen Psychiat 14:631-633, 1966

63. Rickels K, Anderson FL: Attrited and completed lower socioeconomic class clinic patients in psychiatric drug therapy. Compr Psychiat 8:90-99, 1967

64. Lipman RS, Covi L, Derogatis LR, Rickels K, Uhlenhuth EH: Medication, anxiety reduction, and patient report of significant life situation events. Dis Nerv Syst 32:240-244, 1971

65. Lipman RS, Hammer HM, Bernardes JF, Park LC, Cole JO: Patient report of significant life events. (Methodological implications for outpatient drug evaluation.) Dis Nerv Syst 26:586-591, 1965

66. Uhlenhuth EH, Park LC, Lipman RS, Rickels K, Fisher S, Mock J: Dosage deviation and drug effects in drug trials. J Nerv Ment Dis 141:95-99, 1965

67. Rickels K, Hesbacher PT, Weise CC, Gray B, Feldman HS: Pills and improvement: a study of placebo response in psychoneurotic outpatients. Psychopharmacologia 16:318-326, 1970c

68. Hussain MZ, Ahad A: Tablet colour in anxiety states. Brit Med J 3:466, 1970

69. Hussain MZ: Effect of shape of medication in treatment of anxiety states. Brit J Psychiat 120:507-509, 1972

70. Schapira K, McClelland HA, Griffiths NR, Newell DJ: Study of the effects of tablet color in the treatment of anxiety states. Brit Med J 2:446-449, 1970

71. Hartlage LC: Common approaches to the measurement of anxiety. Amer J Psychiat 128:1145-1147, 1972

72. Wittenborn JR: Reliability, validity, and objectivity of symptom-rating scales. J Nerv Ment Dis 154:79-87, 1972

73. Azima H, Arthurs D, Silver A: The effects of chlordiazepoxide (Librium) in anxiety states. A multi-blind study. Canad Psychiat Assoc J 7:44-49, 1962.

74. Chesrow EJ, Kaplitz SE, Vetra H, Breme JT, Marquardt GH: Blind study of oxazepam in the management of geriatric patients with behavioral problems. Clin Med 72:1001-1005, 1965

75. Daneman EA: Double-blind study with diazepam, chlordiazepoxide, and placebo in the treatment of psychoneurotic anxiety. J Med Assoc Georgia 53:55-58 (Feb), 1964

76. Dunlop E, Weisberg J: Double-blind study of prazepam in the treatment of anxiety. Psychosomatics 9:235-238, 1968

77. Hanysova Z, Chloupkova K, Bojanovsky J, Bouchal M, Synkova J: A clinical comparison of placebo, diazepam and diazepoxid at short-time application in neuroses. Activ Nerv Sup 8:438-439, 1966

78. Jenner FA, Kerry, RJ, Parkin D: A controlled trial of methaminodiazepoxide (chlordiazepoxide, "Librium") in the treatment of anxiety in neurotic patients. J Ment Sci 107:575-582, 1961a

79. Kelly D, Brown CC, Shaffer JW: A controlled physiological, clinical, and psychological evaluation of chlordiazepoxide. Brit J Psychiat 115:1387-1392, 1969

80. Lader MH, Wing L: Comparative bioassay of chlordiazepoxide and amylobarbitone sodium therapies in patients with anxiety states using physiological and clinical measures. J Neurol Neurosurg Psychiat 28:414-425, 1965

81. Leedy JJ: What we learned from a double blind study of Librium. Med Times 98:72-79 (Dec), 1970

82. Lipman RS, Park LC, Rickels K: Paradoxical influence of a therapeutic side-effect interpretation. Arch Gen Psychiat 15:462-474, 1966

83. Moriarty JD, Mebane JC: Comparative studies of chlordiazepoxide in office practice. J Neuropsychiat 3:241-245, 1962

84. Rickels K, Baumm C, Raab E, Taylor W, Moore E: A psychopharmacological evaluation of chlordiazepoxide, LA-1 and placebo, carried out with anxious, neurotic medical clinic patients. Med Times 93:238-245, 1965

85. Rickels K, Clyde DJ: Clyde Mood Scale changes in anxious outpatients produced by chlordiazepoxide therapy. J Nerv Ment Dis 145:154-157, 1967

86. Rickels K, Hesbacher PT: Over-the-counter daytime sedatives. A controlled study. JAMA 223:29-33, 1973

87. Shah LP, Shah AV, Shah VD, Bagadia VN, Vahia NS: Librium (Roche)—Its value in certain psychiatric illnesses. Indian J Psychiat 4:23-26, 1962

88. Chien C-P, Tsuang M-T, Rin H: A double-blind test of the effect of chlordiazepoxide (Librium) in anxiety neuroses. J Formosan Med Assoc 62:286-290, 1963

89. Gore CP, McComisky JG: A study of the comparative effectiveness of Librium, amylobarbitone, and a placebo in the treatment of tension and anxiety states. In, *Proceedings of the Third World Congress of Psychiatry,* Vol. II. Toronto, University of Toronto and McGill University Press, 1961, pp 979-982

90. Grosser HH, Ryan E: Drug treatment of anxiety: a controlled study of opipramol and chlordiazepoxide. Brit J Psychiat 111:134-141, 1965

91. McNair DM, Goldstein AP, Lorr M, Cibelli LA, Roth I: Some effects of chlordiazepoxide and meprobamate with psychiatric outpatients. Psychopharmacologia 7:256-265, 1965

92. Rickels K, Weise CC, Whalen EM, Csanalosi I, Jenkins BW, Stepansky W: Haloperidol in anxiety. J Clin Pharmacol 11:440-449, 1971c

93. Rickels K, Hutchison J, Morris RJ, Csanalosi I, Parsia K, Pereira-Ogan JA: Molindone and chlordiazepoxide in anxious neurotic outpatients. Curr Ther Res 14:1-9, 1972a

94. Rickels K, Gratch MI, Gray BM, Laquer KG, Parish LC, Rosenfeld H, Whalen EM: Benzoctamine and chlordiazepoxide in anxious outpatients: a collaborative study. Dis Nerv Syst 33:512-522, 1972b

95. Silver D, Ban TA, Kristof FE, Saxena BM, Bennett J: Prazepam in the treatment of psychoneurotic outpatients: a brief report. Curr Ther Res 11:596-598, 1969

96. Silverstone JT, Carne HJ, Cooper RM, Dell AJ, Salkind MR: The controlled evaluation of a new tranquillizing drug medazepam in the treatment of anxiety. Brit J Clin Prac 25:172-174, 1972

97. Claghorn JL: A comparative study of loxapine succinate, Librium, and placebo in neurotic outpatients. Curr Ther Res 15:8-12, 1973

98. Kingstone E, Villeneuve A, Kossatz I: Double-blind evaluation of prazepam, chlordiazepoxide, and placebo in non-psychotic patients with anxiety and tension: some methodological considerations. Curr Ther Res 11:106-114, 1969

99. Maggs R, Neville R: Chlordiazepoxide (Librium): a clinical trial of its use in controlling symptoms of anxiety. Brit J Psychiat 110:540-543, 1964

100. Oliver JE: Distortions in a psychiatric double-blind trial. Comparing chlordiazepoxide with placebo-with-side-effects. Clin Trials J 5:991-995, 1968

101. Orvin GH: Treatment of the phobic obsessive-compulsive patient with oxazepam, an improved benzodiazepine compound. Psychosomatics 8:278-280, 1967

102. Schwartzberg AZ, Van de Castle RW: A controlled clinical study of chlordiazepoxide. Amer J Psychiat 117:743-745, 1961

103. Scrignar CB, Hornsby L, Bishop MP, Gallant DM: A controlled evaluation of butaperazine in the neurotic anxiety syndrome. Curr Ther Res 9:492-494, 1967

104. Tobin JM, Lorenz AA, Brousseau ER, Conner WR: Clinical evaluation of oxazepam for the management of anxiety. Dis Nerv Syst 25:689-696, 1964

105. Bonn JA, Salkind MR, Rees WL: A technique in the evaluation of psychotropic medication based on a patient demand schedule: comparison of the efficacy of oxypertine, diazepam and placebo in anxiety. Curr Ther Res 13:561-567, 1971

106. Brandsma M: Diazepam in internal medicine. Med Times 95:1048-1054, 1967

107. Cromwell HA: Controlled evaluation of psychotherapeutic drug in internal medicine. Clin Med 70:2239-2244, 1963

108. Eaves D, Jain VK, Swinson RP: A double-blind controlled trial of lorazepam and diazepam in the treatment of anxiety. Curr Med Res Opin 1:265-268, 1973

109. Hare HP: Comparison of diazepam, chlorpromazine, and a placebo in psychiatric practice. J New Drugs 3:233-240, 1963

110. Kellner R, Kelly AV, Sheffield BF: The assessment of changes in anxiety in a drug trial: a comparison of methods. Brit J Psychiat 114:863-869, 1968

111. Okasha A, Sadek A: A comparison of lorazepam, diazepam, and placebo in anxiety states. J Int Med Res 1:162-165, 1973

112. VenkobaRao A: A controlled trial with "Valium" in some psychiatric disorders. Indian J Psychiat 6:188-192, 1964b

113. Zapella DG, Wodinsky A: Diazepam, phenobarbital, and placebo in the treatment of psychiatric patients. (A double-blind study). Dis Nerv Syst 28:30-34, 1967

114. Arfwidsson L, Arn L, Beskow J, Ottosson J-O, Persson G: A comparison between diazepam, dixyrazine, and opipramol, and placebo in anxiety states. Acta Psychiat Scand supp 221:19-32, 1971

115. deLemos GP, Clement WR, Nickels E: Effects of diazepam suspension in geriatric patients hospitalized for psychiatric illness. J Amer Geriat Soc 13:355-359, 1965

116. Itoh H, Ichimaru S, Kawakita Y, et al: A clinical study for the evaluation of anxiolytic drugs. In, Advances in Neuro-Psychopharmacology. Edited by O Vinar, Z Votava, PB Bradley. Amsterdam, North-Holland Publishing Co., 1971, pp 225-235

117. Kearney T, Bonime HC: Problems of drug evaluation in out-patients. Dis Nerv Syst 27:604-606, 1966

118. McLaughlin BE, Chassan JB, Ryan F: Three single-case studies comparing diazepam and meprobamate: an application of intensive design. Compr Psychiat 6:128-136, 1965

119. McLeod WR, Mowbray RM, Davies B: Trials of Ro 5-3350 and diazepam for anxiety symptoms. Clin Pharmacol Ther 11:856-861, 1970

120. McLeod WR: A comparison of diazepam, benzoctamine, and placebo in anxiety states. Curr Ther Res 14:239-245, 1972

121. Ricca JJ: Clorazepate dipotassium in anxiety: a clinical trial with diazepam and placebo controls. J Clin Pharmacol 12:286-290, 1972

122. VenkobaRao A: A controlled trial with "Valium" in obsessive compulsive state. J Indian Med Assoc 42:564-567, 1964a

123. Bonn JA: Some recent advances in the management of anxiety. Postgrad Med J 48(supp 4):24-26 (Sept), 1972

124. Gundlach R, Engelhardt DM, Hankoff L, Paley H, Rudorfer L, Bird E: A double-blind outpatient study of diazepam (Valium) and placebo. Psychopharmacologia 9:81-92, 1966

125. Nesselhof W, Gallant DM, Bishop MP: A double-blind comparison of Wy-3498, diazepam, and placebo in psychiatric outpatients. Amer J Psychiat 121:809-811, 1965

126. Beber CR: Management of behavior in the institutionalized aged. Dis Nerv Syst 16:591-595, 1965

127. Canning JA: Double-blind, controlled trial of oxazepam in the office practice of internal medicine. Psychosomatics 7:364-367, 1966

128. Csillag ER: A sequential trial of Adumbram (oxazepam). Aust New Zealand J Psychiat 1:211-213, 1967

129. LeGassicke J, Harry TVA: The treatment of morbid anxiety. A double-blind cross-over trial of oxazepam (Serenid). Clin Trials J 8(No. 3):19-22, 1971

130. LeGassicke J, McPherson F: A sequential trial of Wy-3498 (oxazepam). Brit J Psychiat 111:521-525, 1965

131. Sanders JF: Evaluation of oxazepam and placebo in emotionally disturbed aged patients. Geriatrics 20:739-746, 1965

132. Janecek J, Vestre ND, Schiele BC, Zimmerman R: Oxazepam in the treatment of anxiety states: a controlled study. J Psychiat Res 4:199-206, 1966

133. McPherson FM, LeGassicke J: A single-patient self-controlled and self-recorded trial of Wy 3498. Brit J Psychiat 111:149-154, 1965

134. Cassano GB, Castrogiovanni P, Gallevi M: Nitrazepam (Ro 4-5360) in the treatment of anxiety states. Double-blind trial. Pharmakopsychiatry 1:195-201, 1968

135. Charalampous KD, Tooley W, Yates C: Clorazepate dipotassium: a new benzodiazepine antianxiety agent. J Clin Pharmacol 13:114-118, 1973

136. Dull TA, Tuzel IH, White RF: The value of worsening rates in psychiatric clinical trials. Psychosomatics 11:50-54, 1970

137. Haider I: Evaluation of a new tranquilizer—WY 4036—in the treatment of anxiety. Brit J Psychiat 119:597-598, 1971a

138. Krakowski AJ: A new benzodiazepine for treatment of anxiety/tension states. Psychosomatics 8:73-78, 1967

139. Sarteschi P, Cassano GB, Castrogiovanni P, Placidi GF, Sacchetti G: Major and minor tranquilizers in the treatment of anxiety states. Arzneim-Forsch 22:93-97, 1972

140. Capstick NS, Corbett MF, Pare CMB, Pryce IG, Rees WL: A comparative trial of diazepam (Valium) and amylobarbitone. Brit J Psychiat 111:517-519, 1965

141. Daneman EA: A comparative trial of medazepam (Nobrium) in anxiety-depressive states. Psychosomatics 10:366-369, 1969

142. Dickel HA, Dixon HH, Shanklin JG, Dixon HH: A clinical double-blind comparison of Librium, meprobamate, and phenobarbital. Psychosomatics 3:129-133, 1962

143. Jenner FA, Kerry RJ, Parkin D: A controlled comparison of methaminodiazepoxide (chlordiazepoxide, "Librium") and amylobarbitone in the treatment of anxiety in neurotic patients. J Ment Sci 107:583-589, 1961b

144. Jenner FA, Kerry RJ: Comparison of diazepam, chlordiazepoxide, and amylobarbitone. (A multidose double-blind crossover study.) Dis Nerv Syst 28:245-249, 1967

145. Kerry RJ, McDermott CM: A double-blind cross-over comparison of Valium and amylobarbitone. Follow-up of five years' clinical experience. Clin Trials J 5:1075-1078, 1968

146. Kerry RJ, McDermott CM: Medazepam compared with amylobarbitone in treatment of anxiety. Brit Med J 1:151-152, 1971

147. McDowall A, Owen S, Robin AA: A controlled comparison of diazepam and amylobarbitone in anxiety states. Brit J Psychiat 112:629-631, 1966
148. General Practitioner Research Group: General practitioner clinical trials. Chlordiazepoxide in anxiety states. Practitioner 195:689-695, 1965
149. Sterlin C, Ban TA, Jarrold L: The place of doxepin among the anxiolytic-sedative drugs. Curr Ther Res 14:195-204, 1972b
150. Stotsky BA, Borzone J: Butisol sodium vs. Librium among geriatric and younger outpatients and nursing home patients. Dis Nerv Syst 33:254-267, 1972
151. DeSilverio RV, Rickels K, Raab E, Jameson J: Oxazepam and meprobamate in anxious neurotic outpatients. J Clin Pharmacol 9:259-263, 1969
152. Goldstein BJ: Double-blind comparison of tybamate and chlordiazepoxide in geriatric patients. Psychosomatics 8:334-337, 1967
153. General Practitioner Research Group: General practitioner clinical trials. Comparative study of a hypnotic and a tranquillizer in anxiety. Practitioner 202:706-709, 1969
154. Bojanovsky J, Chloupkova K: A comparison of the therapeutic effect of smaller and larger doses of chlordiazepoxide (Librium) at a short-time administration. Activ Nerv Sup 6:189-190, 1964
155. Coates H: Lorazepam and diazepam in severe neurotic illness. Curr Med Res Opin 1:74-77, 1972
156. DeBuck R: Clinical experience with lorazepam in the treatment of neurotic patients. Curr Med Res Opin 1:291-295, 1973
157. Gomez G: Double-blind trial of lorazepam for anxiety in general practice. Brit J Clin Prac 26:375, 1972
158. General Practitioner Research Group: General practitioner clinical trials. Oxazepam in anxiety. Practitioner 199:356-359, 1967
159. General Practitioner Research Group: General practitioner clinical trials. Medazepam: a new tranquilizer. Practitioner 206:688-690, 1971a
160. Grozier ML: Motival in the treatment of anxiety, with or without depression. Psychosomatics 13:109-116, 1972
161. Haider I: A comparative trial of lorazepam and diazepam. Brit J Psychiat 119:599-600, 1971b
162. Holmberg G, Livstedt B: Clinical evaluation of a new benzodiazepine derivative, chlorazepate. Arzneim-Forsch 22:916-919, 1972
163. Kerry RJ, Jenner FA, Pearson IB: A double-blind crossover comparison of RO 5-3350, bromazepam, diazepam (Valium) and chlordiazepoxide (Librium) in the treatment of neurotic anxiety. Psychosomatics 13:122-124, 1972
164. Kerry RJ, Jenner FA: A double blind crossover comparison of diazepam (Valium, Ro 5-2807) with chlordiazepoxide (Librium) in the treatment of neurotic anxiety. Psychopharmacologia 3:302-306, 1962
165. Khorana AB, Khorana AS, Nanivadekar AS: Comparison of lorazepam and diazepam in anxiety neurosis. Curr Med Res Opin 1:192-198, 1973
166. Neville R: Chlordiazepoxide (Librium). A controlled comparison of dosage. Clin Trials J 4:739-742, 1967
167. Sherliker J: A comparison of lorazepam and diazepam in general practice. Curr Med Res Opin 1:269-271, 1973
168. Wiersum J: Clorazepate dipotassium in anxiety: a double-blind trial with diazepam controls. Curr Ther Res 14:442-448, 1972
169. Wig NN, Mohan V: A controlled double-blind comparison of lorazepam and diazepam in anxiety neurosis. Curr Med Res Opin 1:199-202, 1973
170. Ban TH, Lehmann HE, Sterlin C, Beaubien J, Jarrold L: Doxepin in the treatment of psychoneurotic patients: a comparison between two clinical settings. Int J Clin Pharmacol 4:236-239, 1971

171. Beaubien J, Ban TA, Lehmann HE, Jarrold L: Doxepin in the treatment of psychoneurotic patients. Curr Ther Res 12:192-194, 1970
172. Bianchi GN, Phillips J: A comparative trial of doxepin and diazepam in anxiety states. Psychopharmacologia 25:85-96, 1972
173. Fielding JM, Mowbray RM, Davies B: A preliminary controlled study of doxepin ("Sinequan") as an antianxiety drug. Med J Aust 2:851-852, 1969
174. Johnstone EE, Claghorn JL: Doxepin vs. chlordiazepoxide: a controlled comparison in neurotic outpatients. Curr Ther Res 10:514-519, 1968
175. Jones BL, Eastgate NO, Downey PG, Davies LJH: A comparison of doxepin with diazepam and amitriptyline in general practice. New Zealand Med J 76:174-179, 1972
176. Kingstone E, Kolivakis T, Kossatz I: Doxepin versus chlordiazepoxide: a double-blind study on anxious outpatients. Curr Ther Res 12:213-222, 1970
177. Krasner EB: Double-blind comparative trial of doxepin and chlordiazepoxide in general practice. Brit J Clin Prac 25:555-556, 1971
178. McLaughlin BE: Management of psychoneurotic anxiety and depression in outpatients. Psychosomatics 10(No. 3, Sect. 2):28-31, 1969
179. Rickels K, Perloff M, Stepansky W, Dion HS, Case WG, Sapra RK: Doxepin and diazepam in general practice and hospital clinic neurotic patients: a collaborative controlled study. Psychopharmacologia 15:265-279, 1969
180. Sim M, Bindman E, Conochie BC, Sandilands DWIM: The treatment of anxiety/depressive states. A comparative trial of doxepin (Sinequan) with chlordiazepoxide (Librium). Clin Trials J 8(No.1):22-27, 1971a
181. Simeon J, Spero M, Nikolovski OT, Fink M: A comparison of doxepin and chlordiazepoxide in the therapy of anxiety. Curr Ther Res 12:201-212, 1970
182. Smith ME: A controlled comparative study of doxepin and chlordiazepoxide in psychoneurotic anxiety. J Clin Pharmacol 11:152-156, 1971
183. Sterlin C, Ban TA, Lehmann HE, Jarrold L: A comparative evaluation of doxepin and chlordiazepoxide in the treatment of psychoneurotic outpatients. Curr Ther Res 12:195-200, 1970
184. Sterlin C, Oliveros R, Ban TA, Jarrold L: Doxepin in the treatment of psychoneurotic inpatients. Curr Ther Res 13:580-583, 1971
185. Sterlin C, Ban TA, Lehmann HE, Jarrold L: Doxepin in the treatment of hospitalized and ambulatory psychoneurotic patients. Int J Clin Pharmacol 5:417-419, 1972a
186. Montgomery BA, Cullinan TR, Bayley AJ: A double-blind comparative trial of doxepin hydrochloride and chlordiazepoxide in anxiety and depression in general practice. Brit J Clin Prac 24:207-209, 1970
186a. Smith ME, Chassan JB: Comparisons of diazepam, chlorpromazine, and trifluoperazine in a double-blind clinical investigation. J Neuropsychiat 5:593-600, 1964
187. Carranza-Acevedo J, Tovar-Acosta H: Clinical evaluation of the efficacy of molindone and chlordiazepoxide in anxious outpatients. Curr Ther Res 14:609-614, 1972
188. Goldstein BJ, Slater V, Miller J, Jones E, Olsen P, Shea GW: Comparison of mesoridazine and chlordiazepoxide in psychoneurotic patients. Curr Ther Res 11:657-662, 1969
189. Itoh H, Ichimaru S, Kawakita Y, et al: A clinical trial of anti-anxiety drugs. Aust New Zealand J Psychiat 3:282-287, 1969
190. Lord DJ, Kidd CB: Haloperidol versus diazepam: a double-blind crossover clinical trial. Med J Aust 1:586-588, 1973
191. Myers WH: A comparative clinical trial of Triptafen-Minor and Librium in anxiety. Med Digest (London) 15:821-824, 1970
192. Rickels K, Raab E, Gordon PE, Laquer KG, DeSilverio RV, Hesbacher P: Differential effects of chlordiazepoxide and fluphenazine in two anxious patient populations. Psychopharmacologia 12:181-192, 1968

193. Donald JF: A study of a recognized antipsychotic agent as a tranquillizer in general practice. Practitioner 203:684-687, 1969

194. McKnight E, Bodger JN: A comparative clinical trial of amitriptyline-perphenazine and chlordiazepoxide in anxious university students. Brit J Clin Prac 25:381-383, 1971

195. Biddy RL, Smith RS, Magrinat GS: Ba-30803 in chronic anxiety states. J Clin Pharmacol 10:29-36, 1970

196. Donald JF, McMillin WP: Oxypertine and medazepam in patients suffering from anxiety neurosis. Report of a double-blind study. J Int Med Res 1:130-135, 1973

197. Forrest AD, Maule M: A controlled trial of oxypertine in patients with anxiety. Postgrad Med J 48(supp 4):30-32, (Sept.) 1972

198. Goldstein BJ, Weiner DM: Comparative evaluation of benzoctamine and diazepam in treatment of anxiety. J Clin Pharmacol 10:194-198, 1970

199. General Practitioner Research Group: General practitioner clinical trials. Anxiolytic effects of oxypertine. Practitioner 206:822-825, 1971b

200. General Practitioner Research Group: General practitioner clinical trials. Pimozide in anxiety neurosis. Practitioner 208:836-839, 1972

201. Gringras M, Beaumont G: A double-blind comparison of opipramol and diazepam in the treatment of anxiety in general practice. Brit J Clin Prac 25:455-458, 1971

202. Jepson K, Beaumont G: A comparative trial of opipramol and chlordiazepoxide in the treatment of anxiety. J Int Med Res 1:145-150, 1973

203. Lo WH, Lo T: Clinical trial of benzoctamine versus chlordiazepoxide in anxiety neurosis. J Clin Pharmacol 13:48-53, 1973

204. Murphy JE, Donald JF, Beaumont G: Opipramol and chlordiazepoxide in the treatment of anxiety in general practice. Practitioner 205:677-683, 1970

205. Murphy JE: The treatment of anxiety neurosis in general practice. A double-blind comparison of benzoctamine (Tacitin) with chlordiazepoxide (Librium). Clin Trials J 8(No. 1):18-21, 1971

206. Murphy JE, Donald JF, Beaumont G: The treatment of anxiety. A comparative clinical trial of opipramol and chlordiazepoxide employing a method of patient self-assessment. Clin Trials J 8(No. 2):28-32, 1971

207. Sim M, Bindman E, Conochie BC, Sandilands DWIM: The treatment of anxiety/depressive states. A comparative trial of benzoctamine (Tacitin) with chlordiazepoxide (Librium). Clin Trials J 8(No. 1):12-17, 1971b

208. Wadzisz FJ: A comparison of oxypertine and diazepam in anxiety neurosis seen in hospital out-patients. Brit J Psychiat 121:507-508, 1972

209. Wheatley D: Comparative effects of propranolol and chlordiazepoxide in anxiety states. Brit J Psychiat 115:1411-1412, 1969

210. Yamamoto J, Kline FM, Burgoyne RW: The treatment of severe anxiety in outpatients: a controlled study comparing chlordiazepoxide and chlorpromazine. Psychosomatics 14:46-51, 1973

211. Zapletalek M, Strnad M, Komenda S, Vackova M, Barborakova E, Stepanova M, Hrbek J, Beran I, Siroka A: Alimenazine, chlordiazepoxide, meprobamate, and placebo in anxious depression therapy. Activ Nerv Sup 8:437-438, 1966

212. Martins JK: Combined amitriptyline-perphenazine (Etrafon) compared with chlordiazepoxide hydrochloride: a double-blind, crossover study. Curr Ther Res 8:17-22, 1966

213. Coleman JM: Comparative evaluation of two psychotropic agents in depression related to organic disease. Illinois Med J 132:819-823, 1967

214. Yamamoto J, Kline FM, Burgoyne RW: Double-blind drug study in depressed outpatients. Rocky Mountain Med J 69:71-74 (April), 1972

215. General Practitioner Research Group: General practitioner clinical trials. Antidepressant effects of tranquillizers. Practitioner 206:146-148, 1971

216. Verner JV: Comparison of imipramine and chlordiazepoxide in treatment of the depressed and anxious patient. J Florida Med Assoc 56:15-21, 1969

217. Beber CR: Treating anxiety and depression in the elderly. A double-blind crossover evaluation of two widely used tranquilizers. J Florida Med Assoc 58:35-38 (March), 1971

218. Claghorn J, Kellner R: When is a tranquillizer an antidepressant? Curr Ther Res 13:575-579, 1971

219. Rosenthal SH, Bowden CL: A double-blind comparison of thioridazine (Mellaril) versus diazepam (Valium) in patients with chronic mixed anxiety and depressive symptoms. Curr Ther Res 15:261-267, 1973

220. Wingfield WL, Pollack D: A double-blind, phase I clinical study of oxazepam and protriptyline combined. Curr Ther Res 15:97-112, 1973

221. Rickels M, Laquer KG, Rial WY, Rosenfeld H, Schneider B, Wagner IG: The combination of protriptyline and oxazepam in depressed neurotic general practice patients. Psychosomatics 12:341-348, 1971

222. Houck JE: Combined therapy in anxiety-depressive syndromes. I. Comparative effects of Limbitrol (chlordiazepoxide-amitriptyline) and placebo. Dis Nerv Syst 31:269-273, 1970

223. Rickels K, Gordon PE, Jenkins BW, Perloff M, Sachs T, Stepansky W: Drug treatment in depressive illness. (Amitripyline and chlordiazepoxide in two neurotic populations.) Dis Nerv Syst 31:30-42, 1970

224. Hare HP: Comparison of chlordiazepoxide-amitriptyline compared with amitriptyline alone in anxiety-depressive states. J Clin Pharmacol 11:456-460, 1971

225. Kellner R, Sheffield BF: A cross-over trial of chlordiazepoxide-with-amitriptyline and amitriptyline alone. Brit J Clin Prac 23:459-461, 1969

226. Harry TVA: The treatment of depressive illness. A comparative study of iprindole (Prondol) with a combination of iprindole and oxazepam. Clin Trials J 6:98-101, 1969

227. Houck J: Combined therapy in anxiety-depressive syndromes. II. Comparative effects of amitriptyline and Limbitrol (chlordiazepoxide-amitriptyline). Dis Nerv Syst 31:421-426, 1970

228. Haider I: A comparative trial of Ro 4-6270 and amitriptyline in depressive illness. Brit J Psychiat 113:993-998, 1967

229. Kay DWK, Fahy T, Garside RF: A seven-month double-blind trial of amitriptyline and diazepam in ECT-treated depressed patients. Brit J Psychiat 117:667-671, 1970

230. Hollister LE, Overall JE, Pokorny AD, Shelton J: Acetophenazine and diazepam in anxious depression. Arch Gen Psychiat 24:273-278, 1971

231. Raskin A: A guide for drug use in depression. Presented at the 126th Annual Meeting of the American Psychiatric Association. Honolulu, Hawaii, May 8, 1973

232. Lehmann HE, Ban TA: Notes from the log-book of a psychopharmacological research unit I. Canad Psychiat Assoc J 9:28-32, 1964

233. Stonehill E: A comparative study with benzodiazepines in chronic psychotic patients. Dis Nerv Syst 27:4ll-413, 1966

234. Smith ME: A clinical study of chlorpromazine and chlordiazepoxide. Connecticut Med 25:153-157, 1961

235. Hankoff LD, Rudorfer L, Paley HM: A reference study of ataraxics. A two-week double-blind outpatient evaluation. J New Drugs 2:173-178, 1962

236. Merlis S, Turner WJ, Krumholz W: A double-blind comparison of diazepam, chlordiazepoxide, and chlorpromazine in psychotic patients. J Neuropsychiat 3(supp 1):sl33-sl38, 1962

237. Maculans GA: Comparison of diazepam, chlorprothixene, and chlorpromazine in chronic schizophrenic patients. Dis Nerv Syst 25:164-168, 1964

238. Vilkin MI: Comparative chemotherapeutic trial in treatment of chronic borderline patients. Amer J Psychiat 120:1004, 1964

239. Hekimian LJ, Friedhoff AJ: A controlled study of placebo, chlordiazepoxide, and

chlorpromazine with thirty male schizophrenic patients. Dis Nerv Syst 28:675-678, 1967

240. Sterlin C, Augustin E, Ban TA, Jarrold L: Doxepin as adjuvant medication in the treatment of chronic schizophrenic patients: a comparative study. Curr Ther Res 13:50-52, 1971

241. Guz I, Morales R, Sartoretto JN: The therapeutic effects of lorazepam in psychotic patients treated with haloperiodol: a double-blind study. Curr Ther Res 14:767-774, 1972

242. Holden JMC, Itil TM, Keskiner A, Fink M: Thioridazine and chlordiazepoxide, alone and combined, in the treatment of chronic schizophrenia. Compr Psychiat 9:633-643, 1968

243. Agallianos DD, Ota KY, Quinn MF, Tepper SR, Kurland AA: Drug combinations in the treatment of newly admitted, acutely ill psychiatric patients. Curr Ther Res 6:626-637, 1964

244. Michaux MH, Kurland AA, Agallianos DD: Chlorpromazine-chlordiazepoxide and chlorpromazine-imipramine treatment of newly hospitalized, acutely ill psychiatric patients. Curr Ther Res 8:117-152, 1966

245. Hanlon TE, Ota KY, Agallianos DD, Berman SA, Bethon GD, Kobler F, Kurland AA: Combined drug treatment of newly hospitalized, acutely ill psychiatric patients. Dis Nerv Syst 30:104-116, 1969

246. Hanlon TE, Ota KY, Kurland AA: Comparative effects of fluphenazine, fluphenazine-chlordiazepoxide, and fluphenazine-imipramine. Dis Nerv Syst 31:171-177, 1970

247. Feldman PE: An analysis of the efficacy of diazepam. J Neuropsychiat 3(supp 1):s62-s67, 1962

248. DiMascio A, Shader RI, Giller DR: Behavioral toxicity. Part III: Perceptual-cognitive functions; and Part IV: Emotional (mood) states. In, *Psychotropic Drug Side Effects: Clinical and Theoretical Perspectives.* By RI Shader, A DiMascio, and associates. Baltimore, Williams and Wilkins, 1970, pp 132-141

249. Feldman PE: Current views on antianxiety agents. Scientific exhibit presented at the Annual Meeting of the American Medical Association, Houston, Texas, November 1967

250. DiMascio A, Shader RI, Harmatz J: Psychotropic drugs and induced hostility. Psychosomatics 10(No. 3, Sect. 2):46-47, 1969

251. Shader RI, DiMascio A, Harmatz JS: Single versus repeated dosage of the minor tranquilizer chlordiazepoxide (Librium). Amer J Psychiat 128: 1576-1577, 1972

252. McDonald RL: The effects of personality type on drug response. Arch Gen Psychiat 17:680-686, 1967

253. Salzman C, Kochansky GE, Shader RI, Porrino L, Harmatz JS: Chlordiazepoxide induced hostility in a small group setting. Psychopharmacol Bull (in press)

254. Guaitani A, Marcucci F, Garattini S: Increased aggression and toxicity in grouped male mice treated with tranquilizing benzodiazepines. Psychopharmacologia 19:241-245, 1971

255. Bayliss SG, Gilbertson MP: Controlled trial of chlordiazepoxide in spastic children. Devel Med Child Neurol 4:597-601, 1962

256. Bladin PF: The use of clonazepam as an anticonvulsant—clinical evaluation. Med J Aust 1:683-688, 1973

257. Dean SR: Librium as an adjuvant in psychotherapy. Dis Nerv Syst 23:27-31, 1962

258. Dean SR: Diazepam as an adjuvant in psychotherapy. Amer J Psychiat 121:389-390, 1964

259. Dean SR: Diazepam as an adjuvant in clinical psychotherapy. Dis Nerv Syst 26:181-183, 1965

260. Rose JT: Phenoxypropazine and chlordiazepoxide in depression. Amer J Psychiat 120:899-900, 1964

261. Brown SG: Chlordiazepoxide: an effective adjunct to psychotherapy of the neurotic states. Amer J Psychiat 119:774-775, 1963

262. Yochelson S: Effect of chlordiazepoxide on specific symptoms of psychiatric patients and facilitation of psychotherapy. J Clin Exp Psychopathol 22:79-88, 1961

263. Lederman SJ, Steinberg M: Observations on the effect of chlordiazepoxide in patients requiring psychiatric treatment. J New Drugs 1:114-117, 1961

264. Cline WB: Treatment of emotional disorders with amobarbital, diazepam, and psychotherapy. Texas State J Med 59:512-517, 1963

265. Kelly D, Pik R, Chen C-N: A psychological and physiological study of intravenous diazepam. Brit J Psychiat 122:419-426, 1973

266. Pecknold JC, Raeburn J, Poser EG: Intravenous diazepam for facilitating relaxation for desensitization. J Behav Ther Exp Psychiat 3:39-41, 1972

267. Farb HH: Intravenous diazepam as pre-interview medication. Dis Nerv Syst 24:233-236, 1963

268. McLaughlin BE, Harris J, Ryan F: A double-blind study involving Listica, Librium and placebo as an adjunct to supportive psychotherapy in a psychiatric clinic. Dis Nerv Syst 22(Sept supp):41-43, 1961

269. Podobnikar IG: Implementation of psychotherapy by Librium in a pioneering rural-industrial psychiatric practice. Psychosomatics 12:205-209, 1971

270. Jacobs MA, Globus G, Heim E: Reduction in symptomatology in ambulatory patients. The combined effects of a tranquilizer and psychotherapy. Arch Gen Psychiat 15:45-53, 1966

271. Jacobs MA, Heim E, Chassan JB: Intensive design in the study of differential therapeutic effects. Compr Psychiat 7:278-289, 1966

272. Bellak L, Chassan JB: An approach to the evaluation of drug effect during psychotherapy: a double-blind study of a single case. J Nerv Ment Dis 139:20-30, 1964

273. Lorr M, McNair DM, Weinstein GJ: Early effects of chlordiazepoxide (Librium) used with psychotherapy. J Psychiat Res 1:257-270, 1963

274. Yeung DPH: Diazepam for treatment of phobias. Lancet 1:475-476, 1968

275. McCormick WO, O'Gorman EC: Declining-dose drug desensitization for phobias. Psychol Med 1:339-342, 1971

276. McCormick WO: Declining-dose drug desensitization for phobias. Clinical and psycho-physiological studies. Canad Psychiat Assoc J 18:33-40, 1973

277. Marks IM, Viswanathan R, Lipsedge MS, Gardner R: Enhanced relief of phobias by flooding during waning diazepam effect. Brit J Psychiat 121:493-505, 1972

278. Silverstone JT: Lorazepam in phobic disorders: a pilot study. Curr Med Res Opin 1:272-275, 1973

279. Bryan WJ: Librium: an aid to hypnosis. J Amer Inst Hypnosis 2:26-35 (Apr) 1961

280. Wehlage DF: Diazepam phlebitis. JAMA 224:128-129, 1973

281. d'Amato G: Chlordiazepoxide in management of school phobia. Dis Nerv Syst 23:292-295, 1962

282. Krakowski AJ: Chlordiazepoxide in treatment of children with emotional disturbances. NY State J Med 63:3388-3392, 1963

283. Breitner C: An approach to the treatment of juvenile delinquency. Arizona Med 19:82-87, 1962

284. Kraft IA, Ardali C, Duffy JH, Hart JT, Pearce P: A clinical study of chlordiazepoxide used in psychiatric disorders of children. Int J Neuropsychiat 1:433-437, 1965

285. Ucer E: Pilot study with Ro 5-4556 in emotionally disturbed retarded children. Curr Ther Res 10:187-195, 1968

286. Pilkington TL: Comparative effects of Librium and Taractan on behavior disorders of mentally retarded children. Dis Nerv Syst 22:573-575, 1961

287. Gleser GC, Gottschalk LA, Fox R, Lippert W: Immediate changes in affect with chlordiazepoxide. Arch Gen Psychiat 13:291-295, 1965

288. Lucas AR, Pasley FC: Psychoactive drugs in the treatment of emotionally disturbed children: haloperidol and diazepam. Compr Psychiat 10:376-386, 1969

289. Bartunkova Z, Cerny L, Drtilova J, Sturma J: Propericiazin, diazepam, chlorpromazine, and placebo in a double blind trial in pedopsychiatric therapy. Activ Nerv Sup 14:83-84 , 1972

290. LaVeck GD, Buckley P: The use of psychopharmacologic agents in children with behavior disorders. J Chronic Dis 13:174-183, 1961

291. Zrull JP, Westman JC, Arthur B, Rice DL: A comparison of diazepam, d-amphetamine, and placebo in the treatment of the hyperkinetic syndrome in children. Amer J Psychiat 121:388-389, 1964

292. Zrull JP, Westman JC, Arthur B, Bell WA: A comparison of chlordiazepoxide, d-amphetamine, and placebo in the treatment of the hyperkinetic syndrome in children. Amer J Psychiat 120:590-591, 1963

293. Saletu B, Itil TM: Digital computer "sleep prints"—an indicator of the most effective drug treatment of somnambulism. Clin Electroenceph 4:33-41, 1973

294. Forsythe WI, Merrett JD, Redmond A: Enuresis and psychoactive drugs. Brit J Clin Prac 26:116-118, 1972

295. Kline AH: Diazepam and the management of nocturnal enuresis. Clin Med 75:20-22 (Dec), 1968

296. Wasz-Hockert O: Nitrazepam in enuresis. Brit Med J 3:433, 1971

297. Davis JM: Efficacy of tranquilizing and antidepressant drugs. Arch Gen Psychiat 13:552-572, 1965

298. Kellner R: Drugs, diagnoses, and outcome of drug trials with neurotic patients. J Nerv Ment Dis 151:85-96, 1970

299. Link RE: The relation of drug trials to chlordiazepoxide and diazepam. Applied Ther 7:978-987, 1965

300. Librium and Valium. Med Lett Drugs Ther 11:81-84, 1969

301. Irwin S: Anti-neurotics: practical pharmacology of the sedative-hypnotics and minor tranquilizers. In, *Psychopharmacology: A Review of Progress 1957-1967.* Edited by DH Efron. Washington, D.C., USPHS publications #1836, 1968, pp 185-204

302. Medical Letter on Drugs and Therapeutics: *Reference Handbook.* New Rochelle, N.Y., The Medical Letter Inc., Jan 1973, pp 3-6

303. Kehoe MJ: I. Minor tranquilizers. Southern Med J 64:366-369, 1971

304. Hollister LE: Clinical use of psychotherapeutic drugs: current status. Clin Pharmacol Ther 10:170-198, 1969

305. Katz RL: Drug therapy. Sedatives and tranquilizers. New Eng J Med 286:757-760, 1972

306. Appleton WS: Psychoactive drugs: a usage guide. Dis Nerv Syst 32:607-616, 1971

307. Hollister LE: Drug therapy. Mental disorders—antianxiety and antidepressant drugs. New Eng J Med 286:1195-1198, 1972

308. Hollister LE: The prudent use of antianxiety drugs. Rational Drug Ther 6:March 1972

309. Hollister LE: Clinical use of psychotherapeutic drugs. II. Antidepressant and antianxiety drugs and special problems in the use of psychotherapeutic drugs. Drugs 4:361-410, 1972

310. Lader MH: Anxiolytic drugs. Brit J Hosp Med 9:79-82, 1973

311. Hollister LE: Uses of psychotherapeutic drugs. Ann Intern Med 79:88-98, 1973

312. Greenblatt DJ, Shader RI: Meprobamate: a study of irrational drug use. Amer J Psychiat 127:1297-1303, 1971

313. Greenblatt DJ, Shader RI: The clinical choice of sedative-hypnotics. Ann Intern Med 77:91-100, 1972

Chapter 5
Basic Neurophysiology
and Neuropharmacology

The clinical importance of the benzodiazepines as antianxiety, anticonvulsant, and muscle-relaxing agents has stimulated a great deal of investigation of possible mechanisms of action. Much has been learned about the effects of the benzodiazepines on the physiology and pharmacology of the central nervous system. Because of the obviously limited possibilities for invasive investigation of human brain function, correlations between experimental observation and clinical effects in humans are, necessarily, conjectural.

THE LIMBIC SYSTEM

For years the limbic system has been implicated by neurophysiologists as the seat of emotion and its behavioral, autonomic, and endocrine sequelae.[1] The circuitry is complex, involving multiple reciprocal projections from amygdala to hippocampus to hypothalamus. The amygdala is thought to enhance hypothalamic activity. In some species, bilateral amygdaloid extirpation results in calm, tranquil animals. The benzodiazepines have been shown to have "limbic system sedative" properties to which their antianxiety effects have been attributed.

Electroencephalographic changes induced in experimental preparations by the benzodiazepines are variable, depending upon the dose, route of administration, and the particular animal preparation used. When the drugs are given in intravenous doses large enough to produce sedation and ataxia, recordings from cortex, cerebellum, or subcortical foci show accentuation of high-voltage slow-wave activity, similar to changes induced by other sedative-hypnotics.[2–6] Smaller doses given intravenously or orally are followed by a shift to low-voltage high-frequency activity.[6–8] Recordings of electrical activity from subcortical structures also reveal profound changes following administration of benzodiazepine derivatives. Spontaneous electrical activity in the hippocampus of the rat is depressed by intraperitoneal chlordiazepoxide and diazepam.[9,10] In the cat, benzodiazepines also depress hippocampal activity or produce a shift toward higher frequencies.[11,12] The response to external stimuli is altered more than spontaneous activity. Nitrazepam, diazepam, and chlordiazepoxide reduce or abolish the hippocampal response to auditory, visual, or tactile stimulation in cats and rabbits.[7,12-15] Visual evoked responses in the tectotegmental area and in the visual cortex are also reduced.[16,17]

A number of authors have studied the influence of amygdaloid activity upon hippocampal response. Schallek and associates[18-21] have demonstrated that the threshold for afterdischarge in the amygdaloid nucleus is elevated by intravenous chlordiazepoxide (10 mg/kg), diazepam (10 mg/kg), and nitrazepam (10 mg/kg). Discharges in the amygdalo-hippocampal projection are also depressed, but by much smaller doses. Electrical stimulation of the amygdaloid nucleus in the untreated cat produces a secondary response in the ipsilateral hippocampus. Benzodiazepines in doses of less than 1 mg/kg depress the hippocampal response to amygdaloid stimulation, while the thresholds for thalamocortical arousal are unaltered.[22-24] These findings suggest, but by no means prove, that the benzodiazepines selectively impair amygdaloid discharge and amygdalo-hippocampal transmission. One may further speculate that their antianxiety activity may in part be explained by this "pharmacologic amygdalectomy."

Significant effects of benzodiazepines on hypothalamic function have also been demonstrated. The rage reaction induced by electrical stimulation of the hypothalamus in cats and monkeys can be abolished by benzodiazepines.[25] Electrostimulation of the hypothalamus may also produce a peripheral pressor response and cardiac arrhythmias. Pretreatment with benzodiazepines produces very little direct effect upon blood pressure, but the pressor response—as a consequence of hypothalamic stimulation—is reduced or abolished.[21,26-31] The central nature of this effect is verified by the observation that the pressor response to norepinephrine infusion or to stimulation of the stellate ganglion is unaltered. Vieth and co-workers[8] have emphasized that this pharmacologic effect attributed to the benzodiazepines may in part be due to the solvent system used to inject the drug. In these studies of nitrazepam, the solvent (propylene glycol) alone produced hypothalamic depression in the *cerveau isolé* cat preparation.

MUSCLE RELAXATION

Numerous clinical studies have suggested that the benzodiazepines produce relaxation of skeletal muscles. Normal volunteers and patients without neuromuscular disease experience muscle relaxation after treatment with benzodiazepines. In patients with spastic musculoskeletal disorders, improvement is usually produced by benzodiazepine treatment. Diazepam has received the most study and trial. Objective electromyographic (EMG) investigations and studies of neuromuscular function using normal humans and patients with neuromuscular diseases have substantiated this impression.[32-43] Parenteral administration of diazepam produces a reduction of EMG activity as well as a reduction of the level of muscle tension corresponding to a given EMG discharge. Similar objective results have been obtained both in normal animals and in those made spastic by decerebration.[44-46] Doppman and associates[46a] showed that intra-arterial diazepam effectively antagonized muscle spasms induced in monkeys and dogs by intra-arterial injections of iodinated contrast media used by radiologists for arteriography. In this study it is unclear whether diazepam exerted its muscle-relaxant action in the muscle itself or elsewhere.

The observation that diazepam appears to depress monosynaptic reflex activity in the intact organism[47,48] has given rise to a brisk controversy, as yet unresolved, regarding the site of muscle-relaxant action of the benzodiazepines. *In vitro* studies have generally shown that high concentrations of benzodiazepines are necessary to produce neuromuscular impairment; clinically relevant concentrations have little effect.[49-51] Dasgupta and associates[52] found that diazepam in concentrations of 20 to 40 μg/ml diminished neuromuscular transmission and the response to direct muscle stimulation in various animal nerve-muscle concentrations; chlordiazepoxide at 50 μg/ml had no effect. Pruett et al.[53] showed slowing of impulse conduction rates in the sciatic nerve of the frog by chlordiazepoxide at 3.4×10^{-3} mM concentrations.

Feldman and Crawley[54,55] noted that the incidence of postoperative respiratory depression in patients receiving curare-like drugs was higher among those who received diazepam preoperatively. This prompted the authors to study the influence of diazepam upon the clinical effect of neuromuscular blocking agents. Diazepam potentiated and prolonged the paralyzing effects of gallamine (a curare-like agent) upon forearm musculature in humans, but did not potentiate the effects of succinylcholine (a depolarizing neuromuscular blocker), producing, if anything, a slight antagonism. Other authors, using both *in vitro* and *in vivo* preparations, have not been able to demonstrate potentiation of gallamine or curare by diazepam.[56-60] Dretchen and associates found that diazepam, given intravenously to humans in doses as high as 1.2 mg/kg, did not augment the effect of various neuromuscular blocking drugs[60] This group also noted a slight antagonism of curare and decamethonium by diazepam when given intra-arterially to dogs. However, this effect was found to be a property of the propylene glycol solvent used to inject diazepam rather than of the drug itself.

It would appear from these studies that the muscle-relaxant properties of the benzodiazepines are due to central rather than peripheral effects. In contrast to the high concentrations of diazepam necessary to depress muscular function and neuromuscular transmission *in vitro,* minute quantities produce central muscle relaxation *in vivo.* Sinha et al.[61] showed that less than 1 mg of chlordiazepoxide injected intracerebroventricularly in cats effectively impairs the linguomandibular reflex. Numerous other studies have also suggested that the benzodiazepines have potent central muscle-relaxing properties as opposed to only weak peripheral effects.[62-70] Authors are largely in agreement as to the pertinent facts. Monosynaptic reflexes such as the patellar reflex (knee jerk) are essentially unaffected by large doses of diazepam and other benzodiazepines, whereas polysynaptic reflexes are depressed by relatively small doses. Investigators at the Department of Pharmacology at Columbia University have demonstrated that the polysynaptic inhibition is a supraspinal rather than a spinal effect.[71-74] This group utilized a cat preparation in which the animal is decerebrated by midcollicular transection. They studied the effects of a number of benzodiazepines (DZ, NTZ, CDX, CNZ, BMZ, FLZ, NTZ) on the patellar reflex (monosynaptic) and the quadriceps extensor response to stimulation of the contralateral sciatic nerve (polysynaptic). Small doses of benzodiazepines depressed the polysynaptic reflex, while the patellar reflex was unchanged. Transection of the spinal cord nullified the reflex-depressing effects of the benzodiazepines. Meprobamate, mephenesin, and tybamate also depressed the polysynaptic reflex, but the effect was unaltered by spinal transection. The results demonstrate that both the benzodiazepines and the propanediols have an influence on interneuronal function. The propanediols produce interneuronal blockade at the spinal cord level, whereas the benzodiazepines operate at a supraspinal level, presumably in the reticular formation of the brainstem. Further studies have shown that the effects of diazepam and picrotoxin are mutually antagonistic.[75,76] Picrotoxin is known to nullify presynaptic inhibition, and diazepam and other benzodiazepines have therefore been postulated to be muscle relaxants on the basis of enhanced presynaptic inhibition at the level of the brainstem.

These results imply that diazepam cannot effectively produce muscle relaxation unless the spinal cord is intact. Some studies, however, have not wholly substantiated this. Cook and Nathan investigated the EMG response to intravenous diazepam in patients with spasticity related to partial or complete transection of the spinal cord.[77,78] Objective muscle relaxation was produced by diazepam whether the spinal cord was totally divided or partly intact. The authors concluded that the drug must act at a site distal to the transection, either in the spinal cord or at the neuromuscular junction. Although experimental evidence suggests that the benzodiazepines are predominately central muscle relaxants, observations such as these imply that diazepam and related drugs may, in addition, have a more distal effect which is not yet well understood.

ANTICONVULSANT ACTIVITY

The benzodiazepines have important anticonvulsant properties. In small animals (mice and rats), seizures are produced experimentally by the methods outlined in Chapter 1: maximal electroshock (MaxES), minimal electroshock (MinES), and parenteral pentylenetetrazol. The potencies of various benzodiazepines in preventing experimental seizures in mice are shown in Table 1-1. Each drug is least effective against MinES convulsions and most effective against pentylenetetrazol seizures, but the relative potencies of given drugs in the three seizure models vary widely. Clonazepam and lorazepam have the highest anti-pentylenetetrazol milligram potency; both drugs have a 2′-chloro substitution on the 5-phenyl ring. Yet lorazepam is 200 times more potent than clonazepam in anti-MaxES activity. In general, the entries in Table 1-1 seem to have no striking clinical correlates. In theory, anti-pentylenetetrazol activity in small animals is associated with anti-petit mal effects in humans; likewise, anti-MaxES and anti-MinES properties correlate with effectiveness in grand mal and psychomotor seizure disorders respectively.[79] The theory predicts that all benzodiazepines should be most effective in petit mal epilepsy, but this has not been consistently observed in humans.

Numerous studies have verified the potent anti-pentylenetetrazol properties of the benzodiazepines in animal preparations, using mice, rats, rabbits, cats, and monkeys.[80-90] The drugs are effective in preventing seizures when given prophylactically and in arresting convulsive activity already in progress. In studies which include EEG monitoring, suppression of epileptiform spike discharges is also noted. Several authors have studied the pharmacokinetics of the anti-pentylenetetrazol effects of benzodiazepines in mice. Coutinho et al.[91] showed that pentylenetetrazol altered the metabolic distribution and disposition of chlordiazepoxide, but that anti-pentylenetetrazol effects correlated better with brain levels of desmethylchlordiazepoxide than with chlordiazepoxide itself. In the case of diazepam, the drug is rapidly metabolized by the mouse, but anticonvulsant effects are long lasting. The accumulated N-1 demethylated metabolites (desmethyldiazepam and oxazepam) are thought to account for the persistent seizure protection.[92] Significant levels of oxazepam are present in mouse brain long after diazepam has been metabolized.[93-95] Anti-pentylenetetrazol effects can be demonstrated as long as brain concentrations of oxazepam exceed 0.1 μg/g of tissue.

Generalized convulsions produced by a variety of other methods are also prevented or arrested by benzodiazepines. Bemegride,[96,97] picrotoxin,[98] strychnine,[99,100] electrical or photic stimulation,[101,102] soman,[103] thiosemicarbazide,[104] and several less well known analeptic drugs[104-107] produce, in animals, seizure activity which can be antagonized by benzodiazepines. Local anesthetic agents given systemically also produce seizures. Diazepam, chlordiazepoxide, clonazepam, and nitrazepam antagonize the convulsant effects of lidocaine, mepivicaine, bupivicaine, cocaine, and procaine in various animal systems.[108-111] deJong and associates[112-114] have extensively studied the influence of diazepam upon lidocaine-induced seizures in the cat. Intramuscular diazepam (0.25 to 0.5 mg/kg) given 60 min before lidocaine infusion raised the dosage threshold for lidocaine seizures from 8.4 to 16.8 mg/kg. General anesthesia with nitrous oxide did not potentiate the diazepam protection. Equivalent seizure protection was afforded by intramuscular pentobarbital (10 mg/kg), but the barbiturate produced profound behavioral and cardiovascular depression in comparison with the minimal adverse effects of diazepam.

The biochemical bases of the seizure-antagonizing effects of the benzodiazepines are unclear. Camerman and Camerman[115,116] have investigated the molecular conformation of diazepam and diphenylhydantoin. Although the two compounds are chemically dissimilar, their conformations are markedly alike, possibly accounting for their similar anticonvulsant properties. Gamma-aminobutyric acid (GABA) has been implicated as a possible neurochemical mediator. Epileptic patients are thought to have low levels of GABA in the central nervous system. GABA levels may be elevated by diphenylhydantoin treatment. Recently, Saad[117] has demonstrated that diazepam elevates brain GABA concentrations in normal mice and in those depleted of GABA by isoniazid. In another study, diazepam was found to have no effect upon spinal cord concentrations of GABA in young chickens.[118] The serotonin system has also been implicated. Seizure thresholds are lower and benzodiazepine anticonvulsant effects are less marked in animals depleted of serotonin by reserpine.[119] Diazepam has been shown to alter serotonin metabolism in rats. Intraperitoneal diazepam (20 mg/kg) increases retention of serotonin and retards efflux of 5-hydroxyindoleacetic acid from the rat brain,[120] suggesting this as a possible biochemical basis of anticonvulsant action. Julien[121] has studied the role of the cerebellum in diazepam antagonism of penicillin-induced focal seizures. Purkinje cells in the cerebellum are known to exert an inhibitory influence upon several subcortical structures. Intravenous diazepam enhances electrical activity of Purkinje cells and suppresses cortical epileptiform activity. The two effects occur simultaneously, and the author suggests that the anticonvulsant effects of diazepam may be related to enhancement of Purkinje cell activity. These studies provide interesting "leads," but the mechanisms of benzodiazepine anticonvulsant properties obviously require further elucidation.

The benzodiazepines are extremely effective in antagonizing generalized seizures induced by systemic administration of various analeptic drugs. Their effects upon focal seizure activity are somewhat different. Seizure foci or scars may be produced experimentally by local application to the brain of such agents as morphine, nicotine, aluminum, cobalt, or penicillin. The benzodiazepines may effectively prevent the propagation and generalization of seizure activity originating from such foci, but they are much less effective in suppressing the foci themselves.[122–128] Sharer and Kutt[129] studied the influence of diazepam upon penicillin-induced focal seizures in the cat. Small intravenous doses (0.25 mg/kg) stopped seizure spread and prevented convulsive motor activity, but had little effect upon spike discharges from the seizure focus itself. Another important observation was the occurrence of bradycardia, hypotension, and respiratory arrest after intravenous diazepam. The three effects were reproducible by infusion of the propylene glycol solvent alone, again suggesting that cardiovascular depression attributed to intravenous diazepam, although rarely significant, may be due more to the solvent system than to the drug itself.

The contrasting effects of the benzodiazepines upon primary as opposed to propagated epileptiform activity have been studied in detail by Guerrero-Figueroa and associates at Tulane University.[130-133] These investigators used a cat preparation with epileptic foci produced by stereotactic placement of chemical irritants. Administration of benzodiazepines (primarily diazepam and clonazepam) had little or no effect on spike discharges originating from the primary focus, nor upon electrical activity recorded from electrodes implanted a short distance from the primary focus. In other areas of the brain, however, local evoked potentials produced and recorded from closely placed electrode pairs were reduced in amplitude, indicating an inhibition of the spread of electrical activity. The development of secondary or "mirror image" epileptogenic foci in the contralateral hemisphere could be prevented by diazepam or clonazepam; the secondary focus, if allowed to develop, could be suppressed by the benzodiazepines although the primary focus was unaffected. The one exception to these general findings occurred in a study of kittens with three-per-second spike-wave foci produced by implantation of chemical irritants. In this study intravenous diazepam suppressed both the spike-wave activity and the petit mal-like manifestations of the seizures.[134] The findings of these investigators provide convincing documentation that benzodiazepines prevent or arrest the spread of generalized seizures but have little effect upon the primary seizure foci.

THE HUMAN ELECTROENCEPHALOGRAM

The effects of the benzodiazepines upon the EEG in humans have been extensively studied, and investigators are largely in agreement as to the important findings. In oral or parenteral doses large enough to produce mild sedation but not large enough to cause obtundation and sleep, benzodiazepines produce a decrease in the integrated mean energy content of the EEG.[135,136] Alpha activity is reduced in amplitude, and there is a shift to low-voltage fast activity, predominantly in the beta range.[137-151] These changes, which can be seen after a single dose, originate in the frontal and temporal regions, and then spread posteriorly. The shift to fast activity, nicknamed "the Librium Effect,"[151] is produced to some degree by all benzodiazepines tested as well as by meprobamate and appropriate doses of barbiturates. Some authors feel that anxiolytic efficacy of a given benzodiazepine correlates well with its ability to produce the shift to fast beta activity.[151a] Because chlordiazepoxide and related drugs are slowly eliminated, characteristic EEG changes may persist for days, and in some cases weeks, after drug discontinuation.[152,153] Benzodiazepine effects upon the sleep EEG in humans are discussed in Chapter 9.

Biphasic cortical somatosensory evoked potentials (SSEP) occur in the human EEG following electrical stimulation of an extremity. Benzodiazepines appear to reduce the amplitude of the SSEP.[154] Saletu and associates[155,156] have studied the effects of benzodiazepines on the latencies of the two peaks of the SSEP. The latency of the early peak is prolonged while that of the late peak is shortened. The authors claim that this combination is characteristic of minor tranquilizers and constitutes an EEG "screening" test for antianxiety agents.

The influence of benzodiazepines upon seizure activity in humans resembles that seen in animals. The spread of seizures is prevented, but spike activity originating from the primary focus continues.[157–160] The EEG effects correspond with the clinical cessation of seizures, as discussed in Chapter 6.

NEUROCHEMICAL EFFECTS

The significance of benzodiazepine-induced changes in brain chemistry is obscure. Many systems have been studied. High concentrations of chlordiazepoxide impair oxidative phosphorylation *in vitro* and *in vivo,* producing swelling of mitochondria and reduction of adenosine triphosphate (ATP) levels.[161–163] ATPase activity is reduced *in vitro.*[164] Studies at the Squibb Institute for Medical Research have suggested that inhibition of cyclic adenosine monophosphate (AMP) phosphodiesterase closely correlates with antianxiety activity in animals and may be the specific biochemical correlate.[165,166] Chlordiazepoxide blocks the lipomobilizing effect of norepinephrine, and Italian workers have speculated that this effect may also be based upon phosphodiesterase inhibition.[167]

Wise, Stein, and associates proposed that serotonin antagonism may account for the antianxiety activity of oxazepam.[168,169] Other studies have documented variable effects upon endogenous amine metabolism, and upon the response to exogenous neurogenic amines in unstressed animals.[170–177] Diazepam and chlordiazepoxide have been noted to increase the brain concentrations of glucose and glycogen in rats and mice.[178,179] The meaning of such findings is unclear. Neurochemical changes associated with experimental stress are discussed in Chapter 8.

Benzodiazepines increase the acetylcholine content of rat brain[180,181] and prevent the pressor response to physostigmine.[182] Tremorogenic activity of tremorine is antagonized in some studies[183] but not in others.[184] Chlordiazepoxide inhibits the behavioral response to yohimbine[185] and magnesium pemoline[186] in animals, but bromazepam and diazepam potentiate aberrant behavior induced in dogs by Ditran, a potent anticholinergic hallucinogen.[187] These findings suggest that certain benzodiazepine derivatives may have cholinergic blocking properties. Indeed, the manufacturers state that glaucoma is a contraindication to the clinical use of diazepam. Yet there is no evidence that benzodiazepines have anticholinergic properties of clinical significance.[188]

COMMENT

The benzodiazepines produce a variety of neurophysiological and neuropharmacological changes in animals and humans. The effects on the cortical EEG are similar to those produced by other minor tranquilizers, but the limbic system "sedative" properties of the benzodiazepines appear to be relatively selective and unique. Limbic system depression may account for the clinical antianxiety action of this group of drugs, but this correlation is largely conjectural. The benzodiazepines have potent muscle-relaxant and anticonvulsant properties as measured by a number of reliable objective parameters. The muscle-relaxant effects seem to occur at the central level rather than at the spinal cord or the neuromuscular junction, but the exact sites of action in humans remain unclear. The benzodiazepines are effective inhibitors of the spread of generalized seizure activity but are less effective against the primary seizure foci. In general there has been good correlation between these extensive experimental observations and the corresponding effects in humans.

REFERENCES

1. Himwich HE, Morillo A, Steiner WG: Drugs affecting rhinencephalic structures. J Neuropsychiat 3(supp 1):s15-s26, 1962
2. Gogolak G, Liebeswar G, Stumpf C: Action of drugs on the electrical activity of the red nucleus. Electroenceph Clin Neurophysiol 27:296-303, 1969
3. Gogolak G, Krijzer F, Stumpf C: Action of central depressant drugs on the electrocerebellogram of the rabbit. Naunyn-Schmeid Arch Pharmakol 272:378-386, 1972
4. Joy RM, Hance AJ, Killam KF: A quantitative electroencephalographic comparison of some benzodiazepines in the primate. Neuropharmacology 10:483-497, 1971
5. Schallek W, Lewinson T, Thomas J: Power spectrum analysis as a tool for statistical evaluation of drug effects on electrical activity of brain. Int J Neuropharmacol 7:35-46, 1968
5a. Guerrero-Figueroa R, Gallant DM, Guerrero-Figueroa C, Gallant J: Electrophysiological analysis of the action of four benzodiazepine derivatives on the central nervous system. In, *The Benzodiazepines*. Edited by S Garattini, E Mussini, LO Randall. New York, Raven Press, 1973 pp 489-511
6. Schallek W, Kuehn A: Effects of benzodiazepines on spontaneous EEG and arousal responses of cats. Progr Brain Res 18: 231-238, 1955
7. Arrigo A, Jann G, Tonali P: Some aspects of the action of Valium and of Librium on the electrical activity of the rabbit brain. Arch Int Pharmacodyn 154:364-373, 1965
8. Vieth JB, Holm E, Knopp PR: Electrophysiological studies on the action of Mogadon® on central nervous structures of the cat. A comparison with pentobarbital. Arch Int Pharmacodyn 171:323-338, 1968

9. Iwahara S, Oishi H, Yamazaki S, Sakai K: Effects of chlordiazepoxide upon spontaneous alternation and the hippocampal electrical activity in white rats. Psychopharmacologia 24:496-507, 1972

10. Olds ME, Olds J: Effects of anxiety-relieving drugs on unit discharges in hippocampus, reticular midbrain, and pre-optic area in the freely moving rat. Int J Neuropharmacol 8:87-103, 1969

11. Schallek W, Thomas J: Effects of benzodiazepines on spontaneous electrical activity of subcortical areas in brain of cat. Arch Int Pharmacodyn 192:321-337, 1971

12. Steiner FA, Hummel P: Effects of nitrazepam and phenobarbital on hippocampal and lateral geniculate neurons in the cat. Int J Neuropharmacol 7:61-69, 1968

13. Steiner FA, Hummel P: Modification of spontaneous and evoked activity of hippocampal and lateral geniculate neurons by nitrazepam and phenobarbital (Abstract). Electroenceph Clin Neurophysiol 27:105, 1969

14. Gogolak G, Pillat B: Effect of Mogadon on the arousal reaction in rabbits. Progr Brain Res 18:229-230, 1965

15. Sherwin I: Differential action of diazepam on evoked cerebral responses. Electroenceph Clin Neurophysiol 30:445-452, 1971

16. Olds ME, Baldrighi G: Effects of meprobamate, chlordiazepoxide, diazepam, and sodium pentobarbital on visually evoked responses in the tectotegmental area of the rat. Int J Neuropharmacol 7:231-239, 1968

17. Zattoni J: Study of the effect of Mogadon on the visual cortical responses to photic stimuli in the cat (Abstract). Electroenceph Clin Neurophysiol 27:103, 1969

18. Schallek W, Kuehn A: Effects of psychotropic drugs on limbic system of cat. Proc Soc Exp Biol Med 105:111-113, 1960

19. Schallek W, Kuehn A, Jew N: Effects of chlordiazepoxide (Librium) and other psychotropic agents on the limbic system of the brain. Ann NY Acad Sci 96:303-314, 1962

20. Schallek W, Kuehn A: An action of Mogadon on the amygdala of the cat. Med Pharmacol Exp 12:204-208, 1965

21. Schallek W, Thomas J, Kuehn A, Zabransky F: Effects of Mogadon on responses to stimulation of sciatic nerve, amygdala, and hypothalamus of cat. Int J Neuropharmacol 4:317-326, 1965

22. Morillo A: Effects of benzodiazepines upon amygdala and hippocampus of the cat. Int J Neuropharmacol 1:353-359, 1962

23. Morillo A, Revzin AM, Knauss T: Physiological mechanisms of action of chlordiazepoxide in cats. Psychopharmacologia 3:386-394, 1962

24. Jalfre M, Monachon MA, Haefely W: Effects on the amygdalo-hippocampal evoked potential in the cat of four benzodiazepines and some other psychotropic drugs. Naunyn-Schmied Arch Pharmakol 270:180-191, 1971

25. Hernandez-Peon R, Rojas-Ramirez JA: Central mechanisms of tranquilizing, anticonvulsant, and relaxant actions of RO 4-5360. Int J Neuropharmacol 5:263-267, 1966

26. Morpurgo C: Pharmacological modifications of sympathetic responses elicited by hypothalamic stimulation in the rat. Brit J Pharmacol 34:532-542, 1968

27. Carroll MN, Hoff EC, Kell JF, Suter CG: The effects of ethanol and chlordiazepoxide in altering autonomic responses evoked by isocortical and paleocortical stimulation (Abstract). Biochem Pharmacol 8:15, 1961

28. Schallek W, Zabransky F, Kuehn A: Effects of benzodiazepines on central nervous system of cat. Arch Int Pharmacodyn 149:467-483, 1964

29. Schallek W, Zabransky F: Effects of psychotropic drugs on pressor responses to central and peripheral stimulation in cat. Arch Int Pharmacodyn 161:126-131, 1966

30. Sigg EB, Sigg TD: Hypothalamic stimulation of preganglionic autonomic activity and its modification by chlorpromazine, diazepam, and pentobarbital. Int J Neuropharmacol 8:567-572, 1969

31. Chai CY, Wang SC: Cardiovascular actions of diazepam in the cat. J Pharmacol Exp Ther 154:271-280, 1966

32. Stern J, Mendell J, Clark K: H reflex suppression by thalamic stimulation and drug administration. J Neurosurg 29:393-396, 1968

33. Matthews WB: Ratio of minimum H reflex to maximum M response as a measure of spasticity. J Neurol Neurosurg Psychiat 29:201-204, 1966

34. Hoyt JL, Gergis SD, Sokoll MD: Studies on muscle rigidity: droperidol, diazepam, and promethazine. Anesth Analg 51:188-191, 1972

35. Arroyo P: Electromyography in the evaluation of reflex muscle spasm. Simplified method for direct evaluation of muscle-relaxant drugs. J Florida Med Assoc 53:29-31, 1966

36. Ludin HP, Dubach K: Action of diazepam on muscular contraction in man. Z Neurol 199:30-38, 1971

37. Couvee LMJ, van der Laarse WD, Oosterveld WJ: Clinical experiences on spasticity with a modification of the Mumenthaler pendulum test. Paraplegia 6:96-102, 1968

38. Long C, Krysztofiak B, Zamir IZ, Lane JF, Koehler ML: Viscoelastic characteristics of the hand in spasticity: a quantitative study. Arch Phys Med Rehab 49:677-691, 1968

39. Erdman WJ, Heather AJ: Objective measurement of spasticity by light reflection. Clin Pharmacol Ther 5:883-886, 1964

40. Holt KS: The use of diazepam in childhood cerebral palsy. Report of a small study including electromyographic observations. Ann Phys Med (supp):16-24, 1964

41. Carlson KE, Alston W: The effect of intramuscular diazepam on sustained ankle clonus: a quantitative study. Arch Phys Med Rehab 47:781-786, 1966

42. Carlson KE, Alston W: Measurement of the duration of effect of long-acting diazepam in spastic disorders. Arch Phys Med Rehab 49:36-38, 1968

43. Carter CH: Evaluation of diazepam in skeletal muscle hypertonicity in cerebral palsy. Arch Phys Med Rehab 49:519-523, 1968

44. Diamantis W, Kletzkin M: Evaluation of muscle relaxant drugs by head-drop and by decerebrate rigidity. Int J Neuropharmacol 5:305-310, 1966

44a. Maxwell DR, Read MA: The effects of some drugs on the rigidity of the cat due to ischaemic or intercollicular decerebration. Neuropharmacology 11:849-855, 1972

45. van Riezen H, Boersma L: A new method of quantitative grip strength evaluation. Eur J Pharmacol 6:353-356, 1969

46. Brausch H, Henatsch H-D, Student C, Takano K: Effect of diazepam on development of stretch reflex tension. In, The Benzodiazepines. Edited by S Garattini, E Mussini, LO Randall. New York, Raven Press, 1973, pp 531-543

46a. Doppman JL, Albertson K, Ramsey R, Saltzstein SL: Intra-arterial Valium: its safety and effectiveness. Radiology 106:335-338, 1973

47. Simpson B, Carlin JA, Abreu BE, Drager GA: Preliminary studies of diazepam (Valium) on the myotatic reflex in human volunteers (Abstract). Texas Rep Biol Med 21:474-475, 1963

48. Baird HW, Pileggi AJ: Diminished corneal reflex after diazepam. Lancet 2:106, 1968

49. Madan BR, Sharma JD, Vyas DS: Actions of methaminodiazepoxide on cardiac, smooth and skeletal muscles. Arch Int Pharmacodyn 143:127-137, 1963

50. Prindle KH, Gold HK, Cardon PV, Epstein SE: Effects of psychopharmacologic agents on myocardial contractility. J Pharmacol Exp Ther 173:133-137, 1970

51. Oetliker H: Action of chlordiazepoxide on contractile mechanism in single fibres of frog muscle. Experientia 26:682, 1970

52. Dasgupta SR, Ray NM, Mukherjee BP: Studies on the effect of diazepam (Valium) on neuromuscular transmission in skeletal muscles. Indian J Physiol Pharmacol 13:79-80, 1969

53. Pruett JK, Williams BB: Effects of some psychotropic drugs on peripheral nerve conduction. J Pharmaceut Sci 55:1139-1141, 1966

54. Feldman SA, Crawley BE: Diazepam and muscle relaxants. Brit Med J 1:691, 1970

55. Feldman SA, Crawley BE: Interaction of diazepam with the muscle-relaxant drugs. Brit Med J 2:336-338, 1970

56. Hunter AR: Diazepam (Valium) as a muscle relaxant during general anaesthesia: a pilot study. Brit J Anaesth 39:633-637, 1967

57. Webb SN, Bradshaw EG: Diazepam and neuromuscular blocking drugs. Brit Med J 3:640, 1971

57a. Webb SN, Bradshaw EG: An investigation, in cats, into the activity of diazepam at the neuromuscular junction. Brit J Anaesth 45:313-318, 1973

58. Moudgil G, Pleuvry BJ: Diazepam and neuromuscular transmission. Brit Med J 2:734-735, 1970

59. Southgate PJ, Wilson AB: Pharmacological interaction of lorazepam with thiopentone sodium and skeletal neuromuscular blocking drugs. Brit J Pharmacol 43:434P-435P, 1971

60. Dretchen K, Ghoneim MM, Long JP: The interaction of diazepam with myoneural blocking agents. Anesthesiology 34:463-468, 1971

61. Sinha JN, Dixit KS, Srimal RC, Bhargava KP: Central muscle relaxant activity of a dozen CNS active agents and a correlation with their psychotropic activity. Jap J Pharmacol 18:48-53, 1968

62. Hudson RD, Wolpert MK: Central muscle relaxant effects of diazepam. Neuropharmacology 9:481-488, 1970

63. Crankshaw DP, Raper C: Some studies on peripheral actions of mephenesin, methocarbamol, and diazepam. Brit J Pharmacol 34:579-590, 1968

64. Crankshaw DP, Raper C: Mephenesin, methocarbamol, chlordiazepoxide, and diazepam: actions on spinal reflexes and ventral root potentials. Brit J Pharmacol 38:148-156, 1970

65. Nakanishi T, Norris FH: Effect of diazepam on rat spinal reflexes. J Neurol Sci 13:189-195, 1971

66. Ghelarducci B, Lenzi G, Pompeiano O: A neurophysiological analysis of the postural effects of a benzodiazepine. Arch Int Parmacodyn 163:403-421, 1966

67. Schlosser W: Action of diazepam on the spinal cord. Arch Int Pharmacodyn 194:93-102, 1971

68. Keary EM, Maxwell DR: A comparison of the effects of chlorpromazine and some related phenothiazines in reducing the rigidity of the decerebrate cat and in some other central actions. Brit J Pharmacol Chemother 29:400-416, 1967

69. Hamilton JT: Muscle relaxant activity of chlordiazepoxide and diazepam. Canad J Physiol Pharmacol 45:191-199, 1967

70. Giurgea C, Moyersoons F: Differential pharmacological reactivity of three types of cortical evoked potentials. Arch Int Pharmacodyn 188:401-404, 1970

71. Ngai SH, Tseng DSC, Wang SC: Effect of diazepam and other central nervous system depressants on spinal reflexes in cats: a study of site of action. J Pharmacol Exp Ther 153:344-351, 1966

72. Pryzbyla AC, Wang SC: Locus of central depressant action of diazepam. J Pharmacol Exp Ther 163:439-447, 1968

73. Tseng T-C, Wang SC: Locus of action of centrally acting muscle relaxants, diazepam and tybamate. J Pharmacol Exp Ther 178:350-360, 1971

74. Tseng T-C, Wang SC: Locus of central depressant action of some benzodiazepine analogues. Proc Soc Exp Biol Med 137:526-531, 1971

75. Stratten WP, Barnes CD: Diazepam and presynaptic inhibition. Neuropharmacology 10:685-696, 1971

76. Barnes CD, Moolenaar G-M: Effects of diazepam and picrotoxin on the visual system. Neuropharmacology 10:193-201, 1971

77. Cook JB, Nathan PW: On the site of action of diazepam in spasticity in man. J Neurol Sci 5:33-37, 1967

78. Nathan PW: The action of diazepam in neurological disorders with excessive motor activity. J Neurol Sci 10:33-50, 1970
79. Boyer PA: Anticonvulsant properties of benzodiazepines. (A review). Dis Nerv Syst 27:35-42, 1966
80. Hudson RD, Wolpert MK: Anticonvulsant and motor depressant effects of diazepam. Arch Int Pharmacodyn 186:388-401, 1970
81. Swinyard EA, Castellion AW: Anticonvulsant properties of some benzodiazepines. J Pharmacol Exp Ther 151:369-375, 1965
82. Banziger RF: Anticonvulsant properties of chlordiazepoxide, diazepam, and certain other 1,4-benzodiazepines. Arch Int Pharmacodyn 154:131-136, 1965
83. Chen G, Ensor CR, Bohner B: Studies of drug effects on electrically induced extensor seizures and clinical implications. Arch Int Pharmacodyn 172:183-218, 1968
84. Kirsten EB, Schoener EP: Antagonism of pentylenetetrazol excitation by anticonvulsants on single brain stem neurons. Neuropharmacology 11:591-599, 1972
85. Vizioli R, Ricci GF, Pastena L, Medolago-Albani L: A neurophysiological appraisal of diazepam. In, *Neuro-Psycho-Pharmacology.* Edited by H Brill. Amsterdam, Excerpta Medica Foundation, 1966, pp 1093-1097
86. Mercier J, Dessaigne S, Manez J: Neurophysiological study of dispotassium chlorazepate (4306 CB). Arzneim-Forsch 20:125-127, 1970
87. Straw RN: The effect of certain benzodiazepines on the threshold for pentylenetetrazol-induced seizures in the cat. Arch Int Pharmacodyn 175:464-469, 1968
88. Marcucci F, Mussini E, Airoldi, ML, Guaitani A, Garattini S: Brain concentrations of lorazepam and oxazepam at equal degree of anticonvulsant activity. J Pharm Pharmacol 24:63-64, 1972
89. Christmas AJ, Maxwell DR: A comparison of the effects of some benzodiazepines and other drugs on aggressive and exploratory behavior in mice and rats. Neuropharmacology 9:17-29, 1970
90. Shibata S, Sasakawa S, Fujita Y: The central depressant profile of carbamate ester of glycerol ether: 3-(1,2,3,4-tetrahydro-7-naphthyloxy)-2-hydroxypropyl carbamate. Toxicol Appl Pharmacol 11:591-602, 1967
91. Coutinho CB, Cheripko JA, Carbone JJ: Relationship between the duration of anticonvulsant activity of chlordiazepoxide and systemic levels of the parent compound and its major metabolites in mice. Biochem Pharmacol 18:303-316, 1969
92. Coutinho CB, Cheripko JA, Carbone JJ: Correlation between the duration of the anticonvulsant activity of diazepam and its physiological disposition in mice. Biochem Pharmacol 19:363-379, 1970
93. Marcucci F, Guaitani A, Kvetina J, Mussini E, Garattini S: Species differences in diazepam metabolism and anticonvulsant effect. Eur J Pharmacol 4:467-470, 1968
94. Marcucci F, Fanelli R, Mussini E, Garattini S: Further studies on the long-lasting antimetrazol activity of diazepam in mice. Eur J Pharmacol 11:115-116, 1970
95. Marcucci F, Mussini E, Guaitani A, Fanelli R, Garattini S: Anticonvulsant activity and brain levels of diazepam and its metabolites in mice. Eur J Pharmacol 16:311-314, 1971
96. Aizawa T, Muramatsu F, Hamaguchi K, Tomita M, Kakimi R, Toyoda M: Study of the cerebral circulation, metabolism, and electrical activity: effects of chlordiazepoxide in the normal and convulsive cats. Japanese Circulation J 30:13-20, 1966
97. vanDuijn H: The action of clonazepam on experimental epilepsy (Abstract). Electroenceph Clin Neurophysiol 33:443, 1972
98. Barrada O, Oftedal S-I: The effect of diazepam (Valium) and nitrazepam (Mogadon) on picrotoxin-induced seizures in rabbits. (Abstract). Electroenceph Clin Neurophysiol 29:220-221, 1970
99. Bertolini M, Canger R, Pietropolli-Charmet G: On the anticonvulsant properties of oxazepam. Experimental study on the cat. Arzneim-Forsch 19:742-748, 1969

100. Canger R, Penati G: Comparison of the anticonvulsant properties of diazepam, nitrazepam and RO 4023: an experimental study on the cat (Abstract). Electroenceph Clin Neurophysiol 31:532, 1971

101. Hernandez-Peron R, Rojas-Ramirez JA, O'Flaherty JJ, Mazzuchelli-O'Flaherty AL: An experimental study of the anticonvulsive and relaxant actions of Valium. Int J Neuropharmacol 3:405-412, 1964

102. Stark LG, Killam KF, Killam EK: The anticonvulsant effects of phenobarbital, diphenylhydantoin, and two benzodiazepines in the baboon, *Papio papio*. J Pharmacol Exp Ther 173:125-132, 1970

103. Lipp JA: Effect of diazepam upon soman-induced seizure activity and convulsions. Electroenceph Clin Neurophysiol 32:557-560, 1972

104. Banziger R, Hane D: Evaluation of a new convulsant for anticonvulsant screening. Arch Int Pharmacodyn 167:245-249, 1967

105. Lassen JB, Christensen JA, Lund J, Squires RF: Pharmacological and biochemical studies on 2-amino-4-phenylsulphonylbenzene-sulphonamide (NSD 3004): a new sulphonamide with anticonvulsant and carbonic anhydrase inhibitory properties. Acta Pharmacol Toxicol 30:1-16, 1971

106. Nishie K, Waiss AC, Keyl AC: Toxicity of methylimidazoles. Toxicol Appl Pharmacol 14:301-307, 1969

107. Yen HCY, Sigg EB, Warner CL: Stimulant action of pyridyl derivatives of benzodioxans and benzodioxepans. Int J Neuropharmacol 2:337-347, 1963

108. Wale N, Jenkins LC: Site of action of diazepam in the prevention of lidocaine induced seizure activity in cats. Canad Anaesth Soc J 20:146-152, 1973

108a. Munson ES, Wagman IH: Diazepam treatment of local anesthetic-induced seizures. Anesthesiology 37:523-528, 1972

109. Wessling H, Bovenhorst GH, Wiers JW: Effects of diazepam and pentobarbitone on convulsions induced by local anaesthetics in mice. Eur J Pharmacol 13:150-154, 1971

110. Feinstein MB, Lenard W, Mathias J: The antagonism of local anesthetic induced convulsions by the benzodiazepine derivative diazepam. Arch Int Pharmacodyn 187:144-154, 1970

111. Eidelberg E, Neer HM, Miller MK: Anticonvulsant properties of some benzodiazepine derivatives. Possible use against psychomotor seizures. Neurology (Minneap) 15:223-230, 1965

112. de Jong RH, Heavner JE, de Oliveira LF: Effects of nitrous oxide on the lidocaine seizure threshold and diazepam protection. Anesthesiology 37:299-303, 1972

113. de Jong RH, Heavner JE: Diazepam prevents local anesthetic seizures. Anesthesiology 34:523-531, 1971

114. de Jong RH, Heavner JE: Local anesthetic seizure prevention: diazepam versus pentobarbital. Anesthesiology 36:449-457, 1972

115. Camerman A, Camerman N: Stereochemical basis of anticonvulsant drug action. II. Molecular structure of diazepam. J Amer Chem Soc 94:268-272, 1972

116. Camerman A, Camerman N: Diphenylhydantoin and diazepam: molecular structure similarities and steric basis of anticonvulsant activity. Science 168:1457-1458, 1970

117. Saad SF: Effect of diazepam on γ-aminobutyric acid (GABA) content of mouse brain. J Pharm Pharmacol 24:839-840, 1972

118. Kudo Y, Ohshima T, Sato S, Watanabe K, Fukuda H: Studies on the centrally acting muscle relaxants: the spinal reflex and the spinal gamma-aminobutyric acid level in young chickens. Chem Pharm Bull 18:591-595, 1970

119. Mennear JH, Rudzik AD: Mechanism of action of anticonvulsant drugs. III. Chlordiazepoxide. J Pharmaceut Sci 55:640-641, 1966

120. Chase TN, Katz RI, Kopin IF: Effect of diazepam on fate of intracisternally injected serotonin-C^{14}. Neuropharmacology 9:103-108, 1970

121. Julien RM: Cerebellar involvement in the antiepileptic action of diazepam. Neuropharmacology 11:683-691, 1972

122. Chusid JG, Kopeloff LM: Chlordiazepoxide as an anticonvulsant in monkeys. Proc Soc Exp Biol Med 109:546-548, 1962

123. Kopeloff LM, Chusid JG: Diazepam as an anticonvulsant in epileptic and normal monkeys. Int J Neuropsychiat 3:469-471, 1967

124. Scotti de Carolis A, Longo VG: Studies on the anticonvulsant properties of some benzodiazepines (chlordiazepoxide, diazepam, oxazepam). Arzneim-Forsch 17:1580-1582, 1967

125. Spehlmann R, Colley B: Effect of diazepam (Valium®) on experimental seizures in unanesthetized cat. Neurology (Minneap) 18:52-60, 1968

126. Giunta F, Ottino CA, Rossi GF, Tercero E: Experimental study of the anti-epileptic action of a new benzodiazepine derivative (Ro 5-4023). (Abstract). Electroenceph Clin Neurophysiol 31:179, 1971

127. van Duijn H, Visser SL: The action of some anticonvulsant drugs on cobalt-induced epilepsy and on the bemegride threshold in alert cats. Epilepsia 13:409-420, 1972

128. Roldan E, Radil-Weiss T, Chocholova L: Influence of chlordiazepoxide on paroxysmal EEG activity induced by hippocampal and/or thalamic colbalt foci. Psychopharmaco)ogia 19:266-272, 1971

129. Sharer L, Kutt H: Intravenous administration of diazepam. Effects on penicillin-induced focal seizures in the cat. Arch Neurol 24:169-175, 1971

130. Guerrero-Figueroa R, Rye MM, Guerrero-Figueroa C: Effects of diazepam on secondary subcortical epileptogenic tissues. Curr Ther Res 10:150-166, 1968

131. Guerrero-Figueroa R, Gallant DM: Electrophysiological study of the action of a new benzodiazepine derivative (ORF-8063) on the central nervous system. Curr Ther Res 13:747-758, 1971

132. Guerrero-Figueroa R, Rye MM, Heath RG: Effects of two benzodiazepine derivatives on cortical and subcortical epileptogenic tissues in the cat and monkey. I. Limbic system structures. Curr Ther Res 11:27-39, 1969

133. Guerrero-Figueroa R, Rye MM, Heath RG: Effects of two benzodiazepine derivatives on cortical and subcortical epileptogenic tissues in the cat and monkey. II. Cortical and centrencephalic structures. Curr Ther Res 11:40-50, 1969

134. Guerrero-Figueroa R, Rye MM, Gallant DM: Effects of diazepam on three per second spike and wave discharges. Curr Ther Res 9:522-535, 1967

135. Pfeiffer CC: Problems in drug development as they relate to the clinical investigator. J New Drugs 4:299-305, 1964

136. Pfeiffer CC, Goldstein L, Murphree HB, Jenney EH: Electroencephalographic assay of anti-anxiety drugs. Arch Gen Psychiat 10:446-453, 1964

137. Gibbs FA, Gibbs EL: Clinical and pharmacological correlates of fast activity in electroencephalography. J Neuropsychiat 3(supp 1):s73-s78, 1962

138. Kameda H, Hidaka Y, Furukawa T: Changes in human electroencephalogram following administration of chlordiazepoxide. Folia Psychiat Neurol Japonica 16:15-24, 1962

139. Enge S, Lechner H, Diemath HE: EEG patterns during stereotaxic operations under the effect of psychotropic drugs. Confin Neurol 27:374-388, 1966

140. Ulett GA, Heusler AF, Ives-Word V, Word T, Quick R: Influence of chlordiazepoxide on drug-altered EEG patterns and behavior. Med Exp 5:386-390, 1961

141. Itil TM: Quantitative pharmaco-electroencephalography in assessing new anti-anxiety agents. In, Advances in Neuro-Psychopharmacology. Edited by O Vinar, Z Votava, PB Bradley. Amsterdam, North-Holland Publishing Co., 1971, pp 199-209

142. Jeavons PM: The effect of chlordiazepoxide on the electroencephalogram. Epilepsia 3:110-116, 1962

143. Montagu JD: Effects of quinalbarbitone (secobarbital) and nitrazepam on the EEG in man: quantitative investigations. Eur J Pharmacol 14:238-249, 1971

144. Montagu JD: Effects of diazepam on the EEG in man. Eur J Pharmacol 17:167-170, 1972

144a. Frost JD, Carrie JRG, Borda RP, Kellaway P: The effects of Dalmane (flurazepam hydrochloride) on human EEG characteristics. Electroenceph Clin Neurophysiol 34:171-175, 1973

145. Ulett GA, Bowers CA, Heusler AF, Quick P, Word T, Word V: A study of the behavior and EEG patterns of patients receiving tranquilizers with and without the addition of chlordiazepoxide. J Neuropsychiat 5:558-565, 1964

146. Keskiner A, Lloyd-Smith DL: Effects of intravenous chlordiazepoxide on the electroencephalogram with some clinical observations. J Nerv Ment Dis 134:218-227, 1962

147. Jeavons PM: Overdosage of chlordiazepoxide. Lancet 2:826, 1961

148. Diemath HE: Bioelectric changes in subcortical areas of the brain during the administration of hypnogenic substances (preliminary report). Progr Brain Res 18:223-225, 1965

149. Volavka JV, Joyce CRB, Maloney MJ, Brawn W, Summerfield J, Topham C, Scott DF: Effect of nitrazepam, amylobarbitone sodium, and placebo on the electroencephalogram of normal subjects. Psychopharmacologia 14:178-183, 1969

150. Itil T, Gannon P, Cora R, Polvan N, Akpinar S, Elveris F, Eskazan E: SCH-12,041, a new antianxiety agent (quantitative pharmacoelectroencephalography and clinical trials). Physicians Drug Manual 3:26-35, (July-Aug), 1971

151. Winfield DL, Aivazian GH: Librium therapy and electroencephalographic correlates. J Nerv Ment Dis 133-240-246, 1961

151a. Itil TM: Personal communication, 1973.

152. Clark TO, Arrowsmith R: Persistent EEG changes in chlordiazepoxide toxic state. A case report. Canad Psychiat Assoc J 13:279-280, 1968

153. Towler ML, Beall BD, King JB: Drug effects on the electroencephalographic pattern, with specific consideration of diazepam. Southern Med J 55:832-838, 1962

154. Gath I: Effect of drugs on the somatosensory evoked potential in myoclonic epilepsy. Arch Neurol 20:354-357, 1969

155. Saletu B, Saletu M, Itil T: Effect of minor and major tranquilizers on somatosensory evoked potentials. Psychopharmacologia 24:347-358, 1972

156. Saletu B, Saletu M, Itil TM: Somatosensory evoked potential: an objective indicator of the therapy efficacy of a new psychotropic drug, clorazepate dipotassium (Tranxene). Curr Ther Res 14:428-441, 1972

157. Niedermeyer E: Electroencephalographic studies on the anticonvulsive action of intravenous diazepam. Eur Neurol 3:88-96, 1970

158. Niedermeyer E: Intravenous diazepam and its anticonvulsive action. Johns Hopkins Med J 127:79-96, 1970

159. Scollo-Lavizzari G: Valium and epilepsy. Lancet 1:422, 1970

160. Bell DS: The effect of diazepam on the EEG of status epilepticus. J Neurol Neurosurg Psychiat 33:231-237, 1970

161. David LF, Gatz EE, Jones JR: Effects of chlordiazepoxide and diazepam on respiration and oxidative phosphorylation in rat brain mitochondria. Biochem Pharmacol 20:1883-1887, 1971

162. Kadenbach B, Luhrs W: Effects of 7-chloro-2-methylamino-5-phenyl-3H-1,4-benzodiazepin-4-oxide on mitochondria from rat liver and brain. Nature 192:174-176, 1961

163. Kaul CL, Lewis JJ: Effects of minor tranquillizers on brain phosphate levels in vivo. Biochem Pharmacol 12:1279-1282, 1963

164. Ueda I, Wada T, Ballinger CM: Sodium- and potassium-activated ATPase of beef brain—effects of some tranquilizers. Biochem Pharmacol 20:1697-1700, 1971

165. Beer B, Chasin M, Clody DE, Vogel JR, Horovitz ZP: Cyclic adenosine monophosphate phosphodiesterase in brain: effect on anxiety. Science 176:428-430, 1972

166. Horovitz ZP, Beer B, Clody DE, Vogel JR, Chasin M: Cyclic AMP and anxiety. Psychosomatics 13:85-92, 1972

167. Arrigoni-Martelli E, Corsico N: On the mechanism of lipomobilizing effect of chlordiazepoxide. J Pharm Pharmacol 21:59-60, 1969

168. Wise CD, Berger BD, Stein L: Benzodiazepines: anxiety-reducing activity by reduction of serotonin turnover in the brain. Science 177:180-183, 1972

169. Stein L, Wise CD, Berger BD: Antianxiety action of benzodiazepines: decrease in activity of serotonin neurons in the punishment system. In, *The Benzodiazepines*. Edited by S Garattini, E Mussini, LO Randall. New York, Raven Press, 1973, pp 299-326

170. Corne SJ, Pickering RW, Warner BT: A method for assessing the effects of drugs on the central actions of 5-hydroxytryptamine. Brit J Pharmacol Chemother 20:106-120, 1963

171. Green H, Erickson RW: Effect of some drugs upon rat brain histamine content. Int J Neuropharmacol 3:315-320, 1964

172. da Prada M, Pletscher A: On the mechanism of chlorpromazine-induced changes in cerebral homovanillic acid levels. J Pharm Pharmacol 18:628-630, 1966

173. Ross SB, Renyi AL: *In vivo* inhibition of ³H-noradrenaline uptake by mouse brain slices *in vitro*. J Pharm Pharmacol 18:322-323, 1966

174. Morpurgo C, Theobald W: Pharmacological modifications of the amphetamine-induced hyperthermia in rats. Eur J Pharmacol 2:287-294, 1967

175. Corrodi H, Fuxe K, Hokfelt T: The effect of some psychoactive drugs on central monoamine neurons. Eur J Pharmacol 1:363-368, 1967

176. Lewander T: Influence of various psychoactive drugs on the *in vivo* metabolism of d-amphetamine in the rat. Eur J Pharmacol 6:38-44, 1969

177. Fennessy MR, Lee JR: The effect of benzodiazepines on brain amines of the mouse. Arch Int Pharmacodyn 197:37-44, 1972

178. Hutchins DA, Rogers KJ: Physiological and drug-induced changes in the glycogen content of mouse brain. Brit J Pharmacol 39:9-25, 1970

179. Gey KF: Effect of benzodiazepines on carbohydrate metabolism in rat brain. In, *The Benzodiazepines*. Edited by S Garattini, E Mussini, LO Randall. New York, Raven Press, 1973, pp 243-255

180. Domino EF, Wilson AE: Psychotropic drug influences on brain acetylcholine utilization. Psychopharmacologia 25:291-298, 1972

181. Ladinsky H, Consolo S, Peri G, Garattini S: Increase in mouse and rat brain acetylcholine levels by diazepam. In, *The Benzodiazepines*. Edited by S Garattini, E Mussini, LO Randall. New York, Raven Press, 1973, pp 241-242

182. Varagic V, Krstic M, Mihajlovic L: The effect of some psychopharmacological agents on the hypertensive response to eserine in the rat. Int J Neuropharmacol 3:273-277, 1964

183. Spencer PJS: Activity of centrally acting and other drugs against tremor and hypothermia induced in mice by tremorine. Brit J Pharmacol Chemother 25:442-455, 1965

184. Yen HCY, Day CA: Evaluation of anti-tremor drugs in tremor-induced rodents. Arch Int Pharmacodyn 155:69-83, 1965

185. Lang WJ, Gershon S: Effects of psychoactive drugs on yohimbine induced responses in conscious dogs. A proposed screening procedure for antianxiety agents. Arch Int Pharmacodyn 142:457-472, 1963

186. Berger HJ: Separation of the effects of magnesium pemoline on avoidance learning and memory from its central nervous system stimulant properties by chlordiazepoxide. Proc Soc Exp Biol Med 138:591-596, 1971

187. Korol B, Brown ML: A behavioral and autonomic nervous system study of RO-5-3350 and diazepam in conscious dogs. Pharmacology 1:115-128, 1968

188. Droppleman LF, McNair DM: Screening for anticholinergic effects of atropine and chlordiazepoxide. Psychopharmacologia 12:164-169, 1968

Chapter 6
The Treatment of Neuromuscular and Seizure Disorders

In the several decades prior to 1960, few if any striking advances were made in the pharmacotherapy of neurological disease. Diphenylhydantoin and phenobarbital had long been recognized as effective prophylactic anticonvulsants in grand mal seizure disorders, but available agents for the parenteral treatment of intractable seizures were unsatisfactory. Patients with status epilepticus receiving various concoctions of barbiturates, paraldehyde, and other sedative-hypnotics often became apneic and comatose at the time when seizure activity ceased. Drugs for the treatment of muscle spasticity were also unsatisfactory. Barbiturates, phenothiazines, meprobamate, mephenesin, methocarbamol, and various other agents were limited in utility because of lack of efficacy, intolerability of side effects, or short duration of action. The benzodiazepines have enhanced the possibilities of effective drug therapy in spastic musculoskeletal diseases and in a variety of seizure disorders.

NEUROMUSCULAR DISORDERS

A number of infectious, traumatic, degenerative, and metabolic diseases of the central nervous system become manifest as spastic disorders of skeletal musculature. In chronic diseases such as cerebral palsy or spastic para- and hemiplegias caused by traumatic or vascular accidents, relaxation of an afflicted extremity increases the possibility of overall rehabilitation even if the extremity itself does not become functional. In acute spastic disorders such as tetanus, rigidity and spasm may become so severe as to impair respiratory function. The benzodiazepines, particularly diazepam, have been used with varying degrees of success in most of the clinically important disorders of this type.

Cerebral Palsy

This term describes a group of heterogeneous clinical syndromes thought to reflect damage to the brain occurring either *in utero*, during birth, or shortly after birth. These syndromes can be subdivided on the basis of site of primary involvement into three groups: (1) the *spastic*, which involves the motor cortex and can be anywhere on the spectrum of severity from mild clumsiness, through severe spasticity (characterized by adduction and internal rotation of the thigh with plantarflexion of the foot), to incapacitating opisthotonus; (2) the *athetoid*, which involves the basal ganglia; and (3) the *ataxic*, which involves the cerebellum. Clinical syndromes frequently overlap. Some are associated with mental retardation, hyperactivity, or behavior problems.

Extensive studies (many uncontrolled) have been done using chlordiazepoxide and diazepam in children with cerebral palsy.[1-19] Approximately 50% of these children showed significant benefit such as reduced spasticity, decreased involuntary movements, and better coordination. In many cases behavior improved and hyperactivity diminished.

Effective doses are variable and usually are relatively high with respect to the patient's body weight. Many children experience drowsiness and ataxia before the effective dose level is reached.

Only a few adequately controlled trials have appeared in the literature. Two groups found diazepam substantially better than placebo in trials with cerebral palsied patients, including adults.[20,21] Engle found only a weak diazepam-placebo difference in a study of children.[22] Bayliss and Gilbertson performed a crossover trial of chlordiazepoxide and placebo in nearly 30 children.[23,24] Chlordiazepoxide was of significantly greater benefit, but the differences were attributable to improvement in behavior and sleep patterns rather than to reduction in spasticity. Five patients developed "paradoxical" increases in aggressiveness while on chlordiazepoxide. Sylvester, on the other hand, found chlordiazepoxide to produce more relief of spasticity than place-bo, but the drug produced no behavioral improvement.[25] Studies comparing benzodiazepines to each other and to meprobamate have shown no striking differences.[26,27]

Spasticity from Trauma or Degenerative Disease

Multiple sclerosis, parkinsonism, amyotrophic lateral sclerosis, cerebrovascular accidents, and spinal cord lesions all may produce increased muscle tone. Oral diazepam has been used with success in all of these diseases.[28-33] Electromyographic (EMG) studies demonstrate objective muscle relaxation. Parenteral diazepam may produce immediate relief of spasm.[34,35]

A summary of controlled trials is given in Table 6-1. All of these studies are crossover in design, and drug-placebo differences are demonstrable in the majority. Several authors comment that effective doses often correspond with those that produce drowsiness. The disease entities afflicting the patients in these studies are chronic, debilitating, and generally incurable. No drug can work miracles for these patients, but diazepam may provide some degree of symptomatic relief and increased comfort.

TABLE 6-1. *Controlled trials of benzodiazepines in spastic neuromuscular disorders**

Reference	Author(s)	Diseases	Drugs (daily oral dose in mg)	Result
36	Cocchiarella et al., 1967	Upper motor neuron disease	DZ (6) vs DZ (15) vs phenobarb (45) vs phenobarb (90) vs placebo	No difference between drugs or placebo
37	Kendall, 1964	Hemiplegia	DZ (6) vs placebo	DZ very slightly superior to placebo
38	Levine et al., 1969	Multiple sclerosis	PRZ (10-20) vs placebo	PRZ superior to placebo by EMG assessment
39	McFarland, 1963	Many	CDX (30) vs placebo	CDX superior to placebo
40	Neill, 1964	Spinal cord lesions	DZ (6-20) vs placebo	DZ superior to placebo
41	Wilson and McKechnie, 1966	Multiple sclerosis Spastic paraplegia	DZ (16) vs DZ (28) vs placebo	Both doses of DZ somewhat superior to placebo

*All are crossover trials.

TABLE 6-2. Controlled trials of benzodiazepines in musculoskeletal disorders

Reference	Author(s)	Drugs (daily oral dose in mg)	Results
54	Cazort, 1964	DZ (10) vs chlormezanone (800) vs carisoprodol (1,400)	DZ superior to chlormezanone and carisoprodol
55	Cooper, 1963[X]	DZ (10) vs chlormezanone (800) vs carisoprodol (1,400)	DZ superior to chlormezanone and carisoprodol
56,57	GPRG, 1965; Wheatley, 1964[X]	DZ (6-8) vs aspirin (2,000-2,650)	DZ equivalent to aspirin
58	Hingorani, 1966	DZ* vs placebo	DZ equivalent to placebo
59	Masterson and White, 1964	CDX (40-60) vs OXZ (40-60)	OXZ equivalent to CDX
60	Payne et al., 1964[X]	DZ (20) vs meprobamate (1,600) vs placebo	Drugs and placebo equivalent
61	Rogers, 1963[X]	DZ (4-12) vs methocarbamol (4,000)	DZ superior to methocarbamol
62	Snell et al., 1965[X]	DZ (10-12) vs carisoprodol (1,400) vs phenobarbital (120)	No difference between drugs
63	Tarpley, 1965[X]	DZ (5-10) vs chlormezanone (400-800) vs carisoprodol (700-1400)	DZ superior to chlormezanone and carisoprodol
64	Wickstrom and Haddad, 1962	CDX (30) vs placebo	CDX superior to placebo

x: Crossover trials
*10 mg i.m. q 6 hr for 24 hr, then 8 mg/day orally

Backache and Muscle Strain

Among the most common problems encountered by the practicing physician are the multitude of aches and pains associated with reversible musculoskeletal disorders. In contrast to the gloomy prognosis facing the patients discussed previously, most individuals with traumatic muscular strain, sprain, or spasm can expect to recover with conservative therapy (rest, analgesics, application of local heat, and subsequent rehabilitative exercise). Uncontrolled studies have suggested that the muscle-relaxing properties of the benzodiazepines may be of considerable benefit to such patients.[42-50] The overall improvement rate in these series is more than 70%. When pain and spasm are particularly severe or disabling, intravenous or intramuscular diazepam may provide immediate, dramatic relief.[50] Excellent results have been reported in the treatment of acute disc lesions,[51] spastic torticollis,[52] and in overriding fractures with muscle spasm.[53] Beneficial effects are less obvious in disorders such as rheumatoid arthritis in which joint pain alone is the primary manifestation.[53a]

Controlled trials are summarized in Table 6-2. In four of six studies, diazepam is superior to other muscle relaxants (chlormezanone, carisoprodol, methocarbamol),[54,55,61,63] but when diazepam is compared with placebo or aspirin, differences are not consistently apparent. A possible inference is that the other muscle-relaxant drugs are less effective, or no more effective, than placebo. None of these studies, however, directly addresses this hypothesis. Chlordiazepoxide and placebo were compared in a single study, in which chlordiazepoxide was significantly more effective.[64]

Much of the favorable result in uncontrolled trials is probably attributable to placebo response, spontaneous remission, or the effect of rest and analgesia. Muscle relaxants do not supplant these other modes of therapy. Among the available muscle relaxants, diazepam is the drug of choice for many physicans, but the possibility that chlordiazepoxide may be as effective as diazepam deserves further study.

Tetanus and Strychnine Poisoning

Hyperirritable and spastic musculature in tetanus are thought to be caused by depression of inhibitory interneuronal function with exaggeration of polysynaptic reflex activity. Diazepam, acting by enhancement of presynaptic inhibition, would seem to be a suitable agent for muscle relaxation in tetanus.[65] Many case reports have documented the successful use of diazepam and chlordiazepoxide in this disease (Table 6-3). In most of these reports the response to an intravenous dose of diazepam is dramatic, producing immediate relief of previously intractable spasm and tetany. For continuous suppression and prevention of spasms, very large doses of diazepam are required—up to several hundred milligrams per day in many reports, and as high as 1,200

TABLE 6-3. *Benzodiazepines in tetanus: Case reports**

Reference	Author(s)	Number of cases	Deaths
66	Bacon, 1968	2	0
67	Cheah et al., 1972	1	0
68	Cordova, 1969	3	0
69	Das et al., 1967	10	3
70	Davis et al., 1972	1	0
71	Femi-Pearse, 1966	42	6
72	Femi-Pearse and Fleming, 1965	1	0
73	Grewal, 1966	3	0
74	Groessler, 1966	1	0
75	Kendall and Clarke, 1972	1	0
76	Lockwood and Allison, 1967	3	1
77	Lowenthal and Lavalette, 1966	2	0
78	Moriarty and Bertolotti, 1965	1	0
79	O'Donohoe, 1967	1	0
80	Phillips, 1965	14	2
81	Shershin and Katz, 1964	1	0
82	Sorabjee, 1967	1	0
83	Stoebner et al., 1970	5	1
65	Weinberg, 1964	1	0

*Chlordiazepoxide used in reports by Phillips[80] and Lowenthal and Lavalette.[77] Diazepam used in all other reports.

mg/day in one. The drug can be given in repeated intravenous boluses or by continuous intravenous infusion. During the recovery phase, oral therapy may be substituted for parenteral. Owing to the tendency of diazepam and its active metabolites to accumulate in the body, prolonged central nervous system depression may follow after cessation of high-dose therapy, especially in the elderly. Davis and associates[70] reported persistent obtundation in a 77-year-old man who received high doses of diazepam for tetanus. Four days after the drug was stopped, the blood level of diazepam was 6.1 μg/ml; hypotonia and semiobtundation persisted for 2 weeks or more. Kendall and Clarke[75] treated a 72-year-old man for tetanus using diazepam. Unconsciousness continued for 12 days after the drug was stopped.

Table 6-3 shows that the mortality in tetanus, in spite of benzodiazepine therapy, is 14%. There are no truly blind or controlled trials of diazepam in tetanus. Norredam and Hainau[84] compared their experience with tetanus before and after January 1967. In 159 cases treated before this date, pentobarbital was used as the sedative and muscle relaxant. The mortality was 67%, and 82% of patients required tracheostomies. After January 1967, when diazepam replaced pentobarbital, the mortality in 142 cases was 39%, and only 15% of patients required tracheostomies. The differences were highly significant, although neonatal tetanus was not studied. In a similar type of survey, Phatak and Shah[85] found that the mortality when phenobarbital and diazepam were combined (19%) was somewhat lower than when phenobarbital was used alone (25%) or combined with paraldehyde and chloral hydrate (33%). Tjoen and co-workers[86] reported that in children, the use of diazepam alone was associated with a lower mortality (9%) than were combinations of phenobarbital, chlorpromazine, and diazepam; in neonatal tetanus, however, the mortality was not lowered by diazepam. Hendrickse and Sherman[87,88] found that diazepam given by nasogastric tube was ineffective in children with tetanus. However, the addition of oral diazepam to a phenobarbital-chlorpromazine-paraldehyde combination reduced tetanus-attributed mortality from 32% to 9% in non-neonates. Again, no benefit could be demonstrated in neonatal tetanus.

Although unequivocal proof is lacking, diazepam appears to be the sedative and muscle relaxant of choice in non-neonatal tetanus. The drug should be given parenterally in high doses. Even with benzodiazepine therapy combined with comprehensive supportive care, tetanus is still associated with a significant mortality.

Strychnine also intereferes with inhibitory interneuronal function, causing hyperreflexia, extensor thrusts, opisthotonus, tonic-clonic convulsions, and paralysis of respiration. In a few reports of strychnine poisoning, intravenous diazepam has provided immediate and dramatic relief from spasms and convulsions.[89-92] Diazepam appears to be a reasonable antidote in poisoning by strychnine.

Stiff-Man Syndrome

This rare disorder is characterized clinically by episodic aching and tightening of axial musculature with insidious progression of muscle stiffness over time.[93-95] Any sudden stimulus may precipitate spasm. During sleep there is relaxation. EMG examination reveals persistent tonic contraction of musculature. As time passes, patients become disabled by myotonia and actually may fracture limbs by force of muscle contraction. Occasionally, the syndrome is antedated by a traumatic injury.[96] Closely similar but nonidentical syndromes have also been described.[97] In a number of reports, diazepam has been of significant benefit to these patients, allowing increased comfort and return of some degree of function.[95-100] The etiology of the syndrome and mechanism by which diazepam produces improvement are unknown.

Other Disorders

The benzodiazepines have been used in a variety of other disorders involving muscle spasm and involuntary movement. Intravenous diazepam has produced relief of acute dystonic reactions induced by phenothiazines and butyrophenones.[101,102] Facial tics in children and adolescents were relieved by diazepam in one report,[103] but in a controlled trial diazepam was indistinguishable from placebo.[104] Isolated case reports and small series have described the use of benzodiazepines in Huntington's chorea,[105–107] dystonia musculorum deformans,[108] myotonia dystrophica,[109] intention myoclonus,[110,111] progressive cerebellar dyssynergia,[111a] the "restless leg" syndrome,[112,113] and post-radiculography muscle spasm.[114] These reports are anecdotal, and the place of the benzodiazepines in the treatment of the various disorders remains to be established.

SEIZURE DISORDERS

The role of the benzodiazepines as anticonvulsants has been subject to a great deal of confusion. "Epilepsy," like "cancer," is a heterogenous family of diseases. Failure to distinguish the distinct entities within the family will confound the assessment of drug efficacy. Many trials of the benzodiazepines in epilepsy involve unselected series of patients with seizures of varying etiologies; in addition, most of the studies are uncontrolled. For this reason, results vary widely from gratifying success to complete failure, depending on the duration of the trial, dosage, chronicity of the disorder, and to some extent the distribution of patients within diagnostic categories. Appendix 4 lists uncontrolled studies in unselected series of patients. In patients who improved clinically, there often was improvement in the EEG with reduction in paroxysmal bursts and spikes. In most cases, the EEG shows the characteristic shift to low-voltage fast activity (see also Chapter 5). Livingston and associates (1961, Appendix 4) added chlordiazepoxide to the anticonvulsant regimen of 40 patients with poorly controlled seizures. There was no improvement in any of the patients. In most of the other studies, some degree of clinical improvement accompanies benzodiazepine therapy.

Chien and Keegan reported a controlled trial involving 42 hospitalized epileptics receiving diphenylhydantoin and phenobarbital.[115] In half the patients, the conventional drugs were replaced with diazepam; in the other half, conventional medications were continued. The total number of seizures occurring in both groups was nearly identical, but in the diazepam group the frequency of grand mal seizures was nearly doubled. Lou[116] investigated the effect of oxazepam and placebo on psychomotor epilepsy. Oxazepam proved to be superior to placebo in reducing the frequency of psychomotor seizures. These are the only controlled trials published to date.

Nitrazepam and Minor Motor Seizures

The exceptional effectiveness of nitrazepam in minor motor seizures (infantile spasms or myoclonic epilepsy) and to some extent petit mal absence seizures was discovered more by trial-and-error and chance than by systematic study. Among unselected groups of patients, it was observed with some consistency that those with minor motor and petit mal epilepsy benefited more from benzodiazepine therapy than did patients with other types of seizure disorders. In studies of selected populations, diazepam was shown to produce considerable improvement in these syndromes.[117,118] Comparisons of diazepam with nitrazepam suggested that nitrazepam was even more effective, producing complete or partial control of seizures in 60 to 80% of patients.[119-121] Since 1964, a number of reports have substantiated the efficacy of nitrazepam in petit mal and particularly in infantile spasms.[119-130] Many of the patients had been previously refractory to other pharmacotherapy, including ACTH. Among those with the classic hypsarrhythmia EEG pattern, suppression of the abnormality usually occurs. Although none of the studies is controlled, nitrazepam is now considered by some to be the agent of first choice in the treatment of infantile spasms.

Large doses of nitrazepam, in the range of 0.5 to 1.0 mg/kg per day, are usually required. At this dose level, drowsiness and oversedation are frequent problems. In small children, increased salivation and bronchial secretion have been noted, occasionally resulting in aspiration pneumonia.[125-128] A degree of tolerance occurs in many patients; some children whose seizures are initially controlled by nitrazepam experience a recurrence of seizures as months pass, and the dose of nitrazepam may have to be increased.[125] A final problem is the apparent precipitation of grand mal seizures by nitrazepam. Several authors have noted that grand mal epilepsy becomes worse or first appears during nitrazepam therapy.[128-130] Two groups of investigators have reported a total of six patients who received intravenous diazepam or nitrazepam for the treatment of petit mal status or intractable myoclonic spasms. Immediately following the administration of the drug, generalized tonic-clonic convulsions appeared.[131-134] This poorly understood "paradoxical" event fortunately appears to be quite unusual.

Status Epilepticus

The benzodiazepines have been extremely effective when given parenterally in the treatment of status epilepticus and intractable seizures. Appendix 5 lists reports describing the treatment of 30 patients with chlordiazepoxide and nearly 500 with diazepam. Control is achieved in well over 50% of cases. Most patients had received barbiturates, paraldehyde, diphenylhydantoin and other anticonvulsants without effect before diazepam was administered. The type of seizure does not appear to influence the response. Control is achieved whether the intractable seizures are grand mal, petit mal, myoclonic, or *partialis continualis* in nature. Some physicians feel that status epilepticus is more likely to respond to intravenous diazepam when patients have no previous history of seizures than when seizures have been previously treated and controlled. This impression, although not well substantiated, may in part reflect greater difficulty of seizure control in those with more advanced disease. Patients who first present with seizures usually are in an early stage of disease; those who "break through" previously adequate drug therapy might be expected to have more severe or advanced disease, with seizures more refractory to pharmacologic control. On the other hand, intractable seizures commonly recur in patients with stable or nonprogressive disease simply because of failure to take anticonvulsant medication. In these individuals, control is usually reestablished with relative ease.

The hazards of intravenous diazepam in status epilepticus are difficult to assess, since intractable seizures in themselves can reflect life-threatening neurological disease. In some patients, seizures are a terminal event and cannot be controlled; in others, death ensues despite control of convulsions. Bell[135] described six episodes of significant hypotension in 25 cases of status epilepticus treated with diazepam. The author attributed the adverse reactions to diazepam, but was criticized for this conclusion.[136-138] Large parenteral doses of other sedative-hypnotics had been administered to these patients in addition to diazepam, and it cannot be determined whether the drug combinations or the underlying disease were responsible for the cardiovascular depression. Other authors have noted cardiovascular and respiratory depression in association with intravenous diazepam, but the setting of multiple causality almost always exists (see Chapter 12). In experimental situations, diazepam consistently produces less cardiopulmonary depression than equipotent doses of barbiturates (see Chapter 7). Any intravenous sedative-hypnotic is hazardous in the severely ill patient with status epilepticus, but the benzodiazepines are the least hazardous of the available agents. Other reviewers support our conclusion that intravenous diazepam at present is the drug of first choice in the treatment of intractable seizures and status epilepticus.[139-142]

Diazepam in Electroconvulsive Therapy

Watson[143,144] noted that patients receiving intravenous diazepam as an anesthetic-amnestic agent before electroconvulsive therapy (ECT) required much more current to produce a seizure. The modification of ECT by parenteral diazepam has been described by a number of investigators.[145-147] Pretreatment with this drug appears to allow an easily modified convulsion with no fractures, no problems with recovery or resuscitation, and amnesia for the period of treatment. In a comparison with thiopental, intravenous diazepam modified convulsions with equal effectiveness but produced hypotension and respiratory depression less frequently than the barbiturate.[148] Another study of fluoroethyl-induced convulsions showed that the tonic phase of the seizures was shorter following intravenous diazepam than after thiopental.[149]

Rousos and associates[150] studied intramuscular diazepam and placebo as premedication for ECT. Diazepam produced more sedation, more amnesia, and a more satisfactory ECT than placebo, but did not increase the incidence of respiratory depression. Ekinci and colleagues[151,152] compared oral diazepam (50 to 150 mg given 1 hr prior to ECT) to oral placebo, and to intravenous succinylcholine plus thiopental as pre-ECT therapy. The parenteral combination proved superior to oral diazepam in reducing the severity of convulsions, whereas oral diazepam proved no better than an oral placebo.

When given intravenously, diazepam produces potent muscle-relaxant, anticonvulsant, sedative, and anterograde amnestic effects of rapid onset and short duration (see Chapters 7 and 10). Intravenous diazepam appears to be a suitable "induction" agent for modified ECT. Injection pain and/or subsequent phlebitis are frequent complications of intravenous diazepam (see Chapter 12). Wehlage[152a] noted that the use of diazepam in place of methohexital significantly reduced the incidence of major morbid events associated with ECT. Phlebitis, however, was greatly increased in frequency, particularly when diazepam was injected into the same vein on successive days. Dilution of injectable diazepam causes precipitation of the drug and is not a suitable prophylactic measure.[152b]

When given by the intramuscular route, diazepam is more satisfactory than placebo as a premedicant, but probably is less effective than by intravenous injection. Oral diazepam by itself is inadequate, even when given in large doses, timed such that the peak of action corresponds with the time of ECT.

Benzodiazepines as Diagnostic Aids

Adequate EEG study requires a cooperative subject. Many patients are unable or unwilling to sit still and cooperate, and in such cases the benzodiazepines are a useful aid in producing muscle relaxation and sedation. Chlordiazepoxide (25 to 100 mg) or diazepam (10 to 40 mg) produces adequate sedation and eliminates muscle artifact in a large percentage of patients.[153–156] These drugs may also be of help in the EEG localization of primary epileptogenic foci when secondary foci are also present. Parenteral diazepam suppresses secondary epileptogenic foci, while spike activity from the primary focus continues[156–158] (see also Chapter 5). Study of the EEG evoked by photic stimulation or pentylenetetrazol may provide important diagnostic information but at the risk of inducing grand mal seizures in some patients. Intravenous diazepam effectively suppresses photosensitive or pentylenetetrazol-induced seizures and reduces the hazard of the procedure.[159,160] Some types of episodic behavioral disorders can be associated with epileptiform activity which is suppressible by benzodiazepine derivatives.[161] Monroe and associates[162,163] have described a group of such patients in whom alpha-chloralose produced EEG activation. Chlordiazepoxide was protective against the alpha-chloralose hypersynchrony. By contrast, phenothiazines enhanced the abnormality. Clinically, improved behavior was noted during chlordiazepoxide therapy. The authors suggest that episodic behavioral disorders associated with these EEG findings represent a form of epilepsy and should be treated with chlordiazepoxide or anticonvulsants rather than phenothiazines. Whether benzodiazepines are preferable to other anticonvulsants such as diphenylhydantoin has not yet been established.

Other Uses

Isolated publications describe the use of the benzodiazepines in other clinical situations associated with seizures. Schimschock and associates[164] report complete control of seizures with diazepam in a 5½-month-old infant having infantile spasms and holoprosencephaly. Two articles describe the use of chlordiazepoxide, diazepam, or nitrazepam in 10 patients with progressive myoclonus and epilepsy.[165,166] Forster[167] studied the effect of diazepam on the EEG in spastic pseudosclerosis (Jacob-Cruetzfeldt's disease). Canger and Penati[168,169] found that both intravenous diazepam and nitrazepam produced paradoxical slowing of the EEG in a patient with subacute sclerosing leukoencephalitis.

Clonazepam

Clonazepam is an analogue of nitrazepam differing only in its 2´-chloro substitution of the 5-phenyl ring (Fig. 1-4), with a resultant increase in milligram potency. Clonazepam is discussed separately because it is in the early stages of investigation and appears to be a highly effective anticonvulsant.[170-179] The most success has been achieved in the treatment of petit mal and variants thereof; some patients with previously intractable seizures of this type have been impressively controlled by clonazepam. The effect upon infantile spasms seems to be less striking. Turner and associates[177] conducted a double-blind trial of clonazepam and placebo in a series of epileptic children, finding significantly better control on the active drug. In several reports, the drug has been used successfully in status epilepticus.[179-181]

Unwanted effects of clonazepam resemble those reported with use of nitrazepam and other benzodiazepines. Drowsiness is frequent when drug therapy is initiated. Precipitation or aggravation of grand mal seizures has been suggested.[179] Bladin[179] noted behavioral changes in 10 of 27 children receiving clonazepam for various seizure disorders. These changes included an increase of irritability, impulsive antisocial behavior, and outbursts of aggressive temper. In two cases, behavior became unmanageable and required discontinuation of clonazepam despite adequate seizure control. Increased hostility and aggression associated with benzodiazepine therapy is discussed in Chapters 1, 3, 4, and 12.

Observations of the anticonvulsant properties of clonazepam are largely preliminary, but the drug appears to hold promise for the treatment of selected seizure disorders.

COMMENT

Because this chapter covers a vast amount of clinical material, generalizations can be made only with reservation. Muscle spasticity associated with progressive or permanent neurological disease cannot be cured by drugs. The benzodiazepines seem to produce symptomatic improvement in many of these patients, but the evidence is not overwhelming. Among patients with pain and spasm due to acute muscle strain or disc disease, conservative regimens of heat, rest, analgesia, and exercise are the most important ingredients of effective therapy. Although there is no consistent evidence that the addition of muscle-relaxant drugs enhances the therapeutic response, diazepam appears to be the most useful of available muscle relaxants. In the treatment of tetanus, diazepam is now the muscle relaxant of choice among many physicians.

The benzodiazepines have not supplanted diphenylhydantoin and phenobarbital as oral maintenance anticonvulsants in grand mal seizure disorders. Intravenous diazepam undoubtedly is the drug of first choice in status epilepticus, but once seizures are controlled, maintenance therapy with other anticonvulsants must be initiated. Nitrazepam is among the most effective agents for controlling infantile spasms, but unfortunately the drug is not available in the United States at present.

The benzodiazepines are relatively new additions to pharmacotherapeutics. Final judgment of their role in neuromuscular and seizure disorders will require more time and further assessment.

REFERENCES

1. Holt KS: Librium. Devel Med Child Neurol 4:665-666, 1962

2. Angara VS, Whittaker JS: Diazepam: a preliminary study of its effects on patients with athetoid cerebral palsy. Canad Med Assoc J 93:364-366, 1965

3. Rudolf GM: The treatment of spasticity with chlordiazepoxide (Librium). Brit J Psychiat 109:554-547, 1963

4. Kanjilal GC: Some observations on clinical trials with diazepam in cerebral palsy. Ann Phys Med (supp):30-32, 1964

5. Phelps WM: Observation of a new drug in cerebral palsy athetoids. Western Med 4(supp 1):5-10, (Oct) 1963

6. Carter CH: Librium in spastic disorders. Clinical evaluation. Arch Pediat 79:22-27, 1962

7. Deberdt R: Librium. Devel Med Child Neurol 4:445, 1962

8. Keats S, Kambin P, Nordlund T: Clinical experiences with chlordiazepoxide (Librium) in infantile cerebral palsy. Devel Med Child Neurol 4:336-337, 1962

9. Thorn I: Primidone and chlordiazepoxide in cerebral palsy. Devel Med Child Neurol 4:325-327, 1962

10. Keats S, Kambin P, Nordlund T: Use of a new relaxant drug in cerebral palsy. (A preliminary report). Dis Nerv Syst 23:399-403, 1962

11. Marsh HO: Diazepam in incapacitated cerebral-palsied children. JAMA 191:797-800, 1965

12. Hiller CJ, Mason JL: Therapeutic test of diazepam (Valium) in cerebral palsy. A comparison study. J South Carolina Med Assoc 62:306-309, 1966
13. Sylvester PE: Effects of chlordiazepoxide. Lancet 1:1006, 1961
14. Bayliss SG, Gilbertson MP: A trial of chlordiazepoxide in spastic children. Lancet 2:995-996, 1962
15. Smith MC, Ferguson WT: Pilot study in the use of diazepam (Valium) in cerebral palsy. Nebraska State Med J 49:662-665, 1964
16. Denhoff E: Diazepam (Valium®) in cerebral palsy. A comparison of uncontrolled office studies versus a controlled team study. Rhode Island Med J 47:429-431, 1964
17. Boelsche A, Danford BH: Drug therapy in cerebral palsy. Current status. Texas State J Med 60:900-903, 1964
18. Carter CH: Diazepam in the management of spasticity and related symptoms in brain-damaged patients. Western Med 4(supp 1):54-60, (Oct) 1963
19. Keats S, Morgese A, Nordlund T: The role of diazepam in the comprehensive treatment of cerebral palsied children. Western Med 4(supp 1):22-25, (Oct) 1963
20. Griffiths APW, Sylvester PE: Clinical trial of diazepam in adult cerebral palsy. Ann Phys Med (supp):25-29, 1964
21. Rapp S, Carter CH: Use of a polygraph to measure spastic activity in athetoid patients. J New Drugs 6:49-54, 1966
22. Engle HA: The effect of diazepam (Valium) in children with cerebral palsy: a double-blind study. Devel Med Child Neurol 8:661-667, 1966
23. Bayliss SG, Gilbertson MP: Controlled trial of chlordiazepoxide in spastic children. Devel Med Child Neurol 4:597-601, 1962
24. Bayliss SG, Gilbertson MP: A trial of chlordiazepoxide in spastic children. Lancet 2:995-996, 1962
25. Sylvester PE: A controlled cross-over trial of chlordiazepoxide (Librium) in mental deficiency. In, *Proceedings of the Second International Congress on Mental Retardation, Vienna, 1961,* Part II. Edited by O Stur. Basel, S Karger, 1963, pp 137-146
26. Fisher FJ, Houtz SJ: Clinical and electromyographic evaluation of chlordiazepoxide, diazepam, and meprobamate in patients with cerebral palsy. Western Med 4(supp 1):26-33, (Oct) 1963
27. Carter CH: A controlled evaluation of two benzodiazepine derivatives in the management of mentally retarded, cerebral-palsied patients. Med Times 92:796-798, 1964
28. Pierson GA, Fowlks EW, King PS: Long-term follow-up on the use of diazepam in the treatment of spasticity. Amer J Phys Med 47:143-149, 1968
29. Jones RF, Burke D, Marosszeky JE, Gillies JD: A new agent for the control of spasticity. J Neurol Neurosurg Psychiat 33:464-468, 1970
30. Simpson CA: Use of diazepam for the relief of spasticity in multiple sclerosis. Ann Phys Med (supp):39-40, 1964
31. Margulies ME, Slade WR: Clinical evaluation of diazepam in spasticity. Clin Med 75:47-51, (Feb) 1968
32. Leavitt LA, Ocampo R, Vallbona C, Spencer WA, Iddings D: Experience with a medical treatment of spasticity in patients with upper motor neuron lesions. Western Med 4(supp 1):16-21, (Oct) 1963
33. Levine IM, Jossmann PB, Friend DG, DeAngelis V, Kane M: Diazepam in the treatment of spasticity. A preliminary quantitative evaluation. J Chronic Dis 22:57-62, 1969
34. Wilson LA: The management of spasticity and rigidity using parenteral diazepam. Gerontol Clin 12:168-174, 1970
35. Fowlks EW, Strickland DA, Peirson GA: Control of spastic states in neurological patients with diazepam. Amer J Phys Med 44:9-19, 1965

36. Cocchiarella A, Downey JA, Darling RC: Evaluation of the effect of diazepam in spasticity. Arch Phys Med Rehab 48:393-396, 1967
37. Kendall KH: The use of diazepam in hemiplegia. Ann Phys Med 7:225-228, 1964
38. Levine IM, Jossmann PB, Friend DG, DeAngelis V: Prazepam in the treatment of spasticity. A quantitative double-blind evaluation. Neurology (Minneap) 19:510-516, 1969
39. McFarland HR: Chlordiazepoxide for spasticity. Dis Nerv Syst 24:296-298, 1963
40. Neill RWK: Diazepam in the relief of muscle spasm resulting from spinal-cord lesions. Ann Phys Med (supp):33-38, 1964
41. Wilson LA, McKechnie AA: Oral diazepam in the treatment of spasticity in paraplegia. A double-blind trial and subsequent impressions. Scottish Med J 11:46-51, 1966
42. Payne RW, Ishmael WK: Clinical evaluation of diazepam in neuromuscular conditions. Western Med 4(supp 1):40-43, (Oct) 1963
43. Wickstrom J, Haddad R: Combined muscle relaxant-tranquilizing therapy in orthopedics. Western Med 4(supp 1):47-50, (Oct) 1963
44. Rogers SP: Clinical observations of diazepam, a new muscle relaxant. Western Med 4(supp 1):51-53, (Oct) 1963
45. McGivney JQ, Cleveland BR: The levator syndrome and its treatment. Southern Med J 58:505-510, 1965
46. Shea PA, Woods WW: The effective use of diazepam (Valium) in the treatment of occipitocervical pain and other neuromuscular lesions. Western Med 4(supp 1): 61-64, (Oct) 1963
47. Blomfield LB: Effects of chlordiazepoxide. Lancet 1:885, 1961
48. Katz RA, Aldes JH, Rector M: A new drug approach to muscle-relaxation. J Neuropsychiat 3(supp 1):s91-s95, 1962
49. Bain LS: The use of diazepam in the treatment of musculo-skeletal disorders. Ann Phys Med (supp):3-6, 1964
50. Pernikoff M: Treatment of acute and chronic muscle spasm with diazepam. Clin Med 71:699-705, 1964
51. Kendall PH: Use of intravenous diazepam in acute skeletal muscle spasm. Preliminary report. Ann Phys Med (supp):14-15, 1964
52. Bianchine JR, Bianchine JW: Treatment of spasmodic torticollis with diazepam. Southern Med J 64:893-894, 1971
53. Kestler OC: The effect of diazepam in the treatment of over-riding fractures. Western Med 4(supp 1):44-46, (Oct) 1963
53a. Vince JD, Kremer D: Double-blind trial of diazepam in rheumatoid arthritis. Practitioner 210:264-267, 1973
54. Cazort RJ: Role of relaxants in treatment of traumatic musculoskeletal disorders: a double-blind study of three agents. Curr Ther Res 6:454-458, 1964
55. Cooper CD: Comparative effects of diazepam, chlormezanone, and carisoprodol in musculoskeletal disorders. Western Med 4(supp 1):34-39, (Oct) 1963
56. General Practitioner Research Group: General practitioner clinical trials. Painful muscular conditions treated with diazepam. Practitioner 194:409-411, 1965
57. Wheatley D: Diazepam in musculo-skeletal spasm. Report on a G.P. research group trial. Ann Phys Med (supp):7-13, 1964
58. Hingorani K: Diazepam in backache. A double-blind controlled trial. Ann Phys Med 8:303-306, 1966
59. Masterson JH, White AE: Benzodiazepin derivatives for relaxation of orthopedic patients. Med Times 92:1194-1198, 1964
60. Payne RW, Sorenson EJ, Smalley TK, Brandt EN: Diazepam, meprobamate, and placebo in musculoskeletal disorders. JAMA 188:229-232, 1964
61. Rogers EJ: Double-blind comparative study of diazepam and methocarbamol in treatment of skeletal muscle spasm. Western Med 4(supp 1):11-15, (Oct) 1963

62. Snell W, Corrigan RF, Zimmerman RC: Comparative drug evaluation in treatment of skeletal muscle spasm. Clin Med 72:957-972, 1965

63. Tarpley EL: Evaluation of diazepam (Valium) in the symptomatic treatment of rheumatic disorders. A controlled comparative study. J Chronic Dis 18:99-106, 1965

64. Wickstrom J, Haddad R: An evaluation of the muscle relaxant properties of chlordiazepoxide: a double-blind study. Amer J Med Sci 244:23-29, 1962

65. Weinberg WA: Control of the neuromuscular and convulsive manifestations of severe systemic tetanus: Case report with a new drug, Valium (diazepam). Clin Pediat 3:226-228, 1964

66. Bacon AK: Diazepam in tetanus. Brit Med J 4:646, 1968

67. Cheah PS, Mah PK, Feng PH: Severe tetanus successfully treated with high dose diazepam (Valium) and propranolol—a case report. Singapore Med J 13:163-165, 1972

68. Cordova AB: Control of the spasms of tetanus with diazepam (Valium). Evaluation of clinical usefulness based upon observations of three childhood cases. Clin Pediat 8:712-716, 1969

69. Das AK, Gupta RK, De S: Diazepam in tetanus. J Indian Med Assoc 49:130-132, 1967

70. Davis LE, Wesley RB, Juan D, Carpenter CCJ: "Locked-in syndrome" from diazepam toxicity in a patient with tetanus. Lancet 1:101, 1972

71. Femi-Pearse D: Experience with diazepam in tetanus. Brit Med J 2:862-865, 1966

72. Femi-Pearse D, Fleming SA: Tetanus treated with high dosage of diazepam. J Trop Med Hyg 68:305-306, 1965

73. Grewal RS: Valium in tetnas (a preliminary report). Punjab Med J 15:461-462, 1966

74. Groessler AJ: Diazepam in tetanus. Brit Med J 2:1456, 1966

75. Kendall MJ, Clarke SW: Prolonged coma after tetanus. Brit Med J 1:354-355, 1972

76. Lockwood WR, Allison F: Injectable diazepam: a new drug for the treatment of tetanus. J Mississippi State Med Assoc 8:66-70, 1967

77. Lowenthal MN, Lavalette J: Chlordiazepoxide in the treatment of tetanus. J Trop Med Hyg 69:157-159, 1966

78. Moriarty J, Bertolotti L: Control of tetanic spasms with diazepam. Case report of severe tetanus. J Med Soc New Jersey 62:403-405, 1965

79. O'Donohoe NV: Tetanus treated with diazepam (Valium). J Irish Med Assoc 60:89-90, 1967

80. Phillips LA: Chlordiazepoxide in the treatment of tetanus. Lancet 1:1097-1098, 1965

81. Shershin PH, Katz SS: Diazepam in the treatment of tetanus: report of a case following tooth extraction. Clin Med 71:362-366, 1964

82. Sorabjee SE: A case of trismus following dental extraction treated with diazepam. E Afr Med J 44:186, 1967

83. Stoebner RC, Kiser RW, Decherd JF, Perry JE: Diazepam (Valium) in the treatment of tetanus: a report of five cases. Southern Med J 63:445-447, 1970

84. Norredam K, Hainau B: Treatment of tetanus in tropical Africa. A comparison between a barbiturate and diazepam in the treatment of non-neonatal tetanus. Ann Soc Belge Med Trop 50:239-246, 1970

85. Phatak AT, Shah SH: Diazepam as adjuvant therapy in childhood tetanus. 477 patients with tetanus in Baroda. Clin Pediat 9:573-576, 1970

86. Tjoen LW, Darmawan S, Ismael S, Sudigbia I, Suradi R, Munthe BG: The effect of diazepam on tetanus. Paediatrica Indonesiana 10:248-258, 1970

87. Hendrickse RG, Sherman PM: Therapeutic trial of diazepam in tetanus. Lancet 1:737-738, 1965

88. Hendrickse RG, Sherman PM: Tetanus in childhood: Report of a therapeutic trial of diazepam. Brit Med J 2:860-862, 1966

89. Jackson G, Ng SH, Diggle GE, Bourke IG: Strychnine poisoning treated successfully with diazepam. Brit Med J 3:519-520, 1971

90. Hardin JA, Griggs RC: Diazepam treatment in a case of strychnine poisoning. Lancet 2:372-373, 1971

91. Maron BJ, Krupp JR, Tune B: Strychnine poisoning successfully treated with diazepam. J Pediat 78:697-699, 1971

92. Herishanu Y, Landau H: Diazepam in the treatment of strychnine poisoning. Brit J Anaesth 44:747-748, 1972

93. Olafson RA, Mulder DW, Howard FM: "Stiff-man" syndrome: review of the literature, report of three additional cases and discussion of pathophysiology and therapy. Mayo Clinic Proc 39:131-144, 1964

94. Gordon EE, Januszko DM, Kaufman L: A critical survey of stiff-man syndrome. Amer J Med 42:582-599, 1967

95. Little SC, Johnson BK, Anhalt MA, Chastain DE: The "stiff-man" syndrome. A report of two additional cases treated with diazepam. Alabama J Med Sci 4:416-421, 1967

96. Hall CD, Haworth CC: "Stiff man syndrome" and trauma. Brit Med J 3:531, 1971

97. Ricker K, Mertens HG, Paal G: Polyneuropathy and stiff-man syndrome. Eur Neurol 5:11-24, 1971

98. Howard FM: A new and effective drug in the treatment of the stiff-man syndrome: preliminary report. Proc Staff Meetings Mayo Clinic 38:203-212, 1963

99. Cohen L: Stiff-man syndrome. Two patients treated with diazepam. JAMA 195:222-224, 1966

100. Kasperek S, Zebrowski S: Stiff-man syndrome and encephalitis. Arch Neurol 24:22-30 1971

101. Schnell RG: Drug induced dyskinesia treated with intravenous diazepam. J Florida Med Assoc 59:22-23, (Jan) 1972

102. Korczyn AD, Goldberg GJ: Intravenous diazepam in drug-induced dystonic reactions. Brit J Psychiat 121:75-77, 1972

103. Frederiks JAM: Facial tics in children: the therapeutic effect of low-dosage diazepam. Brit J Clin Prac 24:17-20, 1970

104. Connell PH, Corbett JA, Horne DJ, Mathews AM: Drug treatment of adolescent tiqueurs. A double-blind trial of diazepam and haloperidol. Brit J Psychiat 113-375-381, 1967

105. Haynes E, Blanchette J, Gericke OL: Experience with chlordiazepoxide in Huntington's chorea. Dis Nerv Syst 23:326-328, 1962

106. Nilsen JA: Valium therapy of Huntington's chorea. Amer J Psychiat 120:1197-1198, 1964

107. Farrell DF, Hofmann WW: A quantitative evaluation of the effect of diazepam in Huntington's chorea. Arch Phys Med Rehab 49:586-591, 1968

108. Keats S: Dystonia musculorum deformans progressiva. Experience with diazepam. Dis Nerv Syst 24:624-629, 1963

109. Lewis I: Trial of diazepam in myotonia. A double-blind, single crossover study. Neurology (Minneap) 16:629-634, 1966

110. Sherwin I, Redmond W: Successful treatment of action myoclonus. Neurology (Minneap) 19:846-850, 1969.

111. Rosen AD, Berenyi KJ, Laurenceau V: Intention myoclonus—diazepam and phenobarbital treatment. JAMA 209:772-773, 1969

111a. Kentsmith DK, Carter TN: Progressive cerebellar dyssynergia. The use of diazepam. J Kansas Med Soc 74:138-139, 1973

112. Morgan L: The symptom of restless legs. Med J Aust 2:134-135, 1967

113. Morgan LK: Restless Limbs: a commonly overlooked symptom controlled by "Valium". Med J Aust 2:589-594, 1967

114. Go KG, Penning L: Favourable effect of intravenous diazepam on muscular spasms in the lower extremities following iothalamate (Conray) radiculography. Eur Neurol 4:253-255, 1970

115. Chien C-P, Keegan D: Diazepam as an oral long-term anticonvulsant for epileptic mental patients. Dis Nerv Syst 33:100-104, 1972
116. Lou HOC: Oxazepam in the treatment of psychomotor epilepsy. Neurology (Minneap) 18:986-990, 1968
117. Weinberg WA, Harwell JL: Diazepam (Valium) in myoclonic seizures. Favorable response during infancy and childhood. Amer J Dis Child 109:123-127, 1965
118. Gastaut H, Roger J, Soulayrol R, Tassinari CA, Regis H, Dravet C, Bernard R, Pinsard N, Saint-Jean M: Childhood epileptic encephalopathy with diffuse slow spike-waves (otherwise known as "petit-mal variant") or Lennox syndrome. Epilepsia 7:139-179, 1966
119. Lance JW: Myoclonic jerks and falls: aetiology, classification and treatment. Med J Aust 1:113-120, 1968
120. Snyder CH: Myoclonic epilepsy in children: short-term comparative study of two benzodiazepine derivatives in treatment. Southern Med J 61:17-20, 1968
121. Killian JM, Fromm GH: A double-blind comparison of nitrazepam versus diazepam in myoclonic seizure disorders. Devel Med Child Neurol 13:32-39, 1971
122. Carson MJ: Treatment of minor motor seizures with nitrazepam. Devel Med Child Neurol 10:772-775, 1968
123. Baldwin R, Kenny TJ, Segal J: The effectiveness of nitrazepam in a refractory epileptic population. Curr Ther Res 11:413-417, 1969
124. Millichap JG, Ortiz WR: Nitrazepam in myoclonic epilepsies. Amer J Dis Child 112:242-248, 1966
125. Jan JE, Riegl JA, Crichton JU, Dunn HG: Nitrazepam in the treatment of epilepsy in childhood. Canad Med Assoc J 104:571-575, 1971
126. Hagberg B: The chlordiazepoxide HCl (Librium) analogue nitrazepam (Mogadon) in the treatment of epilepsy in children. Devel Med Child Neurol 10:302-308, 1968
127. Hagberg B: The Librium-analogue Mogadon in the treatment of epilepsy in children. Acta Neurol Scand 43(supp 31):167, 1967
128. Volzke E, Doose H, Stephan E: The treatment of infantile spasms and hypsarrhythmia with Mogadon. Epilepsia 8:64-70, 1967
129. Gibbs FA, Anderson EM: Treatment of hypsarhythmia and infantile spasms with a Librium® analogue. Neurology (Minneap) 15:1173-1176, 1965
130. Markham CH: The treatment of myoclonic seizures of infancy and childhood with LA-I. Pediatrics 34:511-518, 1964
131. Tassinari CA, Gastaut H, Dravet C, Roger J: A paradoxical effect: status epilepticus induced by benzodiazepines (Valium and Mogadon). (Abstract). Electroenceph Clin Neurophysiol 31:182, 1971
132. Tassinari CA, Dravet C, Roger J, Cano JP, Gastaut H: Tonic status epilepticus precipitated by intravenous benzodiazepine in five patients with Lennox-Gastaut syndrome. Epilepsia 13:421-435, 1972
133. Prior PF, MacLaine GN, Scott DF, Laurance BM: Intravenous diazepam. Lancet 2:434-435, 1971
134. Prior PF, MacLaine GN, Scott DF, Laurance BM: Tonic status epilepticus precipitated by intravenous diazepam in a child with petit mal status. Epilepsia 13:467-472, 1972
135. Bell DS: Dangers of treatment of status epilepticus with diazepam. Brit Med J 1:159-161, 1969
136. Sinha SN: Status epilepticus and diazepam. Brit Med J 1:440, 1969
137. Bowe J: Status epilepticus and diazepam. Brit Med J 1:439-440, 1969
138. Taylor DC, Ounsted C: Status epilepticus and diazepam. Brit Med J 1:440, 1969
139. Mattson RH: The benzodiazepines. In, *Antiepileptic Drugs*. Edited by DM Woodbury, JK Penry, RP Schmidt. New York, Raven Press, 1972, pp 497-518
140. Brett EM: Diazepam—the new wonder drug? Devel Med Child Neurol 12:655-659, 1970

141. Carter S, Gold AP: The critically ill child: management of status epilepticus. Pediatrics 44:732-733, 1969
142. Swash M: Status epilepticus. Brit J Hosp Med 8:269-272, 1972
143. Watson AC: Modifying electroplexy. Lancet 2:511, 1967
144. Watson AC: Diazepam in convulsive therapy. In, *Diazepam in Anaesthesia.* Edited by PF Knight, CG Burgess. Bristol, John Wright and Sons, 1968, pp 77-81
145. Campbell-Young G: Modifying electroplexy. Lancet 2:987, 1967
146. Bethune HC, Burrell RH, Culpan RH, Ogy GJ: Modifying electroplexy. Lancet 2:265, 1967
147. Kuilman M, Luyendijk F: Intravenous administration of Epontol and Valium in electroconvulsive therapy. Psychiat Neurol Neurochirur 72:545-555, 1969
148. Martin DJ, Kaebling R: Diazepam-modified electroconvulsive therapy. Biol Psychiat 3:129-139, 1971
149. Watson AC, Harrison J, Rees L: Anticonvulsant activity of diazepam (Valium) in man. A controlled study. Clin Trials J 7:433-437, 1970
150. Rousos AP, Hazlewood R, Orr R: Intramuscular diazepam as anti-anxiety agent in SCC-modified EST. Dis Nerv Syst 30:752-757, 1969
151. Ekinci M, Hsu JJ, Bruck M, Braun RA: Diazepam as an anti-convulsant agent in ECT. Amer J Psychiat 120:903-904, 1964
152. Ekinci M, Hsu JJ, Bruck M. Braun RA: Diazepam as an anti-convulsant and anti-anxiety agent in ECT. Dis Nerv Syst 26:40-43, 1965
152a. Wehlage DF: Diazepam phlebitis. JAMA 224:128-129, 1973
152b. Friedenberg W, Barker JD: Intravenous diazepam administration. JAMA 224:901, 1973
153. Winfield DL: The use of chlordiazepoxide in clinical electroencephalography. J Neuropsychiat 2:191-194, 1961
154. Winfield DL: The use of diazepam in clinical electroencephalography. Dis Nerv Syst 24:542-547, 1963
155. Metcalf DR, Whitley DJ: Experience with diazepam in an electroencephalography laboratory controlled evaluation. Amer J Psychiat 120:1114-1115, 1964
156. Laguna JF, Korein J: Diagnostic value of diazepam in electroencephalography. Arch Neurol 26:265-272, 1972
157. Torres F, Ellington A, Viera P: Diazepam as a tool for the study of seizure mechanisms in man: I. Inter-ictal spike foci. (Abstract) Electroenceph Clin Neurophysiol 30:164-165, 1971
158. Darby CE, Fung D, Goodin J, Scheaff PC: Diazepam-induced sleep in the investigation of focal epilepsies (Abstract). Electroenceph Clin Neurophysiol 33:448, 1972
159. Ebe M, Meier-Ewert K-H, Broughton R: Effects of intravenous diazepam (Valium) upon evoked potentials of photosensitive epileptic and normal subjects. Electroenceph Clin Neurophysiol 27:429-435, 1969
160. Denhoff E, Shammas E: Diazepam as an aid in the photo-Metrazol activation test. Dis Nerv Syst 29:759-762, 1968
161. Guerrero-Figueroa R, Gallant DM, Guerrero-Figueroa C, Rye MM: Electroencephalographic study of diazepam on patients with diagnosis of episodic behavioral disorders. J Clin Parmacol 10:57-64, 1970
162. Monroe RR, Dale R: Chlordiazepoxide in the treatment of patients with "activated EEG's." Dis Nerv Syst 28:390-396, 1967
163. Monroe RR, Kramer MD, Goulding R, Wise S: EEG activation of patients receiving phenothiazines and chlordiazepoxide. J Nerv Ment Dis 141:100-107, 1965
164. Schimschock JR, Carlson CB, Ojemann LM: Massive spasms associated with holoprosencephaly. Amer J Dis Child 118:520-524, 1969
165. Nixon DW, Mayher WE: Progressive myoclonus with epilepsy. Southern Med J 65:81-85, 1972

166. Hambert O, Petersen I: Clinical, electroencephalographical, and neuropharmacological studies in syndromes of progressive myoclonus epilepsy. Acta Neurol Scand 46:149-186, 1970

167. Forster C: EEG changes in Jacob-Creutzfeldt's disease under the influence of diazepam. (Abstract) Electroenceph Clin Neurophysiol 29:218, 1970

168. Canger R, Penati G: EEG patterns in a case of subacute sclerosing leukoencephalitis after intravenous administration of two benzodiazepine derivatives. (Abstract) Electroenceph Clin Neurophysiol 28:217, 1970

169. Canger R, Penati G: Some aspects of the action of diazepam and nitrazepam on the EEG features in a case of subacute sclerosing leucoencephalitis (SSLE). Acta Neurol 24:767-780, 1969

170. Symposium on clonazepamum NFN, INN, organized by the Danish Society of Epilepsy. Epilepsia 14:77-90, 1973

171. Gastaut H: Exceptional anticonvulsive properties of a new benzodiazepine. In, *Epilepsy. Modern Problems of Pharmacopsychiatry*, Vol 4. Edited by E Niedermeyer. Basel S Karger, 1970, pp 261-269

172. Negrin P, Ravenna C, Semerano A: Antiepileptic properties of RO 5-4023 by mouth; report of 40 cases. (Abstract) Electroenceph Clin Neurophysiol 31:532, 1971

173. Birket-Smith E, Mikkelsen B: Preliminary observations on the effect of a new benzodiazepine (RO 5-4023) in epilepsy. Acta Neurol Scand 48:385-389, 1972

174. Hanson RA, Menkes JH: A new anticonvulsant in the management of minor motor seizures. Devel Med Child Neurol 14:3-14, 1972

175. Hooshmand H: Trial of a new anticonvulsant for uncontrollable minor motor seizures. (Abstract) Epilepsia 12:287-288, 1971

176. Hooshmand H: Intractable seizures. Treatment with a new benzodiazepine anticonvulsant. Arch Neurol 27:205-208, 1972

177. Turner M, Funes JRC, Perea RA, Cantlon B, Fejerman N, Lon JC, Giachetti M: Clinical EEG evaluation of a new benzodiazepine derivative (Ro 5-4023) by oral administration in epileptic patients using the double-blind technique. Electroenceph Clin Neurophysiol 31:628, 1971

178. Rossi GF, DiRocco C, Maira G, Meglio M: Experimental and clinical studies of the anticonvulsant properties of a benzodiazepine derivative, clonazepam (Ro 5-4023). In, *The Benzodiazepines*. Edited by S Garattini, E. Mussini, LO Randall. New York, Raven Press, 1973, pp 461-488

179. Bladin PF: The use of clonazepam as an anticonvulsant—clinical evaluation. Med J Aust 1-683-688, 1973

180. Papini M: The treatment of epilepsy in childhood and of status epilepticus with RO 5-4023 (Abstract). Electroenceph Clin Neurophysiol 31:532, 1971

181. Gastaut H, Courjon J, Poire R, Weber M: Treatment of status epilepticus with a new benzodiazepine more active than diazepam. Epilepsia 12:197-214, 1971

Chapter 7
Organ System Effects:
Experimental and Clinical

The effects of the benzodiazepines upon organ systems and aspects of physiologic function have been the object of considerable study. Several major approaches to investigation are discernible. The first involves the direct pharmacologic action of the drugs upon organ function. The benzodiazepines have been shown in various animal and isolated muscle preparation studies, for example, to alter cardiac contractility, reduce blood pressure, relax uterine musculature, or produce hyperglycemia. Each of these properties is of clinical relevance inasmuch as it can be exploited for therapeutic purposes or is seen as indicative of potential toxic effects. Second, emotional disturbance may be manifest as symptomatology referable to a specific organ system. Many anxious or depressed individuals have somatic complaints such as palpitations, abdominal pain, or dyspareunia which are unaccompanied by demonstrable organic disease. For such psychosomatic disorders the benzodiazepines can be of value by virtue of psychotropic effects rather than by peripheral pharmacologic activity. Surveys of outpatient psychotropic drug use in the United States suggest that benzodiazepines and other minor tranquilizers are more often used by individuals with complaints referable to particular organ systems than in those with primary psychiatric diagnoses.[1] Finally, a number of relatively new diagnostic and therapeutic techniques in medicine are sufficiently discomforting or disquieting to require some sort of psychotropic premedication but not painful enough to warrant the hazard of general anesthesia. The benzodiazepines, particularly diazepam, have become quite popular as psychosedative premedication for procedures such as gastroscopy, bronchoscopy, and direct-current electrical cardioversion.

The organ system approach, although cross-disciplinary, has been selected for this chapter because of its usefulness to the clinician. From reading a single section the gastroenterologist, for example, can be directed to literature on the influence of the benzodiazepines upon gastric and salivary secretion, their potential use in functional bowel complaints, and the use of intravenous diazepam for gastroscopy. Studies specifically dealing with the influence of the benzodiazepines upon stress-induced physiologic changes are discussed in Chapter 8.

CARDIOVASCULAR SYSTEM

The benzodiazepines affect blood pressure and myocardial function through both direct and neurogenic mechanisms, with the observed result depending upon the interaction of the two influences. Clearly, the type of experimental model is of great importance—the denervated heart preparation may behave quite differently than the intact animal or human.

The hypothalamic depressing property of the benzodiazepines is discussed in Chapter 5. The benzodiazepines by themselves have little effect on blood pressure when given intravenously, but the pressor response to hypothalamic stimulation is blocked. The increase in blood pressure produced by norepinephrine infusion or stellate ganglion stimulation, however, is preserved. Hockman and Livingston,[1a] using cats with high spinal cord transections, studied the cardiodepressant response to carotid sinus (afferent) and vagal (efferent) stimulation. The afferent response was inhibited by intravenous diazepam (0.175 to 2.8 mg/kg) while the efferent response was unchanged. When the animal was decerebrated at the midcollicular level, diazepam no longer antagonized the cardiodepression following carotid sinus stimulation. These studies suggest that the benzodiazepines can influence cardiovascular function by effects which are mediated through the central nervous system. The influence is dependent upon the intactness of the nervous system. The work of Vieth and associates[2] indicates that the solvent vehicle in which diazepam and nitrazepam are dissolved may account for some of this pharmacologic activity. This has been observed by other investigators and is further discussed in this chapter and elsewhere (Chapters 5, 6, and 12).

The benzodiazepines have little effect upon measurable parameters of myocardial metabolism in isolated preparations.[3] The contractility of isolated cat papillary muscle was not influenced by chlordiazepoxide or diazepam in clinically relevant concentrations of less than 1 μg/ml. Chlordiazepoxide depressed contractility only when concentrations reached 16 μg/ml or more.[4] Hitch and Nolan[5,6] studied myocardial performance and peripheral resistance in anesthetized dogs with high spinal transection and bilateral cervical vagotomy. Intravenous chlordiazepoxide (200 mg) produced cardiac depression and a transient fall in total peripheral resistance. It was estimated that this dosage would produce chlordiazepoxide blood levels of approximately 13 μg/ml—again considerably above the usual clinical range.

Abel and associates[7-9] studied in some detail the effects of diazepam upon a canine heart-circulation preparation. Intravenous diazepam (0.1 to 0.2 mg/kg) produced an increase in myocardial contractility lasting 1 hr or more, together with a fall in peripheral resistance of less than 10-min duration.[7] Diazepam-induced coronary artery vasodilation and increased coronary blood flow accounted for this finding; the effect was a direct one, requiring that diazepam reach the coronary circulation.[8] Atropine and ganglionic blocking agents inhibited this effect, while vagotomy and alpha-adrenergic blocking drugs did not.[9] These findings suggest that diazepam stimulates postganglionic adrenergic and cholinergic vasodilating mechanisms. None of these effects of diazepam could be reproduced by injection of the propylene glycol solvent alone. Bianco and associates,[10] using an areflexic right heart bypass preparation, found that large doses of diazepam administered directly into the pulmonary artery or left ventricle produced coronary and peripheral vasodilation, but depressed left ventricular function. Infusion of the propylene glycol solvent alone produced an identical response.

In the intact animal, the benzodiazepines produce little if any hemodynamic alterations. Starley and Michie,[11] using conscious unrestrained dogs, infused diazepam (0.5 mg/kg) intravenously, finding no significant effect upon numerous parameters (heart rate, cardiac output, blood pressure, stroke volume, left ventricular work). Rapid intravenous infusion of diazepam (2 mg/kg) to cats produced transient apnea, bradycardia, and hypotension, but a nearly identical effect occurred when the solvent alone was given.[12,13] deJong and Heavner[14] compared the effects of intramuscular diazepam (0.25 mg/kg) and pentobarbital (10 mg/kg) in healthy adult cats. Both drugs were equally effective in preventing lidocaine-induced seizures, but the neurologic, cardiovascular, and respiratory depressant effects produced by pentobarbital were much more profound.

Systematic hemodynamic studies in humans reveal that the benzodiazepines are quite innocuous. Venous tone and venomotor reflexes are impaired by diazepam, but venous pooling is not sufficient to alter arterial pressure.[15] Blood pressure adjustment on the tilt-table is unaffected by intravenous diazepam (10 mg) or chlordiazepoxide (20 mg).[16,17] In healthy subjects, intravenous diazepam (up to 0.2 mg/kg) or chlordiazepoxide (up to 1.5 mg/kg) produced no clinically important changes in blood pressure or cardiac output.[18,19] Of greater importance are the effects in patients with cardiovascular disease. Francisco and Lebowitz[20] administered intravenous diazepam (average dose 16 mg) prior to cardiac catheterization in 25 patients. Three Class IV* cardiac patients had transient episodes of bradycardia and hypotension, while 22 others experienced no cardiopulmonary depression. Dalen and associates[21] noted no cardiovascular or respiratory depression of clinical consequence among 15 patients with organic heart disease receiving diazepam intravenously during catheterization. Abel and Reis[22] used intravenous diazepam (0.1 mg/kg) as a psychosedative in patients who had undergone cardiac surgery within the previous 72 hr. There were no important changes in heart rate, blood pressure, peripheral resistance, or cardiac index. Knapp and Dubow[23,24] used clinically comparable and equally effective doses of intravenous diazepam (0.2 mg/kg) and thiopental (2 mg/kg) as preanesthetic induction agents in Class III and IV cardiac patients. Among 400 diazepam

---

*New York Heart Association Classification. Individuals with Class IV cardiac disease are limited to a bed-and-chair existence.

recipients, only three (less than 1%) experienced a cardiac output reduction of more than 15%, and *none* had a mean blood pressure drop of greater than 15%. By contrast, reductions of 15% or more in cardiac output occurred in 85% of thiopental-treated patients; blood pressure drops were noted in 68% of patients receiving thiopental.

Rao and associates[24a] studied the cardiopulmonary effects of relatively large quantities of intravenous diazepam. Doses averaging 0.77 mg/kg were given to normal subjects and compared with average doses of 0.48 mg/kg in patients with obstructive pulmonary disease. Results were similar in both groups. Modest reductions in blood pressure, cardiac output, and stroke volume were observed, but none were of clinical consequence. Coleman and co-workers[24b] administered flunitrazepam (2 to 3 mg) intravenously to 28 healthy males prior to minor elective surgery. Again, reductions in blood pressure, cardiac output, stroke volume, central venous pressure, and total peripheral resistance were noted. The changes were statistically significant but clinically not important. Comer and colleagues[24c] found that very large doses of intravenous lorazepam (up to 9 mg) produced no changes in blood pressure, cardiac output, or total peripheral resistance in healthy male volunteers.

Cardioversion

Published reports on more than 450 patients receiving diazepam intravenously prior to direct current cardioversion (Table 7-1) underscore the safety of this agent in patients with cardiac disease. The procedure described in most of the articles is similar. Digitalis is withheld for at least 24 hr prior to elective cardioversion and is replaced by quinidine sulfate,

TABLE 7-1. *Diazepam in cardioversion*

Reference	Author(s)	Number of patients
25	Hendrix, 1969	18
26	Kahler et al., 1967	35
27	Kernohan, 1966	25
28	Kernohan, 1968	81
29	Lebowitz, 1969	50
30	Nelson and Sloman, 1967	44
31	Nutter and Massumi, 1965	15
32	Rosenblatt and Nettles, 1970	20
33	Rotem, 1970	40
34	Somers et al., 1971	53
35	Stiles et al., 1968	26
36	Turkel and Lemmert, 1969	32
37	Vinge et al., 1971	85
38	Winters et al., 1968	18

200 mg orally every 6 hr. Occasionally, patients receive other sedative-hypnotics prior to the procedure, but in most reports the only special preparation is assuring that the patient has an empty stomach. Diazepam is given intravenously at approximately 5 mg/min until dysarthria occurs. The usual effective dose is between 10 and 20 mg, but in a few patients more may be required (up to 60 mg). Cardioversion is performed with the patient in a condition of light sleep. In an overwhelming majority of cases, the patient does not remember the shock. Adverse hemodynamic effects are extremely rare among the published cases—pain, and occasionally phlebitis, associated with the injection are the only consistent problems (see also Chapter 12). Recovery is rapid, varying from a few minutes to a few hours. Muenster and associates[39] compared clinically equivalent doses of intravenous diazepam and thiopental prior to cardioversion. The frequency of ventricular extrasystoles was much lower in association with diazepam than with thiopental. In other respects, the two drugs were essentially identical. Similar safety and effectiveness has been reported with diazepam use for coronary angiography and cardiac catheterization.[20,21,40,41]

Cardiodepressant and hypotensive effects of parenteral benzodiazepines in animals are attributable largely to the propylene glycol solvent system. In humans, adverse hemodynamic effects are rare, even in patients with significant cardiac or pulmonary disease. The barbiturates are far more hazardous. These conclusions are supported by observations on the use of parenteral benzodiazepines prior to phobia desensitization (Chapter 4), in the treatment of intractable seizures (Chapter 6), prior to electroconvulsive therapy (Chapter 6), as psychosedatives for endoscopy (this Chapter), as premedication and induction agents for surgery and dentistry (Chapter 10), and in the treatment of alcohol withdrawal (Chapter 11).

Arrhythmias

Diazepam has been reported both to produce and to prevent cardiac arrhythmias. van Loon[42] reported the case of an 88-year-old man with life-threatening ventricular irritability refractory to lidocaine, diphenylhydantoin, and procainamide. On three different occasions, he converted to normal sinus rhythm immediately following intravenous diazepam. Spracklen and associates[43] noted that one of seven patients with paroxysmal atrial tachycardia, and one of eight with ventricular tachycardia, converted to sinus rhythm after intravenous diazepam, obviating the need for cardioversion. These authors also found that diazepam significantly raised the threshold for shock-induced ventricular tachycardia in dogs. In a similar study in dogs, Dunbar and colleagues[44] showed that diazepam has an antiarrhythmic effect by itself and that it also potentiates the effects of lidocaine. Liebeswar[45] investigated the influence of flurazepam on the electrophysiologic properties of isolated guinea pig papillary muscle preparations. Flurazepam prolonged the duration of the action potential and decreased its amplitude and maximum rate of rise. The author suggests that flurazepam might have antiarrhythmic properties similar to quinidine. The concentrations of flurazepam used in the study, however, were well above the clinically relevant range.

Diazepam has been found ineffective against digitalis-induced arrhythmias in dogs.[43,46] Baum and associates[47] studied a number of standard anti-arrhythmics as well as lorazepam and diazepam in anesthetized dogs given toxic doses of ouabain. The benzodiazepines were the least effective antiarrhythmic agents tested.

Two cases of transient ectopic ventricular activity following cardioversion using diazepam sedation were reported by Barrett and Hey.[48] Three correspondents correctly point out that a causal association with diazepam is extremely dubious.[49-51] No other similar reports have been published.

Anxiety and Cardiac Disease

Uncontrolled studies suggest that the benzodiazepines are effective in the treatment of anxiety and depression associated with cardiac disease.[52-57] Symptomatic improvement in anxious patients with the hyperventilation syndrome[58,59] and with peripheral arterial occlusive disease[60] has been reported as well.

Two controlled trials show a clear superiority of benzodiazepine over placebo. George and associates[61] studied medazepam and placebo in anxious cardiac patients in a crossover trial. Medazepam was significantly more effective, although drowsiness was reported four times as often on drug as on placebo. Aronson,[62] in a crossover trial of chlordiazepoxide and placebo, found the active drug significantly more effective among 13 patients with the hyperventilation syndrome. Two double-blind studies have compared benzodiazepines to barbiturates in acute myocardial infarction. Benson[63] found diazepam (6 to 16 mg/day) more effective by all physician ratings (apprehension, depression, restlessness, preoccupation with illness) than phenobarbital (45 to 120 mg/day). Hackett and Cassem[64] compared chlordiazepoxide to amobarbital in anxious patients treated in a coronary care unit. Among patients with confirmed myocardial infarction, opiate analgesia was required less often and in smaller doses in those receiving chlordiazepoxide. No other parameters related to anxiety were reported. Side effects— predominantly oversedation—occurred significantly more frequently in amobarbital-treated patients.

A drug combination containing chlordiazepoxide and pentaerythritol tetranitrate received trial as an antianginal agent in 1964 and 1965. Two trials[65,66] suggested that the combination was more effective than chlordiazepoxide alone, but no comparison was made with pentaerythritol tetranitrate alone. A third study showed no significant differences between placebo, chlordiazepoxide, and the drug mixture.[67] Currently this combination preparation is not commercially available.

Physicans may wish to prescribe benzodiazepines to cardiac patients in whom anxiety or agitation are important components of the disease. It should be emphasized, however, that antianxiety agents do not substitute for the usual pharmacologic modes of pain relief (nitroglycerine, morphine) in patients with pain due to acute cardiac ischemia.

RESPIRATION

All sedative-hypnotics, including the benzodiazepines, are potential respiratory depressants. Florez[68] studied the effect of intravenous diazepam, nitrazepam, and clonazepam (0.1 to 0.5 mg/kg of each) upon the respiratory drive in decerebrate cats. All three drugs reduced tidal volume, elevated arterial carbon dioxide tension (pCO_2), and depressed the respiratory response to carbon dioxide. The degree to which such findings are applicable to humans is obviously of great importance.

In subjects without pulmonary disease, respiratory depression produced by intravenous doses of benzodiazepines is barely detectable. Chlordiazepoxide (0.5 to 1.5 mg/kg), diazepam (0.14 to 0.2 mg/kg), and oxazepam (0.5 to 1.0 mg/kg) have all been studied. In three reports there was no significant change in steady-state alveolar minute ventilation ($\dot{V}_A$), arterial oxygen (pO_2) or carbon dioxide tensions (pCO_2), immediately after the dose[18,19,69] By contrast, meperidine (0.5 mg/kg) and pentobarbital (1.0 mg/kg) significantly reduced $\dot{V}_A$.[18] In two studies of intravenous diazepam (approximately 0.15 mg/kg), small changes in the three parameters occurred.[21,70] The changes were statistically but not clinically significant—the mean pCO_2 rose from 34 to 40 and from 38 to 43 mm Hg, respectively, in the two reports, while the mean pO_2 fell from 92 to 86 and from 90 to 80 mm Hg. Rao and associates[24a] used larger doses of diazepam (averaging 0.77 mg/kg) and likewise found evidence of statistically significant but clinically unimportant respiratory depression.

When normal subjects breathe air mixtures enriched with carbon dioxide, hyperventilation occurs. The response is proportional to the inspired CO_2 concentration and is a sensitive index of the central respiratory drive. A number of studies have demonstrated that intravenous benzodiazepines (chlordiazepoxide, diazepam, oxazepam) do not alter the hyperventilation response to CO_2 challenge.[71-75] Intravenous or intramuscular meperidine, however, produced significant depression in all studies. When benzodiazepines and meperidine are given at the same time, the depressant effect is no greater than with the opiate alone.[73-76] No respiratory depression was produced in healthy subjects by oral meperidine (100 mg), pentobarbital (200 mg), or flurazepam (45 mg).[77]

There are scattered reports in the literature of respiratory failure apparently precipitated by the use of nitrazepam in patients with chronic obstructive pulmonary disease (COPD) who have CO_2 retention.[78-80] Unfortunately, the effect of the benzodiazepines in patients with lung disease has received inadequate study. Catchlove and Kafer[81] administered intravenous diazepam (0.11 mg/kg) to patients with COPD, but without CO_2 retention. The changes in $\dot{V}_A$ and pCO_2 were statistically significant although small in magnitude and clinically unimportant; pO_2 was unchanged as was the response to breathing CO_2. Rao and associates[24a] found that intravenous diazepam (average dose 0.48 mg/kg) produced only slight respiratory depression in patients with COPD. Changes in VA, pH, pO_2, and pCO_2 were estimated to be no greater than those normally occurring during physiologic sleep. Gaddie and associates[82] compared the influence of oral nitrazepam (10 mg) and placebo upon ventilation in six patients with COPD and CO_2 retention (mean pCO_2 approximately 60 mm Hg). Two hours after the dose, nitrazepam significantly depressed forced vital capacity and the 1-sec forced expiratory volume; pCO_2 and pO_2, however, were unchanged in comparison with placebo.

In healthy individuals, the benzodiazepines alone produce no clinically important respiratory depression, and do not potentiate the depressant effects of opiates. Possible interactions with other centrally acting drugs, however, have not been adequately evaluated. Acutely agitated psychotic patients may require parenteral combinations of phenothiazine tranquilizers, barbiturates, and benzodiazepines to control their behavior. The problem of multiple drug use in status epilepticus is discussed in Chapter 6. A reliable estimate of the risks of these combinations cannot be made at present. One can only emphasize that sedative-hypnotics should be used with caution when the respiratory drive is impaired, either by pulmonary disease or by other drugs.

Bronchoscopy

In 1965 Rogers and associates[83] first described the use of diazepam as a psychosedative medication for bronchoscopy. Oral pentobarbital and intramuscular meperidine were adminstered just prior to the procedure in 201 patients. After topical anesthesia, intravenous diazepam was used as a sedative. The results were excellent in 93% of cases, and almost 95% of patients had no recollection of the procedure. Adverse reactions at the time of bronchoscopy were negligible, although many patients had fatigue, weakness, or blurring of vision after the procedure. Several other reports have described similar good results.[84-86] In two studies intravenous diazepam (5 to 20 mg) and meperidine (50 to 100 mg) were compared on a double-blind basis.[87,88] In both studies meperidine was superior to diazepam with respect to the physician's evaluation of patient cooperation. The ease of the procedure was the same or better with meperidine than with diazepam, but patients' recall of the procedure was less when diazepam was used. Diazepam appears to be a suitable adjuvant for bronchoscopy, but does not replace or substitute for opiates.

Asthma

Two groups of investigators have suggested that chlordiazepoxide has antihistaminic properties.[89,90] In studies of guinea pigs and mice, chlordiazepoxide significantly antagonized the lethal effects of histamine, and inhibited bronchoconstriction produced by histamine, acetylcholine, serotonin, and bradykinin. A clinical correlate has not been found. Heinonen and Muittary[91] administered intravenous diazepam (5 mg) to 11 patients with status asthmaticus, and found no change in airway resistance. The use of central depressant drugs in status asthmaticus is hazardous. Sedatives may precipitate carbon dioxide narcosis, coma, and death in such patients. Yet some physicians feel that a parenteral antianxiety agent such as diazepam is appropriate in an individual in whom anxiety is clearly an important factor in perpetuating bronchospasm. If sedative drugs are to be given, resuscitation equipment must be available and the patient must be observed continuously.

Drug combinations containing a benzodiazepine, a xanthine (theophylline or proxiphylline), and ephedrine have been tested as antiasthmatic remedies.[92] The drug combinations provide more relief of bronchospasm than placebo.[93,94] However, replacement of the benzodiazepine with a barbiturate produces an equally effective medication,[95-97] although in some studies the barbiturate-containing preparation appears to produce more side effects.[97] Undoubtedly, the therapeutic benefit of these drug combinations is attributable primarily to the ephedrine and xanthine components. It is not clear if the addition of an antianxiety agent produces further benefit.

THE GASTROINTESTINAL TRACT

Having no clinically significant anticholinergic properties,[98,99] the benzodiazepines have no striking direct effects upon gastrointestinal (GI) function. At very high doses, diazepam (16 mg/kg) and chlordiazepoxide (32 mg/kg) produce bile stasis in dogs.[100] When diazepam (50 μg/ml) is added to the perfusate of an isolated perfused rat liver, the excretion of bromsulphthalein falls threefold.[101] Diazepam also exerts a noncompetitive antagonism of bradykinin in the isolated guinea pig ileum preparation.[102]

The most important effects of the benzodiazepines are indirect, inasmuch as the GI tract is under central nervous influence. In carefully controlled studies, diazepam alone has been shown to reduce resting gastric secretion and acid production in patients with peptic ulcer disease.[103] In normal volunteers, resting and glutamate-evoked salivary secretion is also inhibited.[104] Further radiological observations suggest that diazepam slows gastric emptying and small bowel transit time in patients with previously demonstrated hypermotility.[105] Direct antisecretory and spasmolytic properties of diazepam cannot be ruled out, but they are not supported by experimental evidence. More likely, the above effects are explained by diazepam's central sedative and antianxiety properties which can be observed even in normal individuals.

Emotion and the GI Tract

The benzodiazepines are frequently used to treat organic or functional gastrointestinal disorders in which anxiety is judged to have a precipitating or exacerbating role. Uncontrolled trials with chlordiazepoxide and diazepam suggest that the drugs are as effective in this setting as they are in patients with manifest anxiety alone.[106–108] Kasich[109] studied doxepin, diazepam, and placebo in such patients; both active drugs produced significantly more global improvement than placebo. Chlorazepate, diazepam, and placebo were compared in another study by the same author.[109a] Both drugs were significantly superior to placebo with respect to both global improvement and scores on the Hamilton Anxiety Rating Scale. Chlorazepate produced slightly more global improvement and significantly fewer side effects than diazepam. Deutsch[110] compared diazepam (10 mg/day) and placebo in a group of patients who all received propantheline bromide in addition. Diazepam produced more global improvement than placebo after the first week of treatment, but the differences subsequently disappeared despite continuation of therapy.

Fixed drug combinations containing anticholinergics and tranquilizers are popular "stomachache" remedies. Librax® contains chlordiazepoxide, 5 mg, and clidinium bromide, 2.5 mg, per capsule. This preparation seems to produce fewer side effects than other similar combinations.[111] The usual dosage is three to eight capsules per day. Results of open trials, all of which were published before 1963, are favorable.[112–116] Gastric secretion studies suggest that pretreatment with Librax® reduces both resting and stimulated acid secretion.[117–119] In placebo-controlled clinical trials, Librax® produces significantly more symptomatic improvement than placebo.[119,120] One study comparing Librax® with Triavil® (amitriptyline plus perphenazine) in patients with psychosomatic GI disorders showed Triavil® to produce greater overall improvement.[120a]

It is not clear which component of anxiolytic-anticholinergic drug combinations is responsible for the physiological and clinical effects. Warshaw[121,122] attempted to answer the question in a comparative study of placebo, clidinium, chlordiazepoxide, and Librax® in acute functional GI disorders. After 8 hr of therapy, both chlordiazepoxide and Librax® were superior to placebo and clidinium as measured by patients' estimates of symptomatic improvement. The four drugs were equally effective at 24 hr. A second study compared oxazepam alone to a combination drug containing oxazepam plus hexadiphane, an anticholinergic agent.[123] The combination was superior to oxazepam alone only with respect to symptoms of abdominal pain and epigastric distress; for all other target symptoms (heartburn, abdominal distension, nausea, vomiting, insomnia, and others), the two drugs were equivalent. The symptomatic relief produced by anxiolytic-anticholinergic combinations in anxiety-related GI disturbances seems to be due largely, if not entirely, to the antianxiety agent.

Endoscopy

Intravenous diazepam is now frequently used as a psychosedative for gastroscopy, sigmoidoscopy, peritoneoscopy, and liver biopsy.[124–129] Gastroscopy patients usually are premedicated with intramuscular meperidine and sometimes atropine and barbiturates. Intravenous diazepam is given just prior to the passage of the instrument; nearly always there is adequate sedation without adverse cardiovascular effects, and most patients cannot recall the procedure. Injection-site complications were the only important untoward effects in a series of 1,500 patients receiving intravenous diazepam prior to gastroscopy reported by Langdon and associates.[130] Pain on injection was reported by many patients, and significant thrombophlebitis developed in approximately 3.5%. Size of the vein, speed of injection, and drug dilution appear to be important factors. It is unclear whether diazepam itself or its solvent vehicle is responsible for these local sequelae. Injection-site complications following intravenous diazepam are also discussed in Chapters 4, 6, 10, and 12.

Castiglioni and associates[130a] compared intravenous diazepam (mean dose 8.6 mg) to placebo as a psychosedative prior to esophagogastroscopy. There were 100 patients in each treatment group, and all received intramuscular meperidine prior to the procedure. By the physician's assessment of relaxation, restlessness, and anxiety, diazepam was significantly superior to placebo. Diazepam produced total anterograde amnesia in 16% of patients; none of the placebo recipients had amnesia. Ludlam and Bennett[131] compared subcutaneous morphine (10 to 15 mg) to intravenous diazepam (0.15 to 0.2 mg/kg) as pre-endoscopy medication. All patients received atropine and a lidocaine throat cleansing. Both drugs were equally satisfactory sedatives; a significantly higher proportion of diazepam patients had either no recall of the procedure or did not remember discomfort. Loebel and Danzig[132] studied intravenous diazepam versus meperidine as pre-sigmoidoscopy medication. Diazepam patients were more relaxed and drowsy during the procedure, had fewer side effects, and recalled the procedure less often than the meperidine recipients. Intramuscular diazepam (10 mg) was compared to placebo prior to gastroscopy in a study by Petersen and Myren.[133] The physician's assessment of the patient's status and the ease of the procedure were more often favorable in the diazepam group, but the differences were not statistically significant. In a study of oral premedication for sigmoidoscopy, Ehrlich[134] confirmed the essential equivalence of chlordiazepoxide and Librax®.

Watson and Corke[135] made the interesting observation of yawning as a consequence of intravenous diazepam in a study of 108 patients who received the drug prior to endoscopy. Of these, 33 yawned once, approximately 1 min after receiving the drug; seven patients breathed a single deep sigh, two developed hiccoughs, and one had transient Cheyne-Stokes respirations. Such observations raise the question of laryngeal competence under diazepam sedation. Healy and Vickers[136] administered intravenous diazepam (0.2 mg/kg) to healthy subjects prior to dental work. Twenty-seven subjects were asked to swallow a radio-opaque liquid contrast material within 5 min of receiving the drug. Ten of the 27 subjects were found to have contrast material in the lungs by X-ray. Using a similar method of study, Prout and Metreweli[137] found that the frequency of post-gastroscopy pulmonary aspiration was similar (approximately 20 to 30%) with both diazepam and chlormethiazole premedication. The event probably is not attributable to a particular drug, but is most likely a hazard of oropharyngeal instrumentation with any sedative-hypnotic premedication. Clinically significant aspiration is infrequent. Taylor and colleagues[138] reported only two important instances of aspiration among 1,000 patients receiving diazepam for esophagogastroscopy.

Sedation in Liver Disease

Agitation and combativeness are not infrequently encountered among patients with liver disease and impending hepatic decompensation. Sedatives may precipitate hepatic coma in such patients. Murray-Lyon and associates[139] administered small doses (no more than 5 mg) of intravenous diazepam to 23 individuals with severe parenchymal liver disease from a variety of causes. Adequate sedation was achieved in all, with no clinical deterioration. Electroencephalographic monitoring showed the usual shift to fast frequencies, with no evidence of slowing. Diazepam, cautiously administered, probably is an appropriate psychosedative for patients whose hepatic function is impaired from whatever cause.

OBSTETRICS AND GYNECOLOGY

Diazepam relaxes human uterine musculature *in vitro*,[140] but a prediction of *in vivo* effects is impossible from this observation alone. One could easily rationalize that labor would be hastened, prolonged, or made more or less difficult. Uncontrolled studies dealing with hundreds of patients suggest that the benzodiazepines can be safely used during labor.[141–144] In animal studies using pregnant sheep, Mofid and colleagues[144a] showed that large

TABLE 7-2. *The benzodiazepines in labor: Controlled studies*

Reference	Author(s)	Design	Duration of labor	Effect of benzodiazepine upon		
				Pain or analgesia	Recall	The infant
145	Bepko et al., 1965	DZ (20 mg IM/IV) vs placebo	None	Analgesia enhanced	Amnesia enhanced	None
146	Choksi and Motashaw, 1967	DZ (10 mg IM) vs placebo	Shortened[a]	None	NR[b]	
147	Daftary et al., 1964	CDX (50 mg IM) vs placebo	Shortened[a]	NR	NR	NR
148	Duckman et al., 1964	CDX (50 mg IM) vs placebo	None	None	NR	None
149	Elder and Crossley, 1969	DZ (20 mg IM) vs placebo	None	None	None	None
150	Flowers et al., 1969	DZ (20 mg IV then 10 mg IM q 3 hr) vs placebo	None	Meperidine requirement reduced	Amnesia enhanced	Hypotonicity and hypo-activity noted
151	Friedman et al., 1969	DZ (20 mg IV then 10 mg IM q 3 hr) vs placebo	Shortened[c]	NR	NR	NR
152	Lee, 1968	DZ (10 mg IM) vs placebo	Shortened in multiparous patients only	None	NR	None
153	Mark and Hamel, 1968	CDX (100 mg IM) vs placebo	None	NR	NR	None
154	Nisbet et al., 1967	DZ (10-20 mg IM) vs placebo	None	Analgesia enhanced	None	None
155	Niswander, 1969	DZ (20 mg IV then 10 mg IM q 3 hr) vs placebo	Shortened	Less pain; meperidine requirement reduced	Amnesia enhanced	None

[a]Time from 3 cm dilation to full dilation is the parameter measured.
[b]NR: Not reported.
[c]Duration of labor the same in groups with equal degrees of sedation.

doses of intravenous diazepam given to mother (up to 2.0 mg/kg) or fetus (up to 8 mg/kg) produced no important changes in maternal or fetal circulation, and did not influence placental oxygen transfer.

The effects of benzodiazepines upon the process of labor and delivery in humans are shown in a summary of placebo-controlled trials (Table 7-2). In nearly all of the controlled studies, active drugs and placebo are given by the intramuscular or intravenous routes. The duration of labor is either shortened or unchanged by diazepam and chlordiazepoxide in comparison with placebo. Two groups showed that the time from 3 cm dilation to full dilation was reduced by benzodiazepines.[146,147] Lee[152] showed that the overall duration of labor was reduced by diazepam, but only in multiparous women. Niswander[155] noted a shortening of total labor time by diazepam. Friedman and colleagues,[151] however, showed that this effect was related to the additive sedation produced by diazepam plus meperidine rather than to diazepam alone, suggesting that central sedation rather than peripheral muscle relaxation may underlie the change in total labor time. In other studies, no significant difference in duration of labor between benzodiazepine and placebo groups is demonstrated.[145,148–150,153,154] The effects on analgesia and amnesia are also variable. In approximately half the studies in which these effects were evaluated, benzodiazepine treatment enhanced analgesia or reduced opiate requirements, and decreased the frequency of recall.

Anecdotal reports have suggested that benzodiazepines used during labor may be associated with muscular hypotoxicity and subsequent "failure to thrive" in the neonate.[156] Flowers and associates[150] noted that infants of diazepam-treated mothers tended to be hypoactive and hypotonic for the first 24 hr after delivery. These effects were unassociated with respiratory impairment. None of the other controlled trials (Table 7-2) revealed adverse effects upon the infant attributable to benzodiazepines. Suonio and co-workers,[156a] however, noted that infants of mothers receiving intravenous diazepam (20 mg) just prior to delivery were significantly more acidotic and hypercarbic than neonates born to untreated mothers. Although there was no increase in neonatal morbidity or mortality, the authors emphasize that diazepam has the potential to produce neonatal depression. In two further reports,[157,158] transient impairment of temperature regulation occurred in infants following maternal diazepam administration, causing a period of relative hypothermia.

Experimental and clinical studies have confirmed that benzodiazepines rapidly cross the placental barrier. In pregnant mice and monkeys, significant levels of diazepam are detectable in the placenta and fetus minutes after parenteral administration to the mother.[159] Oxazepam likewise reaches the fetus rapidly in animal studies.[160] In humans, diazepam administered to the mother equilibrates with the infant in less than an hour.[161–163] A finding common to nearly every human study is that benzodiazepine concentrations in cord blood or fetal plasma exceed those in maternal plasma.[153,158,161–167]

The lipid solubility of diazepam may in part explain this finding, with the drug being preferentially taken up by the placenta. It is also possible that immature drug detoxification mechanisms in the fetal liver result in delayed conjugation and excretion.[167a] Diazepam can reach the infant via breast milk,[168,169] but probably not in sufficient quantities to cause sedation.

Toxemia

The benzodiazepines have been used as sedatives in the treatment of toxemia of pregnancy. Table 7-3 summarizes pertinent reports. Chlordiazepoxide and diazepam have no intrinsic antihypertensive activity but may reduce blood pressure when anxiety and agitation contribute to the elevation. In many of these series, the benzodiazepines were used adjunctively with other antihypertensive agents, of which hydralazine was the most popular. Diazepam and chlordiazepoxide when used intravenously have been reported effective against true eclamptic convulsions.[172,173]

In the three series involving 40 or more patients, the perinatal mortality associated with toxemia and benzodiazepine use was in the range of 6 to 10%. There are no controlled studies to indicate whether this frequency is influenced one way or another by the benzodiazepines. Some authors note that the infants of eclamptic mothers receiving diazepam were excessively

TABLE 7-3. *Benzodiazepines in toxemia of pregnancy*

Reference	Author(s)	Number of cases	Drug	Other therapy
170	Elliott, 1970	3	DZ	Protoveratrine
171	El-Zeneiny et al., 1969	40	DZ	Hydrochlorothiazide
172	Gilbert, 1961	1	CDX	Hydralazine
173	Gorbach, 1968	1	DZ	Reserpine Diphenylhydantoin Phenobarbital
157	Joyce and Kenyon, 1972	52	DZ	Hydralazine
174	Lean et al., 1968	90	CDX,DZ	Hydralazine Furosemide
175	Lecart and Cavanagh, 1964	30	CDX, DZ	(not reported)
175a	McCarthy et al., 1973	2	DZ	Phenobarbital Furosemide Chlorpromazine Meperidine
158	Owen et al., 1972	12	DZ	Meperidine Promazine Hydralazine
167	Shannon et al., 1972	13	DZ	Hydralazine Furosemide
175b	Thearle et al., 1973	1	DZ	Meperidine

lethargic, hypotonic, hypothermic, and frequently required resuscitation or endotracheal intubation.[157,158] In these reports it is unclear whether the observed depression of the neonate was related to diazepam, to other drugs administered, or to the disease itself. Three case reports, however, suggest that large doses of diazepam given to eclamptic mothers may be responsible for serious neonatal depression.[175a,175b] Three severely toxemic mothers received more than 100 mg of intravenous diazepam prior to delivery. The infants were hypotonic, apneic, and required assisted ventilation. Exchange transfusion was performed on one infant.[175b] In the other two, high blood levels of diazepam (more than 4.5 μg/ml) were found in the infant, and the drug continued to be detectable for many days after delivery.[175a] No ill effects upon the neonate are noted in other series in which lower doses of diazepam were used.[171,175]

There are insufficient data to evaluate the role of the benzodiazepines in hypertensive and toxemic pregnancies. Very high doses appear to carry the risk of excessive depression of the neonate.

Reproductive Physiology

Boris and associates[176] have carried out extensive endocrine studies of chlordiazepoxide. The test systems used are summarized in Table 7-4. In all systems, chlordiazepoxide had no influence. Khazan et al.[177] studied the mammotropic effect of psychotropic drugs in adult female rats. Drugs were given in single daily subcutaneous doses for 10 consecutive days. In doses of 40 mg/kg per day, both chlordiazepoxide and chlorpromazine produced equal degrees of histologic mammary hypertrophy. Meprobamate (80 mg/kg/day) and phenobarbital (30 mg/kg/day) had slight or negligible effects. Superstine and Sulman[178] administered chlordiazepoxide (10 to 40 mg/kg/day) and diazepam (5 to 10 mg/kg/day) to rats for 100 consecutive days. Both drugs had a slight lactogenic effect and also caused an increase in adrenal gland weight. In humans, there is only one case report of lactation and gynecomastia attributed to chlordiazepoxide.[179]

Whitelaw in 1961 suggested that chlordiazepoxide may influence the reproductive cycle in humans.[180] The drug was given to 17 females on days 9 to 14 of the menstrual cycle. The subjects previously had menstruated normally, but all were patients in an infertility practice. In 12 of 17 women, the midcycle rise in basal body temperature was delayed or did not occur. Kamman[181] subsequently pointed out that the etiologic role of chlordiazepoxide was dubious. In 300 female patients treated with chlordiazepoxide by this author, menstrual irregularities were insignificant and rare. Schwartz and Smith[182] used chlordiazepoxide during two complete menstrual cycles in 35 infertility patients. Anxiety and tension were relieved, but no effect upon the reproductive cycle was noted. Cohn[183] intensively studied the effect of chronic diazepam therapy upon the menstrual cycle in five females. Endometrial biopsy specimens were included in the study.

TABLE 7-4. *Endocrine effects of chlordiazepoxide in rats and rabbits*[a]

Dose	Duration	Test[b]
2.5 to 50 mg/kg/day	10 days	Reduction in weight of testes and prostate in immature rats.
5 mg/day	10 days	Prevention of ovarian hypertrophy
50 to 100 mg/kg/day	5 days	Interruption of estrus cycle
25 to 50 mg	1 hr before mating	Prevention of ovulation in rabbit in response to mating
2.5 mg/day	7 days	Effect upon change in seminal vesicle and prostate weight induced in castrated rats by exogenous testosterone
5 to 10 mg/day	3 days	Effect upon change in uterine weight induced in oöphorectomized rats by exogenous estrogen
5 to 20 mg/day	5 days	Effect of exogenous progesterone in estrogen-primed rabbit

[a] Boris et al.: Proc Soc Exp Biol Med 106:708-710, 1961.
[b] Chlordiazepoxide had no effect in any of the test systems.

No abnormalities or changes were noted. At present, there is no good evidence that the benzodiazepines significantly influence the reproductive cycle in human females.

Anxiety in Obstetrics and Gynecology

A number of uncontrolled studies have suggested that the benzodiazepines may be of benefit for anxious patients seen by obstetricians and gynecologists.[184-191] Included are patients with overt symptomatic anxiety, premenstrual tension, dysmenorrhea, dyspareunia, menopausal symptoms, and a number of other psychosomatic disorders. Fromhagen[192] reported a controlled trial of chlordiazepoxide and placebo in a large number of anxious women seen in a private obstetrics and gynecology practice. The superiority of chlordiazepoxide over placebo with respect to both global improvement and target symptoms (phobic and somatic) was highly significant. Shader and associates[192a] compared diazepam (6 mg/day) and placebo in healthy women with impaired psychosocial functioning due to premenstrual symptoms of anxiety, irritability, depression, fatigue, and abdominal distention. During the follicular phase (days 6 through 13) of the menstrual cycle, diazepam was not distinguishable from placebo as measured by scores on the Scheier-Cattell Anxiety Battery (SCAB). During the luteal or premenstrual phase (days 21 through 28) when symptomatology was greatest, diazepam produced significantly more reduction in SCAB scores than placebo.

Menrium® is a combination product containing chlordiazepoxide, 5 to 10 mg, and conjugated estrogens 0.2 to 0.4 mg, per pill. Sheffery and associates[193] studied the combination product, chlordiazepoxide alone, estrogens alone, and placebo in 100 symptomatic menopausal women. In a crossover design, each patient received each active drug for a period of 3 weeks, with drug-free periods interpolated at the time of crossover. The results strongly suggested that the combination preparation was the most effective. Hazan and Conneely[194] used a similar design to compare Menrium,® estrogens alone, and placebo. Menrium® was significantly more effective than the other treatments. These studies suggest that the chlordiazepoxide-estrogen preparation may be a rational one, but further studies are needed to verify its safety and efficacy.

ALLERGIC DISORDERS

Antihistaminic effects of the benzodiazepines, although suggested in some animal studies,[89,90] have not been confirmed in humans. Jaques and Riesterer[195] found that diazepam had no effect upon an experimentally produced inflammatory reaction in animals. Direct antihistaminic and antiinflammatory actions seem an unlikely explanation for the observed clinical efficacy of the benzodiazepines in a number of allergic disorders exacerbated by anxiety or emotion, including eczema, pruritic dermatoses, asthma, sinusistis, and rhinitis.[196–203] Two controlled trials deal specifically with skin diseases. McCormick[204] compared chlordiazepoxide, oxazepam, and placebo in a double-blind trial involving more than 20 patients per treatment group. Oxazepam produced significantly more relief of emotional symptoms than chlordiazepoxide or placebo, but the response to therapy in all three treatment groups was poor. Wilkinson[205] studied the effects of chlordiazepoxide, amobarbital, and placebo in two different crossover trials. Even with placebo reactors excluded from the study, the chlordiazepoxide-placebo difference was weak. Chlordiazepoxide was not significantly better than the barbiturate. Grater[206] compared chlordiazepoxide to placebo in patients with various allergic disorders, and the active drug was superior to placebo in alleviating anxiety. In a study of patients with allergic rhinitis, a significant chlordiazepoxide-placebo difference was not demonstrated.[207]

In all of these studies, both controlled and uncontrolled, relief of emotional symptoms approximately paralleled improvement in pruritis, rhinitis, or whatever allergic manifestation was under study. Again the efficacy of the benzodiazepines seems attributable to their influence upon the emotional component of disease and the somatic sequelae thereof.

OPHTHALMOLOGY AND OTOLARYNGOLOGY

The muscle-relaxant properties of the benzodiazepines apply to the oculomotor system as well as to large skeletal muscles. Chlordiazepoxide and diazepam prolong the duration and reduce the velocity of saccadic eye movements in man.[208] Nitrazepam in doses of 7.5 and 10.0 mg depresses ocular tracking, but the inhibition is less than that produced by phenobarbital.[209] Uncontrolled studies have suggested that benzodiazepines may be of value in tension headache,[210-212] migraine,[212,213] and strabismus.[214] Beneficial effects are probably attributable to emotional improvement rather than objective muscle relaxation. In three controlled studies involving patients with psychogenic headache, two showed benzodiazepine derivatives to be weakly superior to placebo,[215,216] while a third showed a significant diazepam-placebo difference.[216a]

Roberts[217] used chlordiazepoxide and diazepam in patients with glaucoma. Psychic improvement was noted, but there was no change in ocular tension. The manufacturers of diazepam now suggest that the drug be avoided in glaucoma, but the reasons for this are not clear.

Sekitani and associates[218,219] studied the effect of two drugs upon electrical discharge from the medial vestibular nucleus in cats. Intravenous diazepam (0.4 mg/kg) significantly inhibited rotation-induced vestibular discharge, whereas dimenhydrinate in doses up to 8 mg/kg did not. The results suggest that the benzodiazepines may have vestibular sedative properties, potentially useful in the treatment of motion sickness. However, Miller and Graybiel[220] found that chlordiazepoxide (50 mg/day for 3 days) had no effect upon ocular counterrolling in response to head tilt in humans. At present there is no clinical evidence that the benzodiazepines have significant anti-motion sickness effects.

OTHER METABOLIC EFFECTS

Arrigoni-Martelli and Toth[221] have demonstrated that chlordiazepoxide mobilizes hepatic glycogen and produces hyperglycemia in rats. The effect is prevented by treatment with beta-adrenergic blockers and by adrenalectomy, suggesting that chlordiazepoxide activates adrenergic mechanisms. Two studies by Mehta in humans demonstrate that diazepam does not influence blood glucose in nondiabetic patients.[222,223] These studies were performed in association with surgery, with diazepam given either as premedication or as an intravenous induction agent. Gottschalk and associates[223a] found a single oral dose of chlordiazepoxide (25 mg) in healthy volunteers produced no changes in blood glucose levels, but caused a significant rise in plasma triglycerides and free fatty acids in comparison with placebo. Arrigoni-Martelli and Corsico[223b] noted a similar lipomobilizing effect in animals, further suggesting that chlordiazepoxide enhances cyclic adenosine monophosphate activation through phosphodiesterase inhibition (see also Chapter 5).

Oral or intraperitoneal diazepam in rats produces a rise in plasma cortisol levels in comparison with placebo.[224] A small reduction in the basal metabolic rate has also been noted.[225] In humans, a single dose of diazepam produces a drop in plasma cortisol,[226] but chronic treatment does not alter the diurnal cortisol rhythm, total daily excretion of corticosteroids, or the response to adrenocorticotrophic hormone stimulation.[183,227] Intramuscular diazepam in dogs produces a mild degree of hemodilution and leukocytosis.[228] The reasons for this are unclear. In rats, neither chlordiazepoxide nor diazepam stimulates the release of antidiuretic hormone; the antidiuretic hormone response to dehydration is also unchanged.[229]

The effects of the benzodiazepines upon renal function have not been well studied. A preliminary observation by Fariss and Kolb[230] suggested that chlordiazepoxide reduced urinary crystal formation in six patients with cystinuria. Subsequently, however, a double-blind study showed no effect.[231] Vyden and associates[232] hypothesized that copper depletion might be associated with chlordiazepoxide-induced ataxia. However, a controlled trial failed to demonstrate that chlordiazepoxide influenced urinary copper excretion.

Only trace amounts of active benzodiazepines are excreted unchanged in the urine (see Chapter 2). For this reason, forced diuresis is of little benefit in enhancing drug removal.[233] Chlordiazepoxide is relatively water soluble, whereas diazepam is relatively lipid soluble. Hemodialysis, therefore, might be of benefit in cases of chlordiazepoxide overdosage, and this has been confirmed in one report.[234] Fortunately, dialysis is seldom if ever needed in poisoning with benzodiazepines (see Chapter 12).

COMMENT

The benzodiazepines are relatively devoid of pharmacologic effects outside of the central nervous system. Despite their potent sedative properties, large doses produce only minor changes in cardiovascular and respiratory function. Equally sedating quantities of barbiturates frequently result in significant cardiovascular and respiratory depression. The use of intravenous diazepam as psychosedative premedication for cardioversion and endoscopy almost certainly is sound medical practice. Elective cardioversion, for example, may now be performed with little or no hazard and without the presence of an anesthesiologist. Chapter 10 elaborates upon the use of the benzodiazepines as preanesthetic medication and as induction agents.

The interaction of emotion with somatic sensation and disease is complex. Individuals with anxiety or depression may complain primarily or secondarily of somatic dysfunction when objective abnormalities in organ function cannot be demonstrated at our present level of sophistication. Alternatively, organic disease may produce or exacerbate anxiety and depression. The two processes often merge in a perplexing manner, producing an overtly anxious patient with organic disease present but apparently not severe enough to account for the symptomatology. The physician may wish to intervene with psychotropic medication in such cases, and the benzodiazepines are often a reasonable choice. Documentation of their efficacy in this setting is less substantial than in overt anxiety alone, but the benzodiazepines do appear to be at least as effective as other antianxiety agents in the treatment of psychosomatic disorders. At the very least, the physician may prescribe these drugs with reasonable confidence that they will not directly alter physiologic function of the organ system in question. The same cannot be said of many other classes of psychotropic agents.

REFERENCES

1. Parry HJ, Balter MB, Mellinger GD, Cisin IH, Manheimer DI: National patterns of psychotherapeutic drug use. Arch Gen Psychiat 28:769-783, 1973

1a. Hockman CH, Livingston KE: Inhibition of reflex vagal bradycardia by diazepam. Neuropharmacology 10:307-314, 1971

2. Vieth JB, Holm E, Knopp PR: Electrophysiological studies on the action of Mogadon® on central nervous structures of the cat. A comparison with pentobarbital. Arch Int Pharmacodyn 171:323-338, 1968

3. Moe R, Bagdon RE, Zbinden G: The effects of tranquilizers on myocardial metabolism. Angiology 13:4-12, 1962

4. Prindle KH, Gold HK, Cardon PV, Epstein SE: Effects of psychopharmacologic agents on myocardial contractility. J Pharmacol Exp Ther 173:133-137, 1970

5. Hitch DC, Nolan SP: Myocardial depression and peripheral vasodilation caused by the administration of chlordiazepoxide. Surg Forum 20:162-164, 1969

6. Hitch DC, Nolan SP: Changes in myocardial performance and total peripheral resistance produced by the administration of chlordiazepoxide. J Thorac Cardiov Surg 61:352-358, 1971

7. Abel RM, Staroscik RN, Reis RL: The effects of diazepam (Valium) on left ventricular function and systemic vascular resistance. J Pharmacol Exp Ther 173:364-370, 1970

8. Abel RM, Reis RL, Staroscik RN: Coronary vasodilation following diazepam (Valium). Brit J Pharmacol 38:620-631, 1970

9. Abel RM, Reis RL, Staroscik RN: The pharmacological basis of coronary and systemic vasodilator actions of diazepam (Valium). Brit J Pharmacol 39:261-274, 1970

10. Bianco JA, Shanahan EA, Ostheimer GW, Guyton RA, Powell WJ, Daggett WM: Cardiovascular effects of diazepam. J Thorac Cardiov Surg 62:125-130, 1971

11. Starley JW, Michie DD: Hemodynamic alterations produced by intravenous diazepam in conscious, unrestrained dogs. Curr Ther Res 11:796-801, 1969

12. Sharer L, Kutt H: Intravenous administration of diazepam. Effects on penicillin-induced focal seizures in the cat. Arch Neurol 24:169-175, 1971

13. Louis S, Kutt H, McDowell F: The cardio-circulatory changes caused by intravenous Dilantin and its solvent. Amer Heart J 74:523-529, 1967

14. deJong RH, Heavner JE: Local anesthetic seizure prevention: diazepam versus pentobarbital. Anesthesiology 36:449-457, 1972

15. Zsoter TT, Gospodarowicz M: The effect of diazepam and pentozocine on the venomotor reflexes in man. J Clin Pharmacol 12:89-94, 1972

16. Dobkin AB, Criswick VG: Circulatory response to tilt with some antiemetic and sedative drugs. Canad Anaesth Soc J 8:387-393, 1961

17. Katz J, Finestone SC, Pappas MT: Circulatory response to tilting after intravenous diazepam in volunteers. Anesth Analg 46:243-246, 1967

18. Steen SN, Martinez LR: Some pharmacologic effects of intravenous chlordiazepoxide. Clin Pharmacol Ther 5:44-48, 1964

19. Healy TEJ, Robinson JS, Vickers MD: Physiological responses to intravenous diazepam as a sedative for conservative dentistry. Brit Med J 3:10-13, 1970

20. Francisco N, Lebowitz WB: Intravenous diazepam in the cardiovascular laboratory: a physiologic study. St Vincent's Hosp Med Bull 10:8-12, 1968

21. Dalen JE, Evans GL, Banas JS, Brooks HL, Paraskos JA, Dexter L: The hemodynamic and respiratory effects of diazepam (Valium®). Anesthesiology 30:259-263, 1969

22. Abel RM, Reis RL: Intravenous diazepam for sedation following cardiac operations: clinical and hemodynamic assessments. Anesth Analg 50:244-248, 1971

23. Knapp RB, Dubow H: Comparison of diazepam with thiopental as an induction agent in cardiopulmonary disease. Anesth Analg 49:722-726, 1970

24. Knapp RB, Dubow HS: Diazepam as an induction agent for patients with cardiopulmonary disease. Southern Med J 63:1451-1453, 1970

24a. Rao S, Sherbaniuk RW, Prasad K, Lee SJK, Sproule BJ: Cardiopulmonary effects of diazepam. Clin Pharmacol Ther 14:182-189, 1973

24b. Coleman AJ, Downing JW, Moyes DG, O'Brien A: Acute cardiovascular effects of Ro 5-4200: a new anaesthetic induction agent. South Afr Med J 47:382-384, 1973

24c. Comer WH, Elliott HW, Nomof N, Navarro G, Kokka N, Ruelius H, Knowles JA: Pharmacology of parenterally administered lorazepam in man. J Int Med Res 1:216-225, 1973

25. Hendrix GH: Intravenous use of diazepam in cardioversion. Southern Med J 62:483-484, 1969

26. Kahler RL, Burrow GN, Felig P: Diazepam-induced amnesia for cardioversion. JAMA 200:997-998, 1967

27. Kernohan RJ: Diazepam in cardioversion. Lancet 1:718-719, 1966

28. Kernohan RJ: Intravenous diazepam in cardioversion by direct current countershock. In, Diazepam in Anaesthesia. Edited by PF Knight, CG Burgess. Bristol, John Wright and Sons, 1968, pp 82-84

29. Lebowitz WB: Electrical conversion of arrhythmias under diazepam sedation. Connecticut Med 33:173-174, 1969

30. Nelson Y, Sloman G: Diazepam ("Valium") in direct current counter shock. Med J Aust 1:1052, 1967

31. Nutter DO, Massumi RA: Diazepam in cardioversion. New Eng J Med 273:650-651, 1965

32. Rosenblatt WH, Nettles DC: Direct-current cardioversion with diazepam as sedative agent. J Mississippi State Med Assoc 11:57-60, (Feb) 1970

33. Rotem CE: Diazepam injectable as premedication for electrical cardioversion. Canad Med Assoc J 103:1381-1382, 1970

34. Somers K, Gunstone RF, Patel AK, D'Arbela PG: Intravenous diazepam for direct-current cardioversion. Brit Med J 4:13-15, 1971

35. Stiles CM, Pugh DM, Dunn M: Diazepam in cardioversion. J Kansas Med Soc 69:277-278, 1968

36. Turkel RA, Lemmert WA: The use of diazepam in cardioversion. Southern Med J 62:61-64, 1969

37. Vinge LN, Wyant GM, Lopez JF: Diazepam in cardioversion. Canad Anaesth Soc J 18:166-171, 1971

38. Winters WL, McDonough MT, Hafer J, Dietz R: Diazepam. A useful hypnotic drug for direct-current cardioversion. JAMA 204:926-928, 1968

39. Muenster JJ, Rosenberg MS, Carleton RA, Graettinger JS: Comparison between diazepam and sodium thiopental during DC countershock. JAMA 199:758-760, 1967

40. Hendrix GH, Maloy WC: Intravenous diazepam in coronary arteriography. J South Carolina Med Assoc 67:5-6, (Jan) 1971

41. Healy TEJ: Intravenous diazepam for cardiac catheterisation. Anaesthesia 24:537-540, 1969

42. van Loon GR: Ventricular arrhythmias treated by diazepam. Canad Med Assoc J 98:785-787, 1968

43. Spracklen FHN, Chambers RJ, Schrire V: Value of diazepam ('Valium') in treatment of cardiac arrhythmias. Brit Heart J 32:827-832, 1970

44. Dunbar RW, Boettner RB, Haley JV, Hall VE, Morrow DH: The effect of diazepam on the antiarrhythmic response to lidocaine. Anesth Analg 50:685-692, 1971

45. Liebeswar G: The depressant action of flurazepam on the maximum rate of rise of action potentials recorded from guinea-pig papillary muscles. Naunyn-Schmied Arch Pharmacol 275:445-456, 1972

46. Nevins MA, Mattes LM, Spritzer RC, Weisenseel AC, Donoso E, Friedberg CK: Ineffectiveness of diazepam as an antiarrhythmic agent. J Mt Sinai Hosp 36:408-414, 1969

47. Baum T, Eckfeld DK, Shropshire AT, Rowles G, Varner LL: Observations on models used for the evaluation of antiarrhythmic drugs. Arch Int Pharmacodyn 193:149-170, 1971

48. Barrett JS, Hey EB: Ventricular arrhythmias associated with the use of diazepam for cardioversion. JAMA 214:1323-1324, 1970

49. Nevins MA: Ventricular arrhythmias and diazepam. JAMA 215:643, 1971

50. Chaffee WG: Diazepam for cardioversion. JAMA 215:487, 1971

51. Naney AP: Diazepam for cardioversion. JAMA 215:487, 1971

52. Hirshleifer I, Drago S, Nayak R: Chlordiazepoxide in cardiovascular disease. Clin Med 68:926-931, 1961

53. Reinhardt DJ: Use of chlordiazepoxide as an adjuvant in cardiovascular disorders. Delaware Med J 34:171-175, 1962

54. Alimurung MM: Diazepam (Valium) in cardiovascular diseases. J Philippine Fed Priv Med Prac 14:659-664, 1965

55. Alimurung MM, Grajo MZ: Chlordiazepoxide in cardiovascular diseases. J Philippine Fed Priv Med Prac 13:238-242, 1964

56. Murphy FM, Barber JM: Chlordiazepoxide in angina pectoris. Lancet 1:1114-1115, 1961

57. Davis OF, Beck C, Charles A, Bergal M, Horwitz B: Some clinical observations with chlordiazepoxide in depression associated with somatic illness. Psychosomatics 2:100-102, 1961

58. Aronson PR, Hosbach RE: Chronic hyperventilation syndrome. Clinical results, electro-cardiographic findings with chlordiazepoxide. Angiology 13:23-31, 1962

59. Aronson PR: Hyperventilation syndrome. A comparative study of the effects of tranquilizers and a sedative upon the electrocardiogram. Clin Pharmacol Ther 5:553-560, 1964

60. Kuhn PH, de Marchena G, Shaftel HE: Neurogenic vasopasm. Angiology 13:32-34, 1962

61. George RB, Foreman S, Duke R: A new benzodiazepine for the treatment of emotional distress in cardiovascular disease. J Louisiana State Med Assoc 122:310-313, 1970

62. Aronson PR: Evaluation of psychotropic drug therapy in chronic hyperventilation syndrome: intensive study design. J New Drugs 6:305-307, 1966

63. Benson WH: Comparative evaluation of diazepam (Valium®) and phenobarbital for the relief of anxiety-related symptoms in patients hospitalized for acute myocardial infarction. J Med Assoc Georgia 60:276-278, 1971

64. Hackett TP, Cassem NH: Reduction of anxiety in the coronary-care unit: a controlled double-blind comparison of chlordiazepoxide and amobarbital. Curr Ther Res 14:649-656, 1972

65. Russek HI: Combined vasodilator and tranquilizer therapy in angina pectoris: a comparative study with statistical analysis. Amer J Med Sci 249:420-442, 1965

66. Dougherty ES: Pentrium therapy in angina pectoris. Angiology 16:57-61, 1965
67. Dembo DH, Antlitz AM: Chlordiazepoxide therapy in angina pectoris. A double-blind study. Angiology 15:207-209, 1964
68. Florez J: The action of diazepam, nitrazepam, and chlonazepam [sic] on the respiratory center of decerebrate cats. Eur J Pharmacol 14:250-256, 1971
69. Steen SN, Martinez LR: Some pharmacologic effects of intravenous oxazepam. Anesth Analg 44:358-362, 1965
70. Catchlove RFH, Kafer ER: The effects of diazepam on the ventilatory response to carbon dioxide and on steady-state gas exchange. Anesthesiology 34:9-13, 1971
71. Steen SN, Amaha K, Martinez LR: Effect of oxazepam on respiratory response to carbon dioxide. Anesth Analg 45:455-458, 1966
72. Steen SN, Weitzner SW, Amaha K, Martinez LR: The effect of diazepam on the respiratory response to carbon dioxide. Canad Anaesth Soc J 13:374-377, 1966
73. Steen SN, Amaha K, Weitzner SW, Martinez LR: The effect of chlordiazepoxide and pethidine, alone and in combination, on the respiratory response to carbon dioxide. Brit J Anaesth 39:459-463, 1967
74. Cohen R, Finn H, Steen SN: Effect of diazepam and meperidine, alone and in combination, on respiratory response to carbon dioxide. Anesth Analg 48:353-355, 1969
75. Steen SN, Urban BJ: The effect of oxazepam with meperidine on the respiratory response to carbon dioxide. Acta Anaesth Scand supp 23:59-62, 1966
76. Sadove MS, Balagot RC, McGrath JM: Effects of chlordiazepoxide and diazepam on the influence of meperidine on the respiratory response to carbon dioxide. J New Drugs 5:121-124, 1965
77. Finn H, Cohen R, Steen SN: Comparison of the effects of RO 5-6901, pentobarbital, and meperidine on the respiratory response to carbon dioxide. Anesth Analg 49:297-299, 1970
78. Clark TJH, Collins JV, Tong T: Respiratory depression caused by nitrazepam in patients with respiratory failure. Lancet 2:737-738, 1971
79. Pines A: Nitrazepam in chronic obstructive bronchitis. Brit Med J 3:352, 1972
79a. Model DG: Nitrazepam induced respiratory depression in chronic obstructive lung disease. Brit J Dis Chest 67:128-130, 1973
80. Hilton AM: Sedative drugs in respiratory failure. Lancet 2:922, 1971
81. Catchlove RFH, Kafer ER: The effects of diazepam on respiration in patients with obstructive pulmonary disease. Anesthesiology 34:14-18, 1971
82. Gaddie J, Legge JS, Palmer KNV, Petrie JC, Wood RA: Effect of nitrazepam in chronic obstructive bronchitis. Brit Med J 2:688-689, 1972
83. Rogers WK, Waterman DH, Domm SE, Sunay A: Efficacy of a new psychotropic drug in bronchoscopy. Dis Chest 47:280-283, 1965
84. Straja AM, Munro DD, Gilbert RGB: Bronchoscopy with the aid of diazepam. Canad Anaesth Soc J 16:241-248, 1969
85. Waterman DH, Domm SE, Rogers WK: Total care of the chronic bronchitis patient. An evaluation of twenty years' experience. Dis Chest 53:457-461, 1968
85a. Morales ES, Krumperman LW, Cohen JG: Bronchoscopy under diazepam anesthesia. Anesth Analg 52:414-421, 1973
86. Takita H, Mostert JW, Moore RH: Diazepam anesthesia. Evaluation for bronchoscopy. NY State J Med 71:848-850, 1971
87. Sanderson DR, Olsen AM: Diazepam for bronchoscopic premedication. Anesth Analg 48:906-908, 1969
88. Ecker RR, Sugg WL, Rea WJ: Diazepam as an adjunct to bronchoscopy. Chest 62:259-262, 1972
89. Kovacs IB, Gorog P: Effect of chlordiazepoxide on bronchoconstriction. Arch Int Pharmacodyn 173:27-33, 1968

90. Jaques R, Ruegg M: Some peripheral pharmacological characteristics of benzoctamine. Pharmacology 6:89-98, 1971

91. Heinonen J, Muittari A: The effect of diazepam on airway resistance in asthmatics. Anaesthesia 27:37-40, 1972

92. Thomas JW: Resprium (Librium-theophylline-ephedrine compound) in the treatment of bronchial asthma and respiratory allergy. Ann Allergy 20:789-793, 1962

93. Muittari A, Mattila MJ: Bronchodilator action of drug combinations in asthmatic patients: ephedrine, theophylline, and tranquilizing drugs. Curr Ther Res 13:374-385, 1971

94. Bloom S, Markow H: Evaluation of a chlordiazepoxide, theophylline, ephedrine combination in the treatment of bronchial asthma. Ann Allergy 21:601-604, 1963

95. Lascelles BD: Double-blind trial of a combination of chlordiazepoxide, ephedrine, and theophylline (Brontrium) in bronchospasm. J Royal Coll Gen Prac 20:371-375, 1970

96. General Practitioner Research Group: General practitioner clinical trials. An anti-asthmatic combination. Practitioner 208:554-557, 1972

97. Friedman HT: Librium-theophylline-ephedrine compound in bronchial asthma. A double-blind study in 100 patients. Ann Allergy 21:163-167, 1963

98. Droppleman LF, McNair DM: Screening for anticholinergic effects of atropine and chlordiazepoxide. Psychopharmacologia 12:164-169, 1968

99. Babbini M, Torrielli MV: Investigation on pharmacological properties of hexadiphane, oxazepam hemisuccinate and of their combination. Curr Ther Res 14:311-323, 1972

100. Stefko PL, Zbinden G: Effect of chlorpromazine, chlordiazepoxide, diazepam, and chlorprothixene on bile flow and intrabiliary pressure in cholycystectomized dogs. Amer J Gastroenterol 39:410-417, 1963

101. Kvetina J, Guaitani A, Pugliatti C, Veneroni E: Effect of diazepam on liver function of rats. Pharmacology 2:17-20, 1969

102. Leme JG, Rocha e Silva M: Competitive and non-competitive inhibition of bradykinin on the guinea-pig ileum. Brit J Pharmacol Chemother 25:50-58, 1965

103. Birnbaum D, Karmeli F, Tefera M: The effect of diazepam on human gastric secretion. Gut 12:616-618, 1971

104. Steiner JE, Birnbaum D, Karmeli F, Cohen S: Effect of diazepam on human salivary secretion. Digestion 3:262-268, 1970

105. Birnbaum D, Ben-Menachem J, Schwartz A: The influence of oral diazepam on gastrointestinal motility. A preliminary report. Amer J Proctol 21:263-266, 1970

106. Rider JA, Moeller HC: The use of chlordiazepoxide in the treatment of patients with functional gastrointestinal disorders. Amer J Gastroenterol 36:464-467, 1961

107. Brown CH: Clinical evaluation of Librium in gastrointestinal diseases. A preliminary report. Amer J Gastroenterol 35:30-36, 1961

108. Voegtlin WL: Management of functional gastrointestinal disorders with diazepam. Appl Ther 6:801-805, 1964

109. Kasich AM: Clinical evaluation of doxepin and diazepam in patients with gastrointestinal disease and anxiety. Psychosomatics 10(No. 3, Sect. 2):18-20, 1969

109a. Kasich AM: Chlorazepate dipotassium in the treatment of anxiety associated with chronic gastrointestinal disease. Curr Ther Res 15:83-91, 1973

110. Deutsch E: Relief of anxiety and related emotions in patients with gastrointestinal disorders. Amer J Dig Dis 16:1091-1094, 1971

111. Taylor WJR: A comparative determination of side effects associated with the oral use of three anticholinergic-psychotropic drugs. Int J Clin Pharmacol 3:1-13, 1970

112. Hock CW: Clinical trial of Librax in gastrointestinal disorders. J New Drugs 1:90-95, 1961

113. Holloman JLS: Librax in gastrointestinal disorders. J Nat Med Assoc 53:504-507, 1961

114. General Practitioner Research Group: General practitioner clinical trials. A tranquillizer-anticholinergic drug in gastric disorders. Practitioner 189:217-219, 1962

115. Walker RB: Clinical experience with anticholinergic-tranquilizer in gastrointestinal disorders. Clin Med 69:859-870, 1962
116. Nussbaum HE: A new psychotherapeutic-anticholinergic combination for gastrointestinal disorders. Amer J Gastroenterol 38:575-582, 1962
117. Sanowski R, Groisser VW: Effects of Librax and a placebo on gastric secretion. Curr Ther Res 9:508-513, 1967
118. Head HB, Hammond JB: Antisecretory effects of Librax in patients with duodenal ulcer. Amer J Dig Dis 13:540-550, 1968
119. McHardy G, Sekinger D, Balart L, Cradic HE: Chlordiazepoxide-clidinium bromide in gastrointestinal disorders: controlled clinical studies. Gastroenterology 54:508-513, 1968
120. Wayne HH: A tranquilizer-anticholinergic preparation in functional gastrointestinal disorders: a double-blind evaluation. California Med 111:79-83, 1969
120a. Oren BG: Stress-related gastrointestinal dysfunction and combined antidepressant-tranquilizer therapy. Psychosomatics 10:258-263, 1969
121. Warshaw LJ, Bennett HJ: Evaluation of drugs in industry. A method for comparing the effectiveness of drugs in the treatment of acute functional disorders. Arch Environ Health 6:227-234, 1963
122. Warshaw LJ, Bennett HJ, Chassan JB: Chlordiazepoxide and clidinium bromide in management of acute gastrointestinal upset. NY State J Med 64:405-409. 1964
123. Strumia E, Babbini M: A double-blind study of an oxazepam hemisuccinate-hexadiphane combination in management of gastrointestinal disorders. Curr Ther Res 13:251-256, 1971
124. Mayes GR, Kehoe EL, Friedman EL, Belber J: Pre-endoscopic medication: parenteral diazepam used adjunctively. Gastrointestinal Endoscopy 16:187-193, 1970
125. Ticktin HE, Trujillo NP: Evaluation of diazepam for pre-endoscopy medication. Amer J Dig Dis 10:979-984, 1968
126. Ticktin HE, Trujillo NP: Further experience with diazepam for pre-endoscopic medication. Gastrointestinal Endoscopy 15:91-92, 1968
127. Akdamar K, Lilly JO, Mary CC, Maumus L: Peritoneoscopy facilitated by premedication with diazepam. Southern Med J 64:891-893, 1971
128. Villa F, Maestre M: Injectable Valium in peritoneoscopy. Gastrointestinal Endoscopy 17:74-75, 1970
129. Palmer HM: Diazepam sedation for liver biopsy. Practitioner 208:662-663, 1972
130. Langdon DE, Harlan JR, Bailey RL: Thrombophlebitis with diazepam used intravenously. JAMA 223:184-185, 1973
130a. Castiglioni LJ, Allen TS, Patterson M: Intravenous diazepam: an improvement in pre-endoscopic medication. Gastrointestinal Endoscopy 19:134-136, 1973
131. Ludlam R, Bennett JR: Comparison of diazepam and morphine as premedication for gastrointestinal endoscopy. Lancet 2:1397-1399, 1971
132. Loebel AS, Danzig LS: Comparative effects of diazepam and meperidine as premedication for sigmoidoscopy. A double-blind study. Amer J Proctol 21:430-434, 1970
133. Petersen H, Myren J: Premedication for peroral endoscopy. Two double-blind studies. Scand J Gastroenterol 7:583-587, 1972
134. Ehrlich R: Analysis of premedication for sigmoidoscopy: a comparative study with chlordiazepoxide alone and in combination with clidinium bromide. Amer J Proctol 20:130-133, 1969
135. Watson WC, Corke AM: Diazepam and morphine as premedication for gastrointestinal endoscopy. Lancet 1:490, 1972
136. Healy TEJ, Vickers MD: Laryngeal competence under diazepam sedation. Proc Roy Soc Med 64:85-86, 1971
137. Prout BJ, Metreweli C: Pulmonary aspiration after fibre-endoscopy of the upper gastrointestinal tract. Brit Med J 4:269-271, 1972

138. Taylor PA, Cotton PB, Towey RM, Gent AE: Pulmonary complications after oesophagogastroscopy using diazepam. Brit Med J 1:666, 1972
139. Murray-Lyon IM, Young J, Parkes JD, Knill-Jones RP, Williams R: Clinical and electroencephalographic assessment of diazepam in liver disease. Brit Med J 4:265-266, 1971
140. Landesman R, Wilson KH: Relaxant effect of diazepam on uterine muscle. Obstet Gynecol 26:552-556, 1965
141. de Alvarez RR, Zighelboim I: Diazepam during labor. Penn Med 72:93-98, (Nov) 1969
141a. Aguilar J, Nova A: Continuous intravenous infusion of diazepam during labor. Int J Gynaecol Obstet 8:164, 1970
142. Brown WE, Barnes F, Koch W, Clark RB: The use of Valium in labor. J Arkansas Med Soc 66:92-95, 1969
143. Timonen S, Hagner M: Benzodiazepines in an unselected obstetrical series. Ann Chir Gynaecol Fenn 55:65-68, 1966
144. de Boer CH, Chau SS: Diazepam in labour. Lancet 2:1256-1257, 1967
144a. Mofid M, Brinkman R, Assali NS: Effects of diazepam on uteroplacental and fetal hemodynamics and metabolism. Obstet Gynecol 41:364-368, 1973
145. Bepko F, Lowe E, Waxman B: Relief of the emotional factor in labor with parenterally administered diazepam. Obstet Gynecol 26:852-857, 1965
146. Choksi RH, Motashaw ND: Valium (diazepam) for cervical dilatation during labour. J Obstet Gynaecol India 17:273-277, 1967
147. Daftary SN, Parmar H, Doshi NS: Effect of chlordiazepoxide (Librium) on cervical dilatation in labour. J Postgrad Med 10:121-125, 1964
148. Duckman S, Spina T, Attardi M, Meyer A: Double-blind study of chlordiazepoxide in obstetrics. Obstet Gynecol 24:601-605, 1964
149. Elder MG, Crossley J: A double blind trial of diazepam in labour. J Obstet Gynaecol Brit Comm 76:264-265, 1969
150. Flowers CE, Rudolph AJ, Desmond MM: Diazepam (Valium) as an adjunct in obstetric analgesia. Obstet Gynecol 34:68-81, 1969
151. Friedman EA, Niswander KR, Sachtleben MR: Effect of diazepam on labor. Obstet Gynecol 34:82-86, 1969
152. Lee DT: The effects of diazepam (Valium) on labour. Canad Med Assoc J 98:446-448, 1968
153. Mark PM, Hamel J: Librium for patients in labor. Obstet Gynecol 32:188-194, 1968
154. Nisbet R, Boulas SH, Kantor HI: Diazepam (Valium) during labor. Obstet Gynecol 29:726-729, 1967
155. Niswander KR: Effect of diazepam on meperidine requirements of patients during labor. Obstet Gynecol 34:62-67, 1969
156. Bitnun S: Possible effect of chlordiazepoxide on the fetus. Canad Med Assoc J 100:351, 1969
156a. Suonio S, Kauppila A, Jouppila P, Linna O: The effect of intravenous diazepam on fetal and maternal acid-base balance during and after delivery. Ann Chir Gynaecol Fenn 60:52-55, 1972
157. Joyce DN, Kenyon VG: The use of diazepam and hydrallazine [sic] in the treatment of severe pre-eclampsia. J Obstet Gynaecol Brit Comm 79:250-254, 1972
158. Owen JR, Irani SF, Blair AW: Effect of diazepam administered to mothers during labour on temperature regulation of neonate. Arch Dis Child 47:107-110, 1972
159. Idänpään-Heikkilä JE, Taska RJ, Allen HA, Schoolar JC: Placental transfer of diazepam-14C in mice, hamsters, and monkeys. J Pharmacol Exp Ther 176:752-757, 1971
160. Berte F, Benzi G, Manzo L, Hokari S: Investigation on tissue distribution and metabolism of oxazepam in pregnant guinea-pig and rat. Arch Int Pharmacodyn 173:377-381, 1968

161. Idänpään-Heikkilä JE, Jouppila PI, Puolakka JO, Vorne MS: Placental transfer and fetal metabolism of diazepam in early human pregnancy. Amer J Obstet Gynecol 109:1011-1016, 1971

162. Cavanagh D, Condo CS: Diazepam—a pilot study of drug concentrations in maternal blood, amniotic fluid, and cord blood. Curr Ther Res 6:122-126, 1964

163. Scher J, Hailey DM, Beard RW: The effects of diazepam on the fetus. J Obstet Gynaecol Brit Comm 79:635-638, 1972

164. deSilva JAF, D'Arconte L, Kaplan J: The determination of blood levels and the placental transfer of diazepam in humans. Curr Ther Res 6:115-121, 1964

165. Lean TH, Ratnam SS, Sivasamboo R: The use of chlordiazepoxide in patients with severe pregnancy toxaemia. (A preliminary study of effects on the newborn infants). J Obstet Gynaecol Brit Comm 75:853-855, 1968

166. Decancq HG, Bosco JR, Townsend EH: Chlordiazepoxide in labor. Its effect on the newborn infant. J Pediat 67:836-840, 1965

167. Shannon RW, Fraser GP, Aitken RG, Harper JR: Diazepam in preeclamptic toxaemia with special reference to its effect on the newborn infant. Brit J Clin Prac 26:271-276, 1972

167a. Morselli PL, Principi N, Tognoni G, Sereni F: Diazepam metabolism in premature infants. Pediat Res 6:53, 1972

168. Patrick MJ, Tilstone WJ, Reavey P: Diazepam and breast-feeding. Lancet 1:542-543, 1972

169. Erkkola R, Kanto J: Diazepam and breast feeding. Lancet 1:1235-1236, 1972

170. Elliott PM: The management of eclampsia with intravenous diazepam and protoveratrine. Aust New Zealand J Obstet Gynaecol 10:99-100, 1970

171. El-Zeneiny AH, Ammar AR, Sammour MB, Fikry F: Benzodiazepines in toxaemias of late pregnancy. Ain Shams Med J 20:449-453, 1969

172. Gilbert JE: Relief of eclamptic convulsions with chlordiazepoxide. Clin Med 68:2166-2168, 1961

173. Gorbach AC: Diazepam for eclampsia. Amer J Obstet Gynecol 102:611-612, 1968

174. Lean TH, Ratnam SS, Sivasamboo R: Use of benzodiazepines in the management of eclampsia. J Obstet Gynaecol Brit Comm 75:856-862, 1968

175. Lecart C, Cavanagh D: A clinical evaluation of benzodiazepines in the management of toxemia of pregnancy. Curr Ther Res 6:357-362, 1964

175a. McCarthy GT, O'Connell B, Robinson AE: Blood levels of diazepam in infants of two mothers given large doses of diazepam during labour. J Obstet Gynaecol Brit Comm 80:349-352, 1973

175b. Thearle MJ, Dunn PM, Hailey DM: Exchange transfusion for diazepam intoxication at birth followed by jejunal stenosis. Proc Roy Soc Med 66:349-350, 1973

176. Boris A, Costello J, Gower MM, Welsch JA: Endocrine studies of chlordiazepoxide. Proc Soc Exp Biol Med 106:708-710, 1961

177. Khazan N, Primo C, Danon A, Assael M, Sulman FG, Winnik HZ: The mammotropic effect of tranquillizing drugs. Arch Int Pharmacodyn 136:291-305, 1962

178. Superstine E, Sulman FG: The mechanism of the push and pull principle. VII. Endocrine effects of chlordiazepoxide, diazepam, and guanethidine. Arch Int Pharmacodyn 160:133-146, 1966

179. Lampe WT: Lactation following psychotropic agents. Metabolism 16:257-258, 1967

180. Whitelaw MJ: Menstrual irregularities associated with use of methaminodiazepoxide. JAMA 175:400-401, 1961

181. Kamman GR: Chlordiazepoxide. JAMA 175:1184, 1961

182. Schwartz ED, Smith JJ: The effect of chlordiazepoxide on the female reproductive cycle as tested in infertility patients. Western J Surg Obstet Gynecol 71:74-76, 1963

183. Cahn B: Electrolytes and hormonal balance in human subjects receiving diazepam. Curr Ther Res 8:256-260, 1966

184. Moore SF: Therapy of psychosomatic symptoms in gynecology, an evaluation of chlordiazepoxide. Curr Ther Res 4:249-257, 1962

185. Cromwell HA: Chlordiazepoxide and the management of gynecologic problems. Med Times 90:692-696, 1962

186. McAllister D: Prevalence of common menstrual symptoms. Lancet 2:360, 1963

187. McAllister D: Diazepam in dysmenorrhea. New Zealand Med J 63:448-449, 1964

188. Valenzuela D: Observations on the use of chlordiazepoxide in obstetrics and gynecology. J Philippine Fed Priv Med Prac 13:249-252, 1964

189. Marcos PE: Chlordiazepoxide in the emotional reactions of obstetrical and gynecological patients. J Philippine Fed Priv Med Prac 13:243-248, 1964

190. Pena EF: Psychoneurotic reactions in gynecology and obstetrics. Western Med 3:292-298, 1962

191. Pena EF: Management of the anxious patient in gynecology and obstetrics. J Florida Med Assoc 47:1351-1356, 1961

192. Fromhagen C: Management of emotional disturbances in obstetrical and gynecologic patients. Amer J Obstet Gynecol 87:183-189, 1963

192a. Shader RI, DiMascio A, Harmatz JS: Studies of premenstrual tension. Presented at the 125th Annual Meeting of the American Psychiatric Association. Dallas, Texas, May, 1972

193. Sheffery JB, Wilson TA, Walsh JC: Double-blind, cross-over study comparing chlordiazepoxide, conjugated estrogens, combined chlordiazepoxide and conjugated estrogens and placebo in treatment of the menopause. Med Ann D C 38:433-436, 1969

194. Hazan SJ, Conneely R: The menopause—flush, fantasy, and denial. Western J Surg Obstet Gynecol 72:167-170, 1964

195. Jaques R, Riesterer L: The influence of psychopharmacologically active substances on various models of an inflammatory reaction. Pharmacology 6:29-34, 1971

196. Bluefarb SM: Librium as adjunctive therapy in dermatoses. Skin 1:265-267, 1962

197. Olansky S, Olansky M: Role of chlordiazepoxide in dermatoses. J Med Assoc Georgia 51:349-351, 1962

198. McGovern JP, Haywood TJ, Thomas OC, Fernandez AA: Studies with a benzodiazepine derivative in various allergic diseases. Psychosomatics 4:203-206, 1963

199. Levy SW: A psychosomatic approach to the management of recalcitrant dermatoses. Psychosomatics 4:334-337, 1963

200. Segal AE, Rogin JR: Management of the psychogenic factors in dermatoses by use of chemotherapy. Med Times 92:113-116, 1964

201. Boueri-Atem S, Brahim D, Curi JO: Oxazepam in allergic conditions. Psychosomatics 12:46-48, 1971

202. Musaph H, van Loggem M: Research of chlordiazepoxide (Librium) into normal subjects and neurotics with pathological itching states. Psychiat Neurol Neurochirur 65:402-423, 1962

203. Wexler L: Chlordiazepoxide in selected dermatoses. Curr Ther Res 3:383-386, 1961

204. McCormick GE: Control of the psychogenic factors in skin diseases. J Med Assoc Georgia 55:108-111, 1966

205. Wilkinson DS: Some hazards of trials of tranquillising agents in dermatology, with especial reference to a trial of chlordiazepoxide ('Librium'). In, Proceedings of the XII International Congress of Dermatology. Edited by DM Pillsbury, CS Livingood. Amsterdam, Excerpta Medica Foundation, 1963, pp 1244-1248

206. Grater WC: Allergy symptom survey—evaluation of emotional content in allergy. J Kansas Med Soc 69:479-482, 1968

207. Fennell G: Psychogenic factors in vasomotor rhinorrhea. Brit J Psychiat 109:79-80, 1963

208. Gentles W, Thomas EL: Effect of benzodiazepines upon saccadic eye movements in man. Clin Pharmacol Ther 12:563-574, 1971

209. Norris H: The action of sedatives on brain stem oculomotor systems in man. Neuropharmacology 10:181-191, 1971
210. Ryan RE: Myalgia of the head and its treatment with diazepam. Headache 3:63-66, 1966
211. Ogden HD, Ching C: Librium® in headache relief. Headache 2:99-102, 1962
212. Orbell G: Headaches and eyestrain associated with migraine. Preliminary report of a trial of chlordiazepoxide. Brit J Ophthal 47:246-247, 1963
213. Browning TB: Observations on successful management of the migraine syndrome using chlordiazepoxide. Headache 7:73-76, 1967
214. Fletcher MC: Chlordiazepoxide (Librium) in the treatment of strabismus; a preliminary report. J Amer Med Womens Assoc 16:37-44, 1961
215. Lance JW, Curran DA: Treatment of chronic tension headache. Lancet 1:1236-1239, 1964
216. Okasha A, Ghaleb HA, Sadek A: A double blind trial for the clinical management of psychogenic headache. Brit J Psychiat 122:181-183, 1973
216a. Weber MB: The treatment of muscle contraction headaches with diazepam. Curr Ther Res 15:210-216, 1973
217. Roberts W: The use of psychotropic drugs in glaucoma. Dis Nerv Syst 29 (March supp):40-43, 1968
218. Sekitani T, McCabe BF, Ryu JH: Drug effects on the medial vestibular nucleus. Arch Otolaryngol 93:581-589, 1971
219. Sekitani T, Ryu JH, McCabe BF: Drug effects on the medial vestibular nucleus. Arch Otolaryngol 94:401-405, 1971
220. Miller EF, Graybiel A: Effect of drugs on ocular counterrolling. Clin Pharmacol Ther 10:92-99, 1969
221. Arrigoni-Martelli E, Toth E: Effect of chlordiazepoxide on glucose metabolism in rats. In, *Proceedings of the European Society for the Study of Drug Toxicity. Vol. IX, 1968. Toxicity and Side-Effects of Psychotropic Drugs.* Edited by SBD Baker, JR Boissier, W Koll. Amsterdam, Excerpta Medica Foundation, 1968, pp 73-78
222. Mehta S: The influence of premedication with diazepam on the blood sugar level. Anaesthesia 26:468-472, 1971
223. Mehta S: The influence of anaesthesia with thiopentone and diazepam on the blood sugar level during surgery. Brit J Anaesth 44:75-79, 1972
223a. Gottschalk LA, Noble EP, Stolzoff GE, Bates DE, Cable CG, Uliana RL, Birch H, Fleming EW: Relationships of chlordiazepoxide blood levels to psychological and biochemical responses. In, *The Benzodiazepines.* Edited by S Garattini, E Mussini, LO Randall. New York, Raven Press, 1973, pp 257-280
223b. Arrigoni-Martelli E, Corsico N: On the mechanism of lipomobilizing effect of chlordiazepoxide. J Pharm Pharmacol 21:59-60, 1969
224. Marc V, Morselli PL: Effect of diazepam on plasma corticosterone levels in the rat. J Pharm Pharmacol 21:784-786, 1969
225. Petraitis FP, Hoch FL: The effect of some sedating agents on calorigenesis and its responses to 2,4-dinitrophenol and L-thyroxine in rats. J Pharmacol Exp Ther 177:514-519, 1971
226. Butler PWP, Besser GM, Steinberg H: Changes in plasma cortisol induced by dexamphetamine and chlordiazepoxide given alone and in combination in man. J Endocrinol 40:391-392, 1968
227. Havard CWH, Saldanha VF, Bird R, Gardner R: The effect of diazepam on pituitary function in man. J Endocrinol 52:79-85, 1972
228. Soliman MK, El Amrousi S, Khamis MY: The influence of tranquillisers and barbiturate anaesthesia on the blood picture and electrolytes of dogs. Vet Rec 77:1256-1259, 1965
229. Boris A, Stevenson RH: The effects of some psychotropic drugs on dehydration induced antidiuretic hormone activity in the rat. Arch Int Pharmacodyn 166:486-498, 1967
230. Fariss BL, Kolb FO: Factors involved in crystal formation in cystinuria. JAMA 205:846-848, 1968

231. Ettinger B, Kolb FO: Chlordiazepoxide and cystinuric calculus. JAMA 212:627, 1970
232. Vyden JK, Curnow DH, Beck AB, Boundy CAP: Failure of chlordiazepoxide to influence urinary copper excretion. Lancet 2:1090, 1972
233. Rice AJ, Gruhn SW, Gibson TP, Delle M, DiBona GF: Effect of saline infusion on the renal excretion of secobarbital, meprobamate, and chlordiazepoxide. J Lab Clin Med 80:56-62, 1972
234. Cruz IA, Cramer NC, Parrish AE: Hemodialysis in chlordiazepoxide toxicity. JAMA 202:438-440, 1967

Chapter 8
Experimental Stress and Effects on Performance

In its broadest sense, psychological stress refers to an emotionally disruptive influence. The simplest form of stress in both clinical and experimental settings is a noxious stimulus such as shock, noise, or odor. Forced immobilization is a significant stress for laboratory animals. More sophisticated forms of experimental stress include confrontation with insoluble problems or anxiety-provoking situations. At its most complex, stress occurs outside the laboratory as the subtle pressure to perform and achieve encountered by most civilized human beings. At all levels, stress is relative. A particular electrical stimulus may be an intolerably painful shock for one animal but a mere tingle for another. A 12-hr working day may be welcome to some, whereas 8 hr of work can be profoundly oppressive to others.

Numerous physiological and biochemical correlates of stress have been studied, including changes in metabolism of catecholamines, corticosteroids, glucose, and lipids, as well as alterations in autonomic nervous system function. Excessive and/or chronic stress presumably is bad for the organism, as suggested by the clear association of such stress with gastric erosion and mortality in animals, and by the possible association with such entities as ischemic heart disease, hypertension, peptic ulcer, and inflammatory bowel disease in humans.

Chapter 3 discusses the influence of the benzodiazepines on the behavioral sequelae of stress. Physiologic responses, in both animals and humans, are reviewed in this chapter. Also discussed is the closely related problem of whether the benzodiazepines alter actual performance in the stressful situation; more specifically, what is their effect on intellectual and motor function?

EXPERIMENTAL STRESS IN ANIMALS

Electric shock or immobilization reduces the brain content of norepinephrine and increases its turnover, suggesting that stress activates noradrenergic neuron activity. When rats are pretreated with parenteral chlordiazepoxide or diazepam (10 mg/kg), the stress-induced increase in norepinephrine turnover is prevented.[1-3] Electrical activity in noradrenergic neurons innervating the cortex is reduced, as well as the animal's overall state of agitation. Peripheral responses are also attenuated. Shock stress in rats produces elevations in plasma corticosteroids, free fatty acids, glucose, and lactate. Pretreatment of the animals with intraperitoneal chlordiazepoxide (15 to 50 mg/kg) or diazepam (5 mg/kg) significantly inhibits these biochemical sequelae.[4-7] In rabbits, electric shock is followed by a fall in the peripheral eosinophil count. Administration of chlordiazepoxide prior to the shock prevents this fall, although exogenous cortisol still produces eosinopenia.[8] Centrifugal stress in rats causes depletion of adrenal ascorbic acid and cholesterol which is preventable by pretreatment with chlordiazepoxide (10 mg/kg).[9]

Birnbaum[10] has demonstrated that optic and acoustic stimuli which are noxious to rats produce a high incidence of gastric erosions and increase gastric secretion of acid and fluid. With diazepam pretreatment, gastric erosions are much less frequent and acid secretion is significantly reduced. Daily shock stress to rabbits produces gastric congestion, ulceration, and hemorrhage after 3 weeks. When chlordiazepoxide (50 mg/kg) is administered prior to each daily shock, no hemorrhages or ulcerations are seen.[11]

Other investigators have studied vibration and forced running as experimental models of stress. Aston and Roberts[12] found that 20 min of vibration was lethal to 50% of mice in their test system. Among mice pretreated with intraperitoneal chlordiazepoxide (50 mg/kg), the same duration of vibration was lethal to only 13%. The combination of amphetamine (15 mg/kg) and revolving drum stress was lethal for 100% of untreated rats, but for only 33% of rats receiving chlordiazepoxide (20 mg/kg).[13] Guinea pigs passively sensitized to bovine serum albumin (BSA) have a mortality rate of greater than 90% when challenged with BSA, but this is reduced to 0% by pretreatment with chlordiazepoxide (10 to 40 mg/kg).[14] Diazepam (1 mg/kg) prolongs survival and delays the onset of convulsions in rabbits stressed by exposure to pure oxygen at three atmospheres of pressure.[15]

Noxious olfactory stimuli produce bradycardia and characteristic behavioral responses in rabbits which can be prevented by diazepam (1 to 10 mg/kg).[16] Conditioned physiological responses such as hypertension and hyperthermia are also attenuated by benzodiazepines.[17,18] Kamano and Arp[19] have made a paradoxical observation in a study of rats subjected to chronic nonlethal shock stress. When given a voluntary choice between drug-free and chlordiazepoxide-containing water, the animals' consumption of drugged water diminished.

Two authors have noted paradoxical biochemical effects. Adrenocorticotropic hormone (ACTH) infusion elevates plasma citrate levels and produces hypocalcemia in fasted rabbits. Chlordiazepoxide (2 mg/kg) reduces plasma citrate and causes no change in calcium.[20] When given together with ACTH, chlordiazepoxide potentiates the ACTH-induced rise in citrate levels. Nomura[21] studied rat liver tryptophan pyrrolase (RLTP) activity under various conditions. Forced running, immobilization, and hypothermia increase RLTP activity; diazepam also produces an increase.

With rare exceptions, experimental observations show that the benzo-diazepines attenuate the physiological and biochemical sequelae of stress in laboratory animals.

PAIN

Experimental evidence concerning the analgesic properties of the benzodiazepines is examined in Chapter 3. In general, studies have failed to demonstrate specific analgesic properties but do reveal that high doses of benzodiazepines impair the motor response to painful stimulation. Compo-nents of the response to pain have been examined using the model of tail-shock in rats. Low levels of shock cause a reflex motor response—extension of the hind legs. Slightly higher intensities also produce a vocal reaction during the shock which ceases after termination of the stimulus. High-intensity stimu-lation produces not only motor and vocalization reflexes during the shock but also a vocal "after-discharge"—a persistent vocalization after the shock has ceased. The latter response is thought to represent the emotional impact of the shock. Chlordiazepoxide (15 mg/kg orally) elevates the threshold for all three of these responses,[22] but examination of the dose-effect relationship for each shows that the vocalization after-discharge is the most sensitive to the benzodiazepines while the two reflex responses are relatively insensitive.[23] These results are consistent with the hypothesis that the benzodiazepines are much more potent in attenuating the emotional response to pain than in altering the actual sensation of pain.

Pain tolerance in humans has not been extensively investigated. Some of the studies cited in Chapter 7 suggest that diazepam reduces the opiate requirements in obstetrical patients during labor. In a study of pain induced by anterior tibial pressure, Morrison[24] found that intravenous diazepam (10 mg) produced no changes in sensitivity. The interaction of pain and emotion in humans is complex. Singh and Verma[25] compared chlordiazepoxide (30 to 150 mg/day) to several tricyclic antidepressants in a 1-month study of patients with persistent somatic pain but without demonstrable organic dis-ease. Patients with typical anxiety neuroses were excluded from the study. Improvement was reported in 70% of patients receiving antidepressants but in only 10% of those on chlordiazepoxide. The authors interpret the results as suggesting that in some patients persistent somatic pain of unknown etiology may indicate an underlying depressive illness. The influence of psychotropic drugs on pain can be expected to depend on the etiology of the pain as well as the associated primary and secondary emotional disorders.

STRESS IN HUMANS

A number of methods have been used to create stressful situations for the purposes of laboratory testing. Cutaneous electric shock, venipuncture, unpleasant noise, or the threat of shock as signaled by a conditioned stimulus are among the simplest. Arithmetic and problem-solving stress are also used. Anxiety-provoking movies are a reliable source of experimental stress. Some investigators have utilized intravenous infusions of yohimbine. Occasionally, the experimental setting alone is sufficient. The response to stress can be measured by monitoring vital signs (heart rate, blood pressure, respiratory rate), skin resistance and temperature, or finger pulse volume. Plasma free fatty acids and urinary catecholamines are reliable biochemical parameters. Behavioral responses and changes in mood can be assessed by global ratings or by self-rating scales, as discussed in Chapter 4.

In three reports, "stressor" films were used to induce anxiety and somatic reactions. Pillard and Fisher[26] selected high-anxious normal volunteers using the Taylor Manifest Anxiety Scale. Subjects received either chlordiazepoxide (15 mg), secobarbital (100 mg), or placebo, and completed the Psychiatric Outpatient Mood Scale before and after exposure to the film. Tension and anxiety as measured by this mood scale rose markedly after the film, with no significant difference among treatment groups. Fatigue scores were significantly higher in subjects receiving active sedative drugs than in those receiving placebo. Clemens and Selesnick[27] exposed anxious subjects to a stressful film before and after 1 week of treatment with diazepam or placebo. Heart rate, respiratory rate, finger pulse volume, and skin potential were measured during the film, and from these an overall autonomic reactivity score was calculated. Diazepam-treated patients had lower scores on the second exposure to the film suggesting to the authors that "adaptation" to the stress had occurred. In the placebo group, reaction was greater on the second exposure. The difference was highly significant. The same group reported a similar study using asthmatic patients.[28] In addition to the physiological measures, a respiratory reactivity score was calculated from a combination of vital capacity and expiratory cogwheeling. The film was shown only once, following 1 week of diazepam or placebo therapy. Autonomic scores in response to the film did not significantly differ between groups, but respiratory reactivity was significantly smaller in diazepam recipients than in the placebo group.

Shock-induced stress has been used by several groups. Brown and associates[29] studied heart rate, skin potential, and plasma free fatty acids in subjects receiving one dose of either oxazepam (30 mg) or placebo. Oxazepam significantly attenuated the stress-induced rise in plasma free fatty acids. Frostadt and co-workers[30] report that skin potential responses to shock and to arithmetic problem-solving are reduced in subjects pretreated with diazepam compared with those receiving placebo. Biscaldi and associates[31] used psychic and sensory stimuli to induce skin potential changes. Desmethyldiazepam (5 mg) produced greater inhibition of skin potential response than diazepam (5 mg) or oxazepam (10 mg). In all groups, the drugs influenced the response to psychic stimulation more than to sensory stimulation.

Holmberg and William-Olsson[32] produced stress in normal male subjects by noise, an insoluble problem, and intravenous yohimbine. There were few drug effects upon physiologic parameters, but chlordiazepoxide recipients reported a positive subjective impression of the yohimbine experience more often than did those receiving placebo. Gottschalk and associates[33] studied the anxiety content of spontaneous verbiage in prisoner volunteers. When given in parenteral doses of 5 mg, lorazepam significantly reduced anxiety content. Phenobarbital, placebo, and lorazepam in doses lower or higher than 5 mg had no significant effect. The reasons for this dose-specific association are not clear. The same effect was noted in a subsequent study, although the sample size was small.[33a]

The studies cited above differ considerably in design and in methods of evaluation, yet they suggest with some consistency that the benzodiazepines may attenuate the psychophysiological response to experimental stress in human subjects.

PERFORMANCE

A knowledge of the degree to which the benzodiazepines impair intellectual and motor performance is essential to guide the choice of circumstances in which the drugs may be used clinically. The testing of human performance in the laboratory is a highly developed science. Many approaches have been devised, but most testing systems examine some aspect of intellectual function, motor coordination and performance, and reaction time. The categories overlap considerably. Reaction time may appear to be slowed, for example, if the intellectual ability to discriminate or recognize stimuli is impaired, or if poor motor function precludes a rapid response. Often it is unclear how drug effects upon these laboratory tests extrapolate to the tasks faced in real life situations. Patients and physicians are justifiably concerned that sedative or antianxiety drugs may impair higher intellectual function, capacity for quick recognition and reaction, or ability to safely operate industrial machinery or an automobile. Only a few studies, however, deal with the influence of the benzodiazepines upon such realistic tasks. In general, reliable answers can be provided only in terms of drug effects upon such things as arithmetic, card sorting, tapping speed, or digit recall—admittedly somewhat contrived laboratory tests. Nearly all of the reports cited in this section are single-dose studies, in which performance is assessed within a few hours after drug ingestion. "Hangover" effects—drowsiness or impairment of performance the morning after use of a hypnotic medication—are discussed in Chapter 9. The interaction of benzodiazepines with ethanol are reviewed in Chapter 11.

Critical flicker fusion (CFF) frequency is a quantitative, reproducible test of discriminative cortical function used by many investigators. The CFF frequency falls with fatigue or administration of central depressant drugs. Dose-dependent effects of chlordiazepoxide on CFF frequency are evident. In doses of 10 and 20 mg, chlordiazepoxide-induced changes do not differ significantly from placebo.[34,35] At doses of 40 to 60 mg, chlordiazepoxide significantly lowers the CFF frequency.[35,36] Diazepam (10 mg orally or 0.05 mg/kg intravenously) lowers both CFF and auditory flutter fusion (AFF) frequency, the auditory analogue of CFF.[37-40] Lorazepam in oral doses of 1 and 2 mg significantly reduces CFF frequency.[41] Besser has studied the time course of action of oral diazepam.[38,39] Both AFF and CFF frequencies are maximally depressed 2 hr after a 10-mg oral dose; significant depression disappears at approximately 6 hr. Many of these studies involve comparisons with barbiturates and phenothiazines, which, in usual therapeutic doses, profoundly depress both CFF and AFF frequencies.

Benzodiazepine effects upon other aspects of psychomotor function have been investigated using a variety of laboratory tests. Kissin and associates[42] showed that chlorpromazine (50 mg), meprobamate (800 mg), chlordiazepoxide (50 mg), and pentobarbital (100 mg) significantly improved performance in acutely psychotic patients, suggesting that the drugs temporarily reverse the disruption associated wih acute psychiatric stress. Linnoila and Mattila[43] studied the effects of diazepam (5 and 10 mg orally) on laboratory tests of psychomotor skills related to automobile operation in normal volunteers. In many of the tests, improvement in performance was noted after diazepam, together with subjective reports of mood elevation and increased confidence. In none of the tests did diazepam impair performance in comparison to placebo. Several other controlled trials demonstrate that benzodiazepines neither impair nor improve performance.[44-50] In many studies, however, the benzodiazepines produce a dose-dependent impairment of performance in some or all of the laboratory tests utilized. Clear psychomotor depression is usually seen after single doses of 40 to 50 mg of chlordiazepoxide,[35,36,51] 2 to 4 mg of lorazepam,[41,52,53] 5 to 10 mg of diazepam[52,54,55] or nitrazepam,[56-58] and 15 mg of flurazepam.[58] Depressant doses correlate well with those that significantly lower CFF frequency. Of particular interest is the high milligram potency of lorazepam,[33a,41,52,59] at least five to 10 times that of diazepam. Sedation occurs after 1 mg of lorazepam, sleep after 2.5 mg, and deep sleep after 4 to 5 mg.[33a,59]

Reggiani and associates[60] reported the effects of a single 10-mg dose of chlordiazepoxide upon a number of tests of driving proficiency in experienced automobile drivers. This single dose produced no evidence of impairment. Betts and co-workers,[61] however, administered 50 mg of chlordiazepoxide in divided doses over the 36 hr prior to tests of vehicle handling by normal volunteers. At this dosage, significant impairment of automobile driving performance was demonstrated. Further study of this important problem is needed.

COMMENT

It is hardly a surprise that the benzodiazepines share with other sedative-hypnotics the capacity to impair human intellectual function, motor performance, coordination, and reaction time. Animal studies (Chapter 3) suggested that antianxiety or disinhibitory effects may be seen at smaller doses that those which are neurotoxic. This undoubtedly is true for many human beings as well. Reduction of anxiety often occurs after single doses of 5 to 20 mg of chlordiazepoxide or 2 to 4 mg of diazepam—doses which do not consistently produce intellectual and motor impairment in the laboratory. In some individuals, however, daily doses of 60 to 100 mg of chlordiazepoxide or 30 to 40 mg of diazepam are necessary to reduce anxiety or agitation. Clearly, such patients should be cautioned regarding the possible hazards of high dosage. The possible cumulative effects of chlordiazepoxide and diazepam must always be remembered. Both diazepam and its pharmacologically active metabolite desmethyldiazepam will accumulate in the serum during the first 5 days of therapy with the parent drug (see Chapter 2). Few if any of the studies of psychomotor performance involve chronic benzodiazepine therapy.

The data cited in this chapter suggest that the benzodiazepines may attenuate the psychophysiological responses to stress and anxiety-provoking situations. Many anxious individuals are only intermittently symptomatic, with exacerbations occurring in response to specific personal stressful life events. In such patients, the correspondingly intermittent use of antianxiety agents is a rational approach to therapy. Not only are the hazards of cumulative effects and of long-term psychomotor impairment minimized by this approach, but the effectiveness of the drug is more likely to be preserved. Chapter 4 reviews a number of studies in which benzodiazepines proved superior to placebo early in the investigation but with differences diminishing or disappearing after weeks of continuous therapy. The concept of adjusting drug therapy to meet the needs of the individual patient is a well-worn cliché, but it remains the single most useful guideline to the prescription of antianxiety agents.

REFERENCES

1. Taylor KM: The effect of minor tranquillizers on stress-induced noradrenaline turnover in the rat brain. Proc Univ Otago Med School 47:33-35, 1969

2. Taylor KM, Laverty R: The effect of chlordiazepoxide, diazepam, and nitrazepam on catecholamine metabolism in regions of the rat brain. Eur J Pharmacol 8:296-301, 1969

3. Corrodi H, Fuxe K, Lidbrink P, Olson L: Minor tranquilizers, stress and central catecholamine neurons. Brain Res 29:1-16, 1971

4. Krulik R, Cerny M: Influence of chlordiazepoxide on blood corticosterone under repeated stress. Activ Nerv Sup 14:31-34, 1972

5. Krulik R, Cerny M: Effect of chlordiazepoxide on stress in rats. Life Sci 10(part I):145-151, 1971

6. Khan AU, Forney RB, Hughes FW: Plasma free fatty acids in rats after shock as modified by centrally active drugs. Arch Int Pharmacodyn 151:466-474, 1964

7. Satoh T, Iwamoto T: Neurotropic drugs, electroshock, and carbohydrate metabolism in the rat. Biochem Pharmacol 15:323-331, 1966

8. Dasgupta SR, Mukherjee BP: Effect of chlordiazepoxide on eosinopenia of stress in rabbits. Nature (London) 213:199-200, 1967

9. Pohujani SM, Chittal SM, Raut VS, Sheth UK: Studies in stress-induced changes on rat's adrenals. Part I. Effects of central nervous system depressants. Indian J Med Res 57:1081-1086, 1969

10. Birnbaum D: The influence of psychotropic drugs on gastrointestinal function: experimental and clinical data. In, *Psychotropic Drugs in Internal Medicine.* Edited by A Pletscher, A Marino, P Pinkerton. Amsterdam, Excerpta Medica Foundation, 1969, pp 101-108

11. Dasgupta SR, Mukherjee BP: Effect of chlordiazepoxide on stomach ulcers in rabbit induced by stress. Nature (London) 215:1183, 1967

12. Aston R, Roberts VL: The effect of drugs on vibration tolerance. Arch Int Pharmacodyn 155:289-299, 1965

13. Goldberg ME, Salama AI: Amphetamine toxicity and brain monoamines in three models of stress. Toxicol Appl Pharmacol 14:447-456, 1969

14. Kosunen TU, Visakorpi R: Studies in the prevention of fatal anaphylactic shock in guinea pigs. Ann Med Exp Biol Fenn 42:185-187, 1964

15. Toth S, Ungar B, Szilagyi T: Data to the anticonvulsive effect of Valium® diazepam in experimental hyperoxia and guinea-pig anaphylaxis. Int J Clin Pharmacol 2:139-141, 1969

16. Steiner JE, Goldstein S: Effect of LSD, mescaline, and diazepam on olfactory stimuli in the unanesthetized rabbit. Israel J Med Sci 7:707, 1971

17. Benson H, Herd JA, Morse WH, Kelleher RT: Hypotensive effects of chlordiazepoxide, amobarbital, and chlorpromazine on behaviorally induced elevated arterial blood pressure in the squirrel monkey. J Pharmacol Exp Ther 173:399-406, 1970

18. Delina-Stula A, Morpurgo C: The influence of a fear-evoking situation on the rectal temperature of rats. Int J Psychobiol 1:71-75, 1970

19. Kamano DK, Arp DJ: Chlordiazepoxide (Librium) consumption under stress conditions in rats. Int J Neuropsychiat 1:189-192, 1965

20. Natelson S, Walker AA, Pincus JB: Chlordiazepoxide and diphenylhydantoin as antagonists to ACTH effect on serum calcium and citrate levels. Proc Soc Exp Biol Med 122:689-692, 1966

21. Nomura J: Effect of stress and psychotropic drugs on rat liver tryptophan pyrrolase. Endocrinology 76:1190-1194, 1965

22. Cahn J, Herold M: Pain and psychotropic drugs. In, *Pain.* Edited by A Soulairac, J Cahn, J Charpentier. London and New York, Academic Press, 1968, pp 335-371

23. Hoffmeister F: Effects of psychotropic drugs on pain. In, *Pain.* Edited by A Soulairac, J Cahn, J Charpentier. London and New York, Academic Press, 1968, pp 309-319

24. Morrison JD: Alterations in response to somatic pain associated with anaesthesia. XIX. Studies with the drugs used in neuroleptanaesthesia. Brit J Anaesth 42:838-848, 1970.

25. Singh G, Verma HC: Drug treatment of chronic intractable pain in patients referred to

a psychiatry clinic. J Indian Med Assoc 56:341-345, 1971

26. Pillard RC, Fisher S: Effects of chlordiazepoxide and secobarbital on film-induced anxiety. Psychopharmacologia 12:18-23, 1967

27. Clemens TL, Selesnick ST: Psychological method for evaluating medication by repeated exposure to a stressor film. Dis Nerv Syst 28:98-104, 1967

28. Selesnick ST, Malmstrom EJ, Younger J, Lederman AR: Induced somatic reactions in asthmatic adults. (Their reduction by use of a psychotropic drug). Dis Nerv Syst 30:385-391, 1969

29. Brown ML, Sletten IW, Kleinman KM, Korol B: Effects of oxazepam on psychological responses to stress in normal subjects. Curr Ther Res 10:543-553, 1968

30. Frostadt AL, Forrest GL, Bakker CB: Influence of personality type on drug response. Amer J Psychiat 122:1153-1158, 1966

31. Biscaldi GP, Hattab J, Montanaro N, Scoz R: Quantitative polygraphic evaluation of emotional tension in the study of a new benzodiazepine. Curr Ther Res 13:606-615, 1971

32. Holmberg G, William-Olsson U: Effects of benzquinamide, in comparison with chlordiazepoxide and placebo, on subjective experiences and autonomic phenomena in stress experiments. Psychopharmacologia 5:147-157, 1964

33. Gottschalk LA, Elliott HW, Bates DE, Cable CG: Content analysis of speech samples to determine effect of lorazepam on anxiety. Clin Pharmacol Ther 13:323-328, 1972

33a. Comer WH, Elliott HW, Nomof N, Navarro G, Ruelius HW, Knowles JA: Pharmacology of parenterally administered lorazepam in man. J Int Med Res 1:216-225, 1973

34. Lind NA, Turner P: The effect of chlordiazepoxide and fluphenazine on critical flicker frequency. J Pharm Pharmacol 20:804, 1968

35. Idestrom C-M, Cadenius B: Chlordiazepoxide, dipiperon, and amobarbital. Dose effect studies on human beings. Psychopharmacologia 4:235-246, 1963

36. Holmberg G, William-Olsson U: The effect of benzquinamide, in comparison with chlordiazepoxide and placebo, on performance in some psychological tests. Psychopharmacologia 4:402-417, 1963

37. Healy TEJ, Lautch H, Hall N, Tomlin PJ, Vickers MD: Interdisciplinary study of diazepam sedation for outpatient dentistry. Brit Med J 3:13-17, 1970

37a. Besser GM: Auditory flutter fusion as a measure of the actions of centrally acting drugs: modification of the threshold for fusion and the influence of adapting stimuli. Brit J Pharmacol Chemother 30:329-340, 1967

38. Besser GM: Time course of action of diazepam. Nature (London) 214:428, 1967

39. Besser GM, Duncan C: The time course of action of single doses of diazepam, chlorpromazine, and some barbiturates as measured by auditory flutter fusion and visual flicker fusion thresholds in man. Brit J Pharmacol Chemother 30:341-348, 1967

40. Grove-White IG, Kelman GR: Critical flicker frequency after small doses of methohexitone, diazepam, and sodium 4-hydroxybutyrate. Brit J Anaesth 43:110-112, 1971

41. Hedges A, Turner P, Harry TVA: Preliminary studies on the central effects of lorazepam, a new benzodiazepine. J Clin Pharmacol 11:423-427, 1971

42. Kissin B, Tripp CA, Fluckiger FA, Weinberg GH: Effect of ataractic drugs on motor control in acute hospitalized psychiatric patients. J Neuropsychiat 4:409-412, 1963

43. Linnoila M, Mattila MJ: Drug interaction on psychomotor skills related to driving: diazepam and alcohol. Eur J Clin Pharmacol 5:186-194, 1973

44. Austen DP, Gilmartin BA, Turner P: The effect of chlordiazepoxide on visual field, extraocular muscle balance, colour matching ability, and hand-eye co-ordination in man. Brit J Physiol Optics 26:161-165, 1971

44a. Gendreau P, Sherlock D, Parsons T, McLean R, Scott GD, Suboski MD: Effects of methamphetamine on well-practiced discrimination conditioning of the eyelid response. Psychopharmacologia 25:112-116, 1972

45. Mulero R, Kelley JW, Fauth DL: The effects of Valium on psychological testing. Nebraska State Med J 48:499-505, 1963

46. Ogle M, Ditman KS: Librium (chlordiazepoxide) and mental functioning in normal subjects. In, *Neuro-Psycho-Pharmacology*. Edited by H Brill. Amsterdam, Excerpta Medica Foundation, 1966, pp 1235-1239

47. Hughes FW, Forney RB, Richards AB: Comparative effects in human subjects of chlordiazepoxide, diazepam, and placebo on mental and physical performance. Clin Pharmacol Ther 6:139-145, 1965

48. Bernstein ME, Hughes FW, Forney RB: The influence of a new chlordiazepoxide analogue on human mental and motor performance. J Clin Pharmacol 7:330-335, 1967

49. Lawton MP, Cahn B: The effects of diazepam (Valium®) and alcohol on psychomotor performance. J Nerv Ment Dis 136:550-554, 1963

50. Newman MG, Trieger N, Loskota WJ, Jacobs AW: A comparative study of psychomotor effects of intravenous agents used in dentistry. Oral Surg Oral Med Oral Pathol 30:34-40, 1970

51. Brimer A, Schnieden H, Simon A: The effect of chlorpromazine and chlordiazepoxide on cognitive functioning. Brit J Psychiat 110:723-725, 1964

52. Harry TVA, Richards DJ: Lorazepam—a study in psychomotor depression. Brit J Clin Prac 26:371-373, 1972

53. Bell RW, Dickie DS, Stewart-Jones J, Turner P: Lorazepam on visuomotor co-ordination and visual function in man. J Pharm Pharmacol 25:87-88, 1973

54. Masuda M, Bakker CB: Personality, catecholamine metabolites, and psychophysiological response to diazepam. J Psychiat Res 4:221-234, 1966

55. Jaattela A, Mannisto P, Paatero H, Tuomisto J: The effects of diazepam or diphenhydramine on healthy human subjects. Psychopharmacologia 21:202-211, 1971

56. Malpas A, Joyce CRB: Effects of nitrazepam, amylobarbitone, and placebo on some perceptual, motor and cognitive tasks in normal subjects. Psychopharmacologia 14:167-177, 1969

57. Malpas A: Subjective and objective effects of nitrazepam and amylobarbitone in normal human subjects. Psychopharmacologia 27:373-378, 1972

58. Sambrooks JE, MacCulloch MJ, Birtles CJ, Smallman C: Assessment of the effects of flurazepam and nitrazepam on visuo-motor performance using an automated assessment technique. Acta Psychiat Scand 48:443-454, 1972

59. Elliott HW, Nomof N, Navarro G, Ruelius HW, Knowles JA, Comer WH: Central nervous system and cardiovascular effects of lorazepam in man. Clin Pharmacol Ther 12:468-481, 1971

60. Reggiani G, Hurlimann A, Theiss E: Some aspects of the experimental and clinical toxicology of chlordiazepoxide. In, *Proceedings of the European Society for the Study of Drug Toxicity*, Vol. 9. *Toxicity and Side-Effects of Psychotropic Drugs*. Edited by SBD Baker, JR Boissier, W Koll. Amsterdam, Excerpta Medica Foundation, 1968, pp 79-97

61. Betts TA, Clayton AB, MacKay GM: Effects of four commonly-used tranquillizers on low-speed driving performance tests. Brit Med J 4:580-584, 1972

Chapter 9
Sleep

The pharmacologic approach to disorders of sleep is a matter of great medical and social importance. Patients with disturbed sleep, like those with overt anxiety, are symptomatic for a reason. The etiology of the disorder sometimes can be elicited by brief history-taking, but it also may be exceedingly complex and time-consuming to determine. Far too often physicians prescribe hypnotic drugs for patients with disordered sleep without making an attempt to uncover the cause.

Insomnia frequently results from somatic pain. Rheumatoid arthritis, dental caries, traumatic injuries, surgery, metastatic malignancy, peptic ulcer, and ischemic heart disease are among numerous entities notorious for producing nocturnal pain and disordered sleep. For such patients, analgesics or other specific therapy are more rational than hypnotics. When congestive heart failure causes nocturnal dyspnea or cough, hypnotics make little sense. Nocturia and polyuria sufficient to interfere with sleep may occur in cases of prostatic hypertrophy, urinary tract infection, or uncontrolled diabetes mellitus. Patients with ulcerative colitis and regional enteritis frequently are awakened by rectal urgency and the need to defecate. In cases such as these, it is usually evident that therapeutic efforts are best directed at the underlying disease. Insomnia is common in old age. Elderly individuals who complain that they "can't sleep like they used to" can be reassured that their need for sleep decreases with age, so that reduced sleep time is a normal phenomenon.

The relation of insomnia to anxiety may not be so obvious. During periods of emotional stress, anxious individuals may have difficulty falling asleep because of overalertness or preoccupation with life events. Consecutive nights of poor sleep tend to reinforce worry and frustration, creating a self-perpetuating cycle. Eventually, the cycle breaks when the stressful situation remits or when extreme fatigue supervenes. The physician may intervene beneficially simply by listening to the patient's problems or by discussing the feelings which keep him awake. Many patients are helped by traditional sleep aids such as a hot bath or a glass of warm milk at bedtime. If these measures fail, a few nights of hypnotic drug therapy or a short course of antianxiety medication with half or two-thirds of the daily dose given at bedtime, will usually restore sleep habits to their pre-crisis norm.

The association of disordered sleep with depression and melancholia is

important to recognize. In anxious or neurotic depressive states, the disturbance may be one of inability to fall asleep. In patients with more severe
endogenous illnesses, early morning awakening is a classic symptom. Central
depressant drugs may not only fail to improve sleep but may also contribute
to the vegetative aspects of depression, such as inanition, lethargy, and withdrawal from outside activity. At worst, the prescription of hypnotic drugs
for such patients can even provide them with a convenient, painless means
of self-destruction. Physicians should carefully consider the patient's pattern
of insomnia and the possibility that depression is the etiologic basis, in which
case hypnotic medications should be used only with the utmost caution.
"Refill p.r.n." prescriptions for short-acting barbiturates or glutethimide are
seldom rational; for depressed patients, they are certainly unjustified.

A number of recent reviews have discussed clinical and pharmacologic
considerations underlying the choice and sound use of hypnotic drugs.[1-7]
Assuming there is a rational indication for the prescription of a sleeping
medication, harm is seldom done regardless of the choice of hypnotic agent
provided it is used only occasionally or for short periods of time. In the
absence of obvious contraindications such as impending respiratory failure
or hepatic precoma, most hospitalized patients receive hypnotic drugs.[8-10]
The combination of suspected or documented organic disease together with
the nature of the hospital setting is extremely stressful and anxiety-provoking,
and a substantial proportion of hospitalized patients would be sleepless without
pharmacologic assistance. Among outpatients, hypnotic use in isolated
circumstances, such as during an overnight train ride, is not unreasonable
provided the possibility of "hangover" is recognized. The long-term use of
hypnotics, however, is not likely to be so benign. True physiologic habituation
and addiction to these drugs in their usual dosage range is probably
uncommon, but a more subtle kind of dependence—the inability to sleep
without medication—*is* common. This type of hypnotic dependence is in
part related to the physician's prescribing practice and the frequency of his
follow-up.[11,12] "Refill p.r.n." prescriptions with scant follow-up are associated
with hypnotic dependence in nearly one-third of patients after 1 year. When
the physician sees the patient and reviews the problem at frequent intervals
before renewing prescriptions, dependence occurs in less than 10% of patients.
From a purely medical standpoint, long-term hypnotic prescription makes
no more sense than treating persisting fever of unknown etiology with
salicylates alone. Unexplained, continuing insomnia deserves thorough medical
and psychiatric valuation.

Why certain benzodiazepines are promoted and used exclusively as hypnotics rather than antianxiety agents is a mystery. Nitrazepam, flurazepam,
and flunitrazepam are primarily sleep-inducing medications. Reexamination
of the basic pharmacologic properties of flurazepam, for example, reveals
no characteristics which would predict this drug to be more or less useful
as a hypnotic agent than other benzodiazepines.[13,14] The probable explantion,

mentioned in Chapter 2, is a pharmacokinetic rather than a neuropharmacologic one—benzodiazepines which are slowly detoxified and excreted are unsuitable as hypnotics. Adequate doses of chlordiazepoxide and diazepam will induce sleep, but the rates of metabolism and excretion are such that drowsiness and psychomotor impairment are likely to persist well into the next day. Additionally, repeated use may lead to accumulation of the drugs and their active metabolites. With flurazepam, hypnotic doses appear to be "washed out" by the next day.

Benzodiazepine-induced sleep is postulated to differ from sleep produced by older hypnotic drugs such as the barbiturates and glutethimide. Animal studies have suggested that the barbiturates impair the cortical response to stimulation and elevate the mesencephalic reticular arousal threshold.[15] The benzodiazepines, on the other hand, have little effect upon the arousal threshold but depress the hippocampus, thereby reducing vigilance and allowing physiologic sleep to supervene. Electroencephalographic (EEG) studies in humans have documented further differences between barbiturate and benzodiazepine sleep, as will be discussed subsequently. The degree to which these differences are of concern to the practicing physician and his patient is far from clear.

NITRAZEPAM

Experimental evaluations of hypnotic drug efficacy have utilized many subject populations, including normal or asymptomatic volunteers, insomniac volunteers, hospitalized medical or surgical patients, and hospitalized psychiatric patients. Drug effects on total duration of sleep and the time for onset of sleep can be determined by interview, observation, or by continuous EEG recordings. The number of spontaneous awakenings can likewise be quantitated. Subjects may be asked for a retrospective evaluation of the quality of sleep and, in crossover trials, for a drug preference. Evaluation of "hangover" or residual effects upon awakening is included in most studies. The sleep laboratory clearly allows objective measurement of many parameters of sleep; however, sleep laboratory studies are expensive, and therefore usually involve a relatively small number of subjects. Studies can be carried out in the home with no investigator interference at the time of sleep, but unless special equipment is available, evaluations are limited to self-rated subjective judgments. The suggestion that subjects' sleep patterns in a laboratory setting differ from those in the normal home environment appears not to be tenable. Kales and associates[16] used telemetric physiologic recording devices to show that home and laboratory sleep patterns are very similar. Their results suggest that objective sleep analysis can be performed either in the laboratory or by telemetric recording at home with essentially equal validity.

Despite the great differences between subject populations and the difficulties inherent in sleep research, placebo-controlled studies show with almost complete uniformity that nitrazepam is superior to a placebo as a sleep-inducing agent.[17-28] Compared to inactive medication, nitrazepam lengthens total sleep time, shortens the onset of sleep, reduces awakenings, and improves the subjective quality of sleep. Oral doses of either 5 or 10 mg are effective. leRiche and associates[24] compared the two dose levels in a study of patients hospitalized in a chronic disease institution. Both 5 mg and 10 mg of nitrazepam were equally effective in improving sleep, but the large dose produced morning drowsiness far more frequently.

When compared to other hypnotic agents, nitrazepam is almost always equally effective. Comparison drugs have included amobarbital (100 to 200 mg),[18,21-23,26,29] secobarbital (100 to 200 mg),[19,24] phenobarbital (100 mg),[20] butabarbital (50 to 200 mg),[23,27,30] glutethimide (250 to 500 mg),[25,30] and Mandrax.*[21,28] In two studies, nitrazepam was marginally superior to barbiturate[18] and glutethimide,[30] but in all others nitrazepam and other active medications were found to be essentially equivalent. Morgan and Scott[21] reported that nitrazepam more frequently produced residual effects than comparison drugs (amobarbital, dichloralphenazone, Mandrax). In two other comparisons with barbiturates, hangover and side effects occurred more often with the barbiturate hypnotic than with nitrazepam.[18,19] In the remaining studies, active drugs produced residual effects with equal frequencies. Anecdotal reports have described the use of nitrazepam in the treatment of narcolepsy,[31] but further investigation will be needed to establish the value of nitrazepam in this disorder.

Hypnotic drugs occasionally produce unwanted responses in older patients.[32,33] Confusion and disorientation, sometimes associated with agitation, delirium, or combativeness, is the observed clinical syndrome. How frequently hypnotics produce this "paradoxical" response is difficult to determine, inasmuch as nocturnal confusion and agitation may occur spontaneously in elderly patients, especially while they are hospitalized. Barbiturates and chloral hydrate are most often implicated,[34,35] but the syndrome will probably occur in a susceptible patient regardless of the particular hypnotic drug used. The entity has been reported in association with nitrazepam.[36,37] Evans and Jarvis[37] described a 75-year-old woman who precipitously developed confusion, dysarthria, ataxia, and incontinence, all of which disappeared when nitrazepam was discontinued.

The basis for these paradoxical responses is unclear. Impaired cognition produced by central depressant drugs appears to frighten some elderly individuals, and results in an increase of vigilance rather than sedation and sleep. Organic brain disease and impaired drug-metabolizing capacities have been suggested as possible associated factors. Some physicians feel that such reactions may be avoided if nitrazepam is given to elderly patients in reduced

---

*Hypnotic preparation containing methaqualone, 250 mg, plus diphenhydramine, 25 mg, in each pill.

dosage,[37] but this has not been conclusively proven. Kramer,[35] for example, has reported that paradoxical responses to chloral hydrate occur frequently in geriatric patients even after relatively low doses (500 mg). It may well be that *increased* quantities of hypnotic medication are, in fact, appropriate. Nonetheless, it is clear that hypnotics should be used with caution in the elderly.

An association of nitrazepam with nightmares and vivid dreams has been suggested in several reports.[36,38,39] Taylor[38] states that the dreams are most intense during the first few nights of therapy, then subside in intensity with continued drug use. In a number of cases, the content of the dreams involved emotionally traumatic events which had occurred in the subject's past. It appears from these reports that the nightmares are causally related to the use of nitrazepam. Goossens and associates[40] suggest that nitrazepam allows distressing subconscious processes to enter the field of dreams because of its disinhibiting properties (see Chapters 3 and 4). Hallucinations and disturbing, intrusive thoughts have also been attributed to chlordiazepoxide and diazepam. This is discussed in Chapter 12.

FLURAZEPAM

Except for a difference in milligram potency, flurazepam appears to be clinically equivalent to nitrazepam as a hypnotic. Studies using similar subject populations and methods of evaluation uniformly demonstrate flurazepam to be more effective than a placebo and equally effective as other active comparison drugs.

The superiority of flurazepam over placebo in terms of sleep onset, duration of sleep, and quality of sleep has been demonstrated in a number of controlled trials.[41–47] Both 15 mg and 30 mg are effective, and the larger dose does not seem to provide greater benefit.[46,48] Kales and associates have found that there is good correlation between objective EEG findings and subjective reports of improved quality and duration of sleep.[47,49] These investigators also note that flurazepam has a "carryover" effect following drug discontinuation.[45,47] Subjective and objective improvement in sleep parameters persists for several days after flurazepam is replaced by placebo.

Insomnia is a syndrome defined by a subject's assessment of his own sleep habits rather than by objectively evaluated sleep parameters. Some individuals claim they "can't sleep" if they require 30 min to fall asleep; in others, a 30-min sleep latency is accepted as normal. Drug effects can depend upon the degree of symptomatology as well as the absolute value of these parameters. Kales et al.[47] administered flurazepam (30 mg) to a series of subjects complaining of insomnia. In one subgroup, the mean sleep latency was reduced from 30 to 13 min by flurazepam treatment—a significant improvement. In a group of more severe insomniacs in the study, flurazepam reduced the mean sleep latency from 63 to 27 min. As in the first subgroup, this improvement was significant, demonstrating that flurazepam is more effective than placebo. Yet the *absolute value* of flurazepam-induced latency in the second group differs only slightly from the *pre*-drug value of 30 min in the less symptomatic subjects. The work of Vogel and associates[50] has suggested that objective improvement in sleep parameters may be more difficult to demonstrate among individuals who have no symptoms of disordered sleep. In a group of "good" sleepers—asymptomatic subjects who sleep well without medication—30 mg of flurazepam produced no change in sleep onset or duration in comparison with placebo. Among "poor" sleepers, 15 mg of flurazepam reduced the time to sleep onset and prolonged total sleep time.

Flurazepam (15 to 30 mg) has been compared to secobarbital (100 mg),[42,43] pentobarbital (100 mg),[44] amobarbital (50 mg),[51] glutethimide (500 mg),[48,52] chloral hydrate (0.5 to 1.0 g),[48,52,53] and methaqualone (150 to 300 mg)[53] in controlled trials. These studies show the drugs to be similar in hypnotic efficacy during short-term administration. Kales and associates[52] found that flurazepam, chloral hydrate, and glutethimide were effective in reducing sleep latency during the first 3 nights of drug administration. After 2 weeks of nightly administration, flurazepam remained effective, whereas chloral hydrate and glutethimide were no longer effective. Similar findings were replicated in a 4-week comparison of flurazepam, chloral hydrate, glutethimide, methaqualone, and secobarbital.[54] Flurazepam was the only drug found continuously effective during the entire 4 weeks of study.

OTHER BENZODIAZEPINES AS HYPNOTICS

Provided adequate doses are used, a number of other benzodiazepines are adequate sleep-inducers. Kales and Scharf[45] have found diazepam (10 mg) to be an effective hypnotic, although chlordiazepoxide (25 to 50 mg) appeared to be less useful. Hartmann[44] showed that chlordiazepoxide (100 mg) prolonged sleep in normal volunteers in a manner similar to flurazepam (30 mg) and pentobarbital (100 mg). Lower doses are less effective. In a study of hospitalized psychiatric patients, Bordeleau and associates[19] found that neither chlordiazepoxide (50 mg) nor diazepam (10 mg) was more effective than placebo, whereas nitrazepam (10 mg) and secobarbital (200 mg) were significantly better than placebo. Ananth and co-workers[55] also found that diazepam (10 mg) was an ineffective hypnotic when tested in hospitalized schizophrenic individuals with symptomatic insomnia. A limited number of controlled trials have documented that temazepam,[56] chlorazepate,[57] desmethyldiazepam,[58] flunitrazepam,[45,46,59,61] and lorazepam[62] are effective hypnotic agents. A combination preparation (methyprylon, 200 mg, and chlordiazepoxide, 10 mg, per tablet) was tested in 1962,[63] but this preparation is not currently available.

HANGOVER

The ideal hypnotic agent would rapidly induce physiological sleep but produce no unwanted drowsiness or heavy-headedness upon awakening. The benzodiazepines approach this ideal no more closely than other hypnotics. The studies cited previously in general show that hangover occurs as frequently after nitrazepam and flurazepam as it does following barbiturates.

Several investigations have documented objective "morning-after" effects of hypnotics. Typical benzodiazepine-induced EEG changes, consisting of a shift to low-voltage high-frequency activity, continue to be visible 12 to 18 hr after single doses of nitrazepam (5 to 10 mg)[26,27,64] or flurazepam (15 to 30 mg).[65] Impairment of performance in tests of intellectual and motor function identical to that produced by barbiturates is evident as long as 12 to 13 hr after administration of the benzodiazepines.[26,27,64,65] Higher doses cause more marked impairment. By 18 hr following administration, performance returns to normal despite persistence of EEG changes. Bixler and associates[66] have not confirmed these findings. This group reported that flurazepam (30 mg) taken at bedtime caused no impairment of performance on the following morning. Harrer[67] was unable to demonstrate psychomotor impairment 12 hr after oral nitrazepam in doses of 10 mg or less.

Impairment of intellectual and motor function following flurazepam and nitrazepam is more easily detected when testing is performed shortly after the drug is ingested (Chapter 8). Nevertheless, psychomotor and EEG changes are demonstrable in many subjects on the morning after use of a benzodiazepine hypnotic, even though symptomatic hangover may not be recognized. Patients using hypnotic drugs should be warned of this fact by their physicians.

NEUROPHYSIOLOGY OF SLEEP

EEG studies of sleep and dreaming have recently attracted a great deal of attention. The consistent association of subjective reports of dreaming with electromyographically detected rapid eye movements (REM) is striking. Normal subjects spend 20 to 25% of their sleep time in the REM or dreaming stage of sleep. Certain hypnotic drugs significantly reduce this percentage, indicating that hypnotic-induced sleep may differ from undrugged sleep in an objectively measurable way.

The consequences of dream deprivation—even when deprivation is complete—are not established. Hypnotic drugs which reduce dreaming time do not eliminate it completely. Our knowledge of the clinical significance of drug-induced REM deprivation is derived from both fact and speculation.

In some circumstances, dream deprivation can be beneficial. Ischemic heart disease and peptic ulcer may be exacerbated during dreaming when the associated sympathetic nervous system discharge results in anginal pain, arrhythmias, or increased acid secretion. A few nights of REM suppression during "flare-ups" of these diseases could in theory be therapeutically useful. In some patients with endogenous depression or narcolepsy, inhibition of dreaming by drugs is accompanied by clinical improvement.[68] For most individuals, however, the sequelae of drug-induced interference with dreaming are subjectively unpleasant, particularly after the drug is discontinued. Prolonged REM suppression seems to be followed by a "rebound" phenomenon in which total dreaming time is increased, as if the dreaming debt were being repaid. REM rebound is often associated with nightmares and insomnia. A subtle type of hypnotic dependence can be perpetuated, in which the REM-suppressing drug continues to be taken to prevent the rebound phenomenon. Ethanol is a potent dream depressor, and sleep disturbance can be an important aspect of chronic alcoholism. Many of the unpleasant symptoms of alcohol withdrawal may be due to REM rebound, and may be a potent stimulus for the newly abstinent alcoholic to return to drinking.[69]

A number of reviews discuss in detail the neurophysiology of sleep and the influence of hypnotic drugs on dreaming.[6,7,68,70-73] The barbiturates and glutethimide consistently depress REM sleep, with rebound observed upon drug withdrawal. With chloral hydrate and methaqualone, the effects vary from study to study; dream depression by methaqualone seems to be dose dependent.

The Benzodiazepines and REM Sleep

Animal investigations have demonstrated that the benzodiazepines depress REM sleep in a dose-dependent manner.[74] This has been in part confirmed in human studies. Oswald and Priest[75] reported in 1965 that nitrazepam given in doses of 15 mg to two subjects for 14 consecutive nights significantly depressed REM sleep during the drug administration period. After drug withdrawal, REM rebound appeared and persisted for 5 weeks or more. Amobarbital produced a similar result. In other controlled studies, nitrazepam (10 mg) depressed dreaming as much or more than secobarbital (100 mg) or amobarbital (200 mg).[22,61,76] Other authors have reported no apparent dream depression by nitrazepam.[77] Tissot[78] found that 30 to 40 mg of nitrazepam did not alter the percentage of sleep time spent in the REM stage.

Flurazepam has been more extensively investigated. Kales and associates[53] found that 60 mg of flurazepam did reduce REM time, but there was no rebound upon drug withdrawal. Some controlled trials have demonstrated that usual clinical doses of flurazepam (15 to 30 mg) produce minor or insignificant changes in REM sleep time.[44-47,50,52,53] Others reveal significant REM depression by flurazepam.[79,80] Bixler et al.[81] and Allen and associates[82] divided total REM time into 10-sec epochs and calculated the percentage of these epochs in which at least one eye movement occurred. This parameter was termed "REM density." In these studies, flurazepam administration significantly reduced REM density. The results suggest that density or intensity of REMs may be a more sensitive indicator of drug effects on sleep than is total dreaming time.

Greenberg[83] reported in 1967 a study of five patients with an unusual type of insomnia in which multiple awakenings occurred in association with dreaming. Using chlordiazepoxide (50 to 125 mg) or diazepam (20 to 25 mg) as hypnotic medication, he noted a decrease in REM time together with clinical improvement in sleep in all of these patients. Itil and Saletu[79] suggest that all benzodiazepines depress REM time, although several investigations of chlordiazepoxide and diazepam have revealed no dream depression by these drugs.[44,57,84,85] In one animal study, diazepam actually produced an increase in REM sleep time.[86] Chlorazepate[57] and temazepam[56] also appear not to influence dreaming time in clinically effective doses. The effects of flunitrazepam vary from study to study,[45,59–61,77] but in doses of 1 mg this drug probably does not alter dreaming time.[45] Two to 4 mg of lorazepam depresses REM sleep.[87]

Slow-Wave Sleep

The benzodiazepines influence stage IV or slow-wave sleep much more consistently than REM sleep. In essentially all sleep studies involving this EEG parameter, the benzodiazepines depress the time spent in stage IV.[45-47,50,53,56,57,60,61,87-89] This property may have therapeutic implications, since nocturnal enuresis, sleepwalking, and night terrors are thought to occur during stage IV slow-wave sleep. The possible efficacy of diazepam and nitrazepam in the treatment of enuresis is discussed in Chapter 4. Glick and associates[90] reported seven children, ages 7 to 11 years, having combinations of somnambulism, enuresis, and pavor nocturnus, who were successfully treated with diazepam, 2.5 to 5.0 mg nightly. Saletu and Itil[91] found that diazepam (10 mg nightly) produced clinical improvement and reduced stage IV sleep time in a 52-year-old woman with somnambulism. Fisher and associates[92,93] used diazepam (5 to 20 mg nightly) to treat seven individuals with night terrors. Clinical improvement occurred in all subjects, and EEG investigation revealed a marked suppression of slow-wave sleep. The benzodiazepines appear to have promise as stage IV sleep depressants in disorders associated with slow-wave activity. The long-term effects of slow-wave suppression, however, remain to be determined. One subject reported by Fisher and associates[93] had a displacement of night terrors to "day terrors," experiencing extremely disturbing obsessions with self-destructive thoughts. It may be that this displacement effect underlies the ego-alien suicidal ideation reported by some subjects receiving diazepam. This is discussed further in Chapter 12.

COMMENT

Most of the controlled studies cited in this chapter are "multi-crossover" in design—each patient is exposed consecutively to each treatment condition in a systematic sequence. For each drug condition, a treatment mean is generated. Authors statistically test whether, for example, the mean for Drug A differs significantly from the corresponding means for Drug B and placebo. Frequently, multiple paired comparisons are made (e.g., Drug A with placebo, Drug A with Drug B, Drug B with placebo). In so doing, the means for treatments are used multiply with interdependent estimates of the role of chance (sampling error). Statistical considerations dictate that when a single mean value is used for multiple comparisons, the criterion for statistical significance becomes more stringent, although the method of calculating the test statistic may not change.[94-96] In a number of the studies cited, it is not clear whether such considerations or adjustments were made. The critical observer should be aware of this possible shortcoming in the evidence discussed herein. It may be, for example, that some of the significant drug-placebo differences reported would not reach significance were the limits adjusted properly. Conceptually one can contrast this to an experimental design in which six groups were used—two each for Drug A, Drug B, and placebo. In such a design, independent groups could be used for each paired comparison.

Despite these reservations, the evidence reviewed in this chapter suggests that, in usual therapeutic doses, the benzodiazepines are effective hypnotic agents. When compared to other traditional sleep-inducing drugs in short-term studies, the benzodiazepines are equally effective and also equally likely to produce hangover and persistent psychomotor impairment. Both flurazepam and nitrazepam have the potential to depress dreaming, although the effects of flurazepam are less marked than those of barbiturates or glutethimide. The significance of these differences is based as much on theory and speculation as on fact. Flurazepam appears to be unique, however, in that its hypnotic efficacy persists during long-term administration.

A major advantage of benzodiazepine hypnotics is their relative safety. These drugs are quite innocuous when taken in suicidal or accidental overdosage. In addition, benzodiazepines do not cause significant enzyme induction in man and, therefore, do not interact with other drugs such as oral anticoagulants (see Chapter 12). These are substantial reasons for choosing benzodiazepines over other hypnotics in situations where sleep-inducing medication is indicated, despite the relatively high dollar cost of flurazepam.

REFERENCES

1. Lasagna L: The pharmacological basis for the effective use of hypnotics. Pharmacol Physicians 1:1-4, (Feb) 1967

2. Hinton J: Sedatives and hypnotics. Practitioner 200:93-101, 1968
3. Today's drugs. Hypnotics. Brit Med J 2:409-411, 1968
4. Miller RR, DeYoung DV, Paxinos J: Hypnotic drugs. Postgrad Med J 46:314-317, 1970
5. Way WL, Trevor AJ: Sedative-hypnotics. Anesthesiology 34:170-182, 1971
6. Greenblatt DJ, Shader RI: The clinical choice of sedative-hypnotics. Ann Intern Med 77:91-100, 1972
7. Kales A, Kales J: Evaluation, diagnosis, and treatment of clinical disorders related to sleep. JAMA 213:2229-2235, 1970
8. Shapiro S, Slone D, Lewis GP, Jick H: Clinical effects of hypnotics. II. An epidemiological study. JAMA 209:2016-2020, 1969
9. Greenblatt DJ, Shader RI: Psychopharmacologic management of anxiety in the cardiac patient. Psychiatry in Medicine 2:55-66, 1971
10. Johns MW, Hepburn M, Goodyear MDE: Use of hypnotic drugs by hospital patients. Med J Aust 2:1323-1327, 1971
11. Johnson J, Clift AD: Dependence on hypnotic drugs in general practice. Brit Med J 4:613-617, 1968
12. Clift AD: Factors leading to dependence on hypnotic drugs. Brit Med J 3:614-617, 1972
13. Randall LO, Schallek W, Scheckel CL, Stefko PL, Banziger RF, Pool W, Moe RA: Pharmacological studies on flurazepam hydrochloride (RO 5-6901), a new psychotropic agent of the benzodiazepine class. Arch Int Pharmacodyn 178:216-241, 1969
14. Frost JD, Carrie JRG, Borda RP, Kellaway P: The effects of Dalmane (flurazepam hydrochloride) on human EEG characteristics. Electroenceph Clin Neurophysiol 34:171-175, 1973
15. Soulairac A, Cohn J, Gottesman C, Alano J: Neuropharmacological aspects of the action of hypnogenic substances on the central nervous system. Progr Brain Res 18:194-220, 1965
16. Kales A, Bixler EO, Scharf MB: A comparison of home telemetry and sleep laboratory recordings with insomniac subjects. Presented at the Annual Meeting of the Association for the Psychophysiological Study of Sleep. San Diego, Calif, May, 1973
17. Kullander NE: A double-blind clinical trial of a new sleep-inducing combination of methaqualone and etodroxizine compared with nitrazepam and placebo. Arzneim-Forsch 19:1530-1532, 1969
18. Haider I: A double-blind controlled trial of a non-barbiturate hypnotic—nitrazepam. Brit J Psychiat 114:337-343, 1968
19. Bordeleau JM, Charland P, Tetreault L: Hypnotic properties of nitrazepam (Mogadon). Dis Nerv Syst 31:318-323, 1970
20. Andersen T, Lingjaerde O: Nitrazepam (Mogadon) as a sleep-inducing agent. Brit J Psychiat 115:1393-1397, 1969
21. Morgan H, Scott DF, Joyce CRB: The effects of four hypnotic drugs and placebo on normal subjects' sleeping and dreaming at home. Brit J Psychiat 177:649-652, 1970
22. Haider I, Oswald I: Effects of amylobarbitone and nitrazepam on the electrodermogram and other features of sleep. Brit J Psychiat 118:519-522, 1971
23. Matthew H, Proudfoot AT, Aitken RCB, Raeburn JA, Wright N: Nitrazepam—a safe hypnotic. Brit Med J 3:23-25, 1969
24. leRiche WH, Csima A, Dobson M: A clinical trial of four hypnotic drugs. Canad Med Assoc J 95:300-302, 1966
25. Gore CP, McComisky JG: A comparative study of the hypnotic effectiveness of nitrazepam ("Mogadon"), glutethimide, and a placebo. In, *Proceedings of the Fourth World Congress of Psychiatry.* Edited by JJL Ibor. Amsterdam, Excerpta Medica Foundation, 1968, pp 2181-2183
26. Malpas A, Rowan AJ, Joyce CRB, Scott DF: Persistent behavioral and electroencephalographic changes after single doses of nitrazepam and amylobarbitone. Brit Med J 2:762-764, 1970

27. Bond AJ, Lader MH: Residual effects of hypnotics. Psychopharmacologia 25:117-132, 1972
28. Meares R, Mills JE, Oliver LE: A clinical comparison of two non-barbiturate hypnotics, Mogadon and Mandrax. Med J Aust 1:266-268, 1972
29. Davies C, Levine S: A controlled comparison of nitrazepam ("Mogadon") with sodium amylobarbitone as a sleep-inducing agent. Brit J Psychiat 113:1005-1008, 1967
30. General Practitioner Research Group: General practitioner clinical trials. Sedation with a new non-barbiturate compound. Practitioner 195:366-368, 1965
31. Pateiksy K: EEG investigations in the treatment of narcolepsy with nitrazepam and imipramine. (Abstract) Electroenceph Clin Neurophysiol 30:167-168, 1971
32. Dawson-Butterworth K: The chemopsychotherapeutics of geriatric sedation. J Amer Geriat Soc 18:97-114, 1970
33. Lamy PP, Kitler ME: Drugs and the geriatric patient. J Amer Geriat Soc 19:23-33, 1971
34. Gibson IIJM: Barbiturate delirium. Practitioner 197:345-347, 1966
35. Kramer CH: Methaqualone and chloral hydrate: preliminary comparison in geriatric patients. J Amer Geriat Soc 15:455-461, 1967
36. Fraser AG, Shepherd FGG: Trial of a new hypnotic in general practice. Practitioner 196:829-833, 1966
37. Evans JG, Jarvis EH: Nitrazepam and the elderly. Brit Med J 4:487, 1972
38. Taylor F: Nitrazepam in the elderly. Brit Med J 1:113-114, 1973
39. Girdwood RH: Nitrazepam nightmares. Brit Med J 1:353, 1973
40. Goossens T, Bulckaert M, Wakeling E: Nitrazepam and the subconscious. Brit Med J 2:488, 1973
41. Zimmerman AM: Comparative effects of flurazepam hydrochloride (Dalmane) and placebo in patients with insomnia. Curr Ther Res 13:18-22, 1971
42. Jick H, Slone D, Dinan B, Muench H: Evaluation of drug efficacy by a preference technic. New Eng J Med 275:1399-1403, 1966
43. Boston Collaborative Drug Surveillance Program: A clinical evaluation of flurazepam. J Clin Pharmacol 12:217-220, 1972
44. Hartmann E: The effect of four drugs on sleep patterns in man. Psychopharmacologia 12:346-353, 1968
45. Kales A, Scharf MB: Sleep laboratory and clinical studies of the effects of benzodiazepines on sleep: flurazepam, diazepam, chlordiazepoxide, and RO 5-4200. In, *The Benzodiazepines.* Edited by S Garattini, E Mussini, LO Randall. New York, Raven Press, 1973, pp 577-598
46. Dement WC, Zarcone VP, Hoddes E, Smythe H, Carskadon M: Sleep laboratory and clinical studies with flurazepam. In, *The Benzodiazepines.* Edited by S Garattini, E Mussini, LO Randall. New York, Raven Press, 1973, pp 599-611
47. Kales J, Kales A, Bixler EO, Slye ES: Effects of placebo and flurazepam on sleep patterns in insomniac patients. Clin Pharmacol Ther 12:691-697, 1971
48. Jick H: Comparative studies with a hypnotic (RO 5-6901) under current investigation. Curr Ther Res 9:355-357, 1967
49. Kales JD, Bixler EO, Slye ES, Baker M, Kales A: Comparison of subjective reports and EEG findings under conditions of placebo or flurazepam (Dalmane) administration and withdrawal. (Abstract). Psychophysiology 9:92, 1972
50. Vogel GW, Hickman J, Thurmond A, Barrowclough B, Giesler D: The effect of Dalmane (flurazepam) on the sleep cycle of good and poor sleepers. (Abstract). Psychophysiology 9:96, 1972
51. Fisher S, Gal P: Flurazepam versus amobarbital as a sedative-hypnotic for geriatric patients: double-blind study. J Amer Geriat Soc 17:397-399, 1969
52. Kales A, Allen C, Scharf MB, Kales JD: Hypnotic drugs and their effectiveness. All-night EEG studies of insomniac patients. Arch Gen Psychiat 23:226-232, 1970
53. Kales A, Kales JD, Scharf MB, Tan T-L: Hypnotics and altered sleep-dream patterns.

II. All-night EEG studies of chloral hydrate, flurazepam, and methaqualone. Arch Gen Psychiat 23:219-225, 1970

54. Kales A, Kales JD, Leo LA, Bixler EO: Evaluation of the effectiveness of hypnotic drugs under conditions of prolonged use. Presented at the Annual Meeting of the Association for the Psychophysiological Study of Sleep. San Diego, Calif, May, 1973

55. Ananth JV, Bronheim LA, Klinger A, Ban TA: Diazepam in the treatment of insomnia in psychiatric patients. Curr Ther Res 15:217-222, 1973

56. Maggini C, Murri M, Sacchetti G: Evaluation of the effectiveness of temazepam on the insomnia of patients with neurosis and endogenous depression. Arzneim-Forsch 19:1647-1652, 1969

57. Itil TM, Saletu B, Marasa J: Digital computer analyzed sleep electroencephalogram (sleep prints) in predicting the anxiolytic properties of clorazepate dipotassium (Tranxene). Curr Ther Res 14:415-427, 1972

58. Tosi GC, Tosi EC, Hattab JR: The use of N-demethyldiazepam in outpatients suffering from insomnia. Curr Ther Res 15:460-464, 1973

59. Monti J, Trenchi HM, Morales F: Effects of RO 5-4200, a benzodiazepine derivative, on the EEG and the sleep cycle in man (Abstract). Electroenceph Clin Neurophysiol 32:583, 1972

60. Munari C, Gastaut H, Tassinari CA: A double-blind study of a new benzodiazepine (RO 5-4200), compared with Mogadon and a placebo, on nocturnal sleep of normal subjects. (Abstract). Electroenceph Clin Neurophysiol 31:180, 1971

61. Oswald I, Lewis SA, Tagney J, Firth H, Haider I: Benzodiazepines and human sleep. In, *The Benzodiazepines*. Edited by S Garattini, E Mussini, LO Randall. New York, Raven Press, 1973, pp 613-625

62. Imlah NW: Clinical experience with lorazepam in hospital patients. Curr Med Res Opin 1:276-281, 1973

63. Pena EF: Management of insomnia in gynecologic patients. Clin Med 69:1351-1355, 1962

64. Walters AJ, Lader MH: Hangover effects of hypnotics in man. Nature (London) 229:637-638, 1971

65. Bond AJ, Lader MH: Residual effects of a new benzodiazepine: flurazepam. Brit J Pharmacol 44:343P-344P, 1972

66. Bixler EO, Kales A, Tan T-L, Kales JD: The effects of hypnotic drugs on performance. Curr Ther Res 15:13-24, 1973

67. Harrer G: Experience with Mogadon. Progr Brain Res 18:228-229, 1965

68. Pearlman CA, Greenberg R: Medical-psychological implications of recent sleep research. Psychiatry in Medicine 1:261-276, 1970

69. Greenblatt DJ, Greenblatt M: Which drug for alcohol withdrawal? J Clin Pharmacol 12:429-431, 1972

70. Oswald I: Drugs and sleep. Pharmacol Rev 20:274-303, 1968

71. King CD: The pharmacology of rapid eye movement sleep. Adv Pharmacol Chemother 9:1-91, 1971

72. Hartmann E: Pharmacological studies of sleep and dreaming: chemical and clinical relationships. Biol Psychiat 1:243-258, 1969

73. Heuser G, and discussants: Clinical neurophysiology. Newer diagnostic and therapeutic methods in neurological disease and behavior disorders. Ann Intern Med 71:619-645, 1969

74. Lanoir J, Killam EK: Alteration in the sleep-wakefulness patterns by benzodiazepines in the cat. Electroenceph Clin Neurophysiol 25:530-542, 1968

75. Oswald I, Priest RG: Five weeks to escape the sleeping-pill habit. Brit Med J 2:1093-1095, 1965

76. Lehmann HE, Ban TA: The effect of hypnotics on rapid eye movement (REM). Int J Clin Pharmacol 1:424-427, 1968

77. Shliapochnik J, Perea RA, Turner M, Morgan JJ: Observations on eight cases of insomnia

in therapeutic trial with Mogadon and Ro 05-4200 with electroencephalographic control. (Abstract) Electroenceph Clin Neurophysiol 31:630, 1971

78. Tissot R: The effects of certain drugs on the sleep cycle in man. Progr Brain Res 18:175-177, 1965

79. Itil TM, Saletu B: Computer analyzed sleep, REM and EEG characteristics of anxiolytics and hypnotics. In, *Pharmacology of Sleep and Treatment of Sleep Disorders.* Edited by I Karacan. New York, Wiley-Interscience (in press)

80. Itil TM, Saletu B, Marasa J, Mucciardi AN: Digital computer analyzed awake and sleep EEG (sleep prints) in predicting the effects of a triazolobenzodiazepine (U-31,889). Pharmakopsychiatrie Neuro-Psychopharmakologie 5:225-240, 1972

81. Bixler EO, Scharf MB, Kales A: The effect of prolonged use of flurazepam (Dalmane) on eye movement density. Presented at the Annual Meeting of the Association for the Psychophysiological Study of Sleep. San Diego, Calif, May, 1973

82. Allen C, Scharf MB, Kales A: The effect of flurazepam (Dalmane) administration and withdrawal on REM density. (Abstract) Psychophysiology 9:92-93, 1972

83. Greenberg R: Dream interruption insomnia. J Nerv Ment Dis 144:18-21, 1967

84. Itil TM: Effects of psychotropic drugs on computer "sleep prints" in man. In, *The Present Status of Psychotropic Drugs. Pharmacological and Clinical Aspects.* Edited by A Cerletti, FJ Bové. Amsterdam, Excerpta Medica Foundation, 1969, pp 84-89

85. Hartmann E, Cravens J, Stanford G, Zwilling G, Bernstein J: Long-term effects of drugs on sleep: reserpine, amitriptyline, chlorpromazine, chloral hydrate, chlordiazepoxide, placebo. (Abstract) Psychophysiology 9:94, 1972.

86. Loizzo A, Longo VG: A pharmacological approach to paradoxical sleep. Physiol Behav 3:91-97, 1968

87. Globus GG, Phoebus EC, Fishbein W, Boyd R, Leventhal T: The effect of lorazepam on sleep. J Clin Pharmacol 12:331-336, 1972

88. Cornu F: Drug-induced sleep without typical EEG changes. In, *Neuro-Psycho-Pharmacology.* Edited by H Brill. Amsterdam, Excerpta Medica Foundation, 1966, pp 960-961

89. Schallek W, Kuehn A, Kovacs J: Effects of chlordiazepoxide hydrochloride on discrimination responses and sleep cycles in cats. Neuropharmacology 11:69-79, 1972

90. Glick BS, Schulman D, Turecki S: Diazepam (Valium) treatment in childhood sleep disorders. Dis Nerv Syst 32:565-566, 1971

91. Saletu B, Itil TM: Digital computer "sleep prints"—an indicator of the most effective drug treatment of somnambulism. Clin Electroenceph 4:33-41, 1973

92. Fisher C, Kahn E, Edwards A, Davis D: Effects of Valium on NREM night terrors. (Abstract) Psychophysiology 9:91, 1972.

93. Fisher C, Kahn E, Edwards A, Davis DM: A psychophysiological study of nightmares and night terrors. The suppression of stage 4 night terrors with diazepam. Arch Gen Psychiat 28:252-259, 1973

94. Dunnett CW: A multiple comparison procedure for comparing several treatments with a control. J Amer Statistical Assoc 50:1096-1121, 1955

95. Dunn MJ: Multiple comparisons among means. J Amer Statistical Assoc 56:52-64, 1961

96. Games PA: Multiple comparisons of means. Amer Educational Res J 8:531-565, 1971

Chapter 10
Anesthesia and Surgery

Major surgery almost always is severely stressful, both from psychic and physiological points of view. The use of psychotropic drugs is an important means by which physicians can make the situation more tolerable for the patient. Over the last 20 years, a wide variety of agents have been introduced for purposes of preoperative medication, induction, and postoperative sedation. These include propanediols, phenothiazines, butyrophenones, short-acting opiates, and benzodiazepines. Through some combination of tradition and common sense, decisions regarding psychotropic medications in association with surgery are usually made by the anesthesiologist. The availability of numerous psychotropic agents as well as the many newer volatile general anesthetics requires that anesthesiologists be adept clinical pharmacologists.

The patient's apprehension about an elective surgical procedure understandably may begin days or weeks before the scheduled date of the operation. When little or no preparation is needed, the patient can be admitted to the hospital on the evening before or the morning of surgery. For more complicated procedures involving organ transplantation, cardiopulmonary bypass, or vascular repair, several days of hospitalization for special studies or preparation may be required. In such cases, the patient can be extremely anxious, and daytime antianxiety medication is advisable or necessary. Hypnotic medication is usually needed to produce sleep, particularly on the night prior to operation. On the day of surgery, before stretcher transport to the operating area, the patient usually receives a traditional triad of premedication, consisting of an anticholinergic, an analgesic, and a psychosedative. Despite heavy sedation upon arrival at the induction room, few patients willingly accept the application of a face mask for volatile general anesthetic administration. For this reason, short-acting sedative-hypnotics are given intravenously to render the patient unconscious during induction of general anesthesia. If endotracheal intubation is contemplated, adequate sedation is a requisite. By the time surgery actually begins, the patient has a large number of central depressant drugs in his body.

Psychotropic drug administration continues to be necessary in the postoperative period. Patients usually cannot do without opiate analgesia. Emergence from general anesthesia in itself is frequently associated with agitation and delirium requiring sedative medications to control. Nausea and vomiting caused by the anesthetic gases and by opiate analgesics are a common problem, usually treated with any of a variety of parenteral antiemetics including antihistamines, anticholinergics, or phenothiazines. Postoperative delirium and psychoses in association with open-heart surgery are being reported with increasing frequency. It is unclear whether these reactions are related to drugs, to confinement in an intensive care unit, to the actual surgical manipulation of the heart, or to some combination of these factors. Psychotropic medication is often used to manage these problems, for the sake of both the patient and the medical staff.

The problem of anesthesia in dental medicine deserves special attention. Nature has unfortunately arranged that sensation associated with teeth is usually perceived as pain. It is hardly surprising, therefore, that a substantial proportion of humanity equates dental manipulation with pain. The filling of uncomplicated carious teeth now can almost always be done painlessly. However, for procedures involving pulp and root manipulation, tooth extraction, or other dental surgery, local anesthesia is often inadequate. The use of systemic adjuvants to local anesthesia is limited by the fact that most dental work must be done on an outpatient basis. The drug must be effective enough that the patient will tolerate the procedure, but agents that require intensive intra- and postoperative monitoring or that produce prolonged incapacity are unacceptable. Methohexital and/or nitrous oxide are commonly used, but each has significant disadvantages. Intravenous diazepam has fewer disadvantages, and is becoming the psychosedative agent of choice for many dentists.

PREMEDICATION

Evaluation of the efficacy of preoperative medication is both subjective and objective.[1] The patient's anxiety, apprehension, state of consciousness, and cooperation can be rated by both observer and patient. The anesthesiologist can determine the ease of induction and the apparent requirements for anesthetics and muscle relaxants. Vital signs, arterial blood gas tensions, and plasma corticosteroids are among numerous objective parameters. Emetic sequelae, recovery time, analgesic requirements, and the frequency of complications can be rated postoperatively. An important subjective measure is the patient's degree of recall of the event, and his overall impression of the experience.

Uncontrolled series have suggested that chlordiazepoxide and diazepam can be used as preoperative sedatives, given either orally[2-5] or parenterally.[6-11] Controlled trials testing these impressions fortunately are easy to perform, since they are without special risk and do not interfere with the routine of anesthesia and surgery. On busy surgical services, data on large numbers of patients can be gathered in a relatively short period of time.

Oral Premedication

The benzodiazepines have been studied as oral preoperative medications in adults. Brandt and associates[12,13] compared chlordiazepoxide (20 to 50 mg) and diazepam (20 mg) to pentobarbital (100 mg) and placebo. The drugs were given at bedtime on the night before surgery, and again 90 min before anesthesia. All three drugs allowed a better night's sleep than placebo. The 50-mg dose of chlordiazepoxide was comparable to pentobarbital according to the anesthesiologist's global evaluation,[12] whereas diazepam was superior to both pentobarbital and placebo.[13] More than half of diazepam recipients had amnesia for the induction period—a desirable effect of premedication—while less than one-fourth of barbiturate- and placebo-treated patients reported lack of recall. All active drugs were superior to placebo by observer and patient evaluation. Wordsworth[14] confirmed that both diazepam (10 mg) and chlordiazepoxide (20 mg) were effective sleep-inducers on the night before surgery. Three studies compared oral lorazepam (4 mg)[15,15a] and flunitrazepam (2 mg)[16] to placebo and to standard doses of other hypnotics (barbiturates, glutethimide) given on the preoperative night. Both benzodiazepine compounds were superior to comparison drugs and placebo by several patient and observer criteria.

Murray and associates[17] studied a number of medications given orally prior to surgery. Ratings were made according to observed patient apprehensiveness and drowsiness, and acceptance by patient and anesthetist. By all measures, pentobarbital (200 mg), diazepam (10 to 20 mg), and ethchlorvynol (1.0 gm) were approximately equivalent, and superior to hydroxyzine (200 mg) and oxazepam (60 mg), which were no better than placebo. There were no significant differences among any of the drugs and placebo with respect to the frequency of side effects. Moore and Hollis[18] found that oral premedication with diazepam (in doses averaging 0.33 mg/kg) was as effective as the traditional parenteral combination of morphine and scopolamine. Norris and associates[19,20] compared nitrazepam (5 to 10 mg), lorazepam (2 to 4 mg), and Mandrax* in female patients prior to minor gynecological procedures. The degree of sedation produced by all drugs was approximately equivalent. Postoperative vomiting was observed somewhat more frequently after the higher dose of nitrazepam.[19] Wilson[20a] found that oral lorazepam (3 mg) and diazepam (10 mg) were equally effective preoperative sedatives. More than 50% of lorazepam recipients were judged to have poor recall of the preoperative period when interviewed after surgery, whereas poor recall was not reported by *any* of the patients on diazepam. Similar findings were noted by Turner,[20b] who compared oral lorazepam

---

*Hypnotic preparation containing methaqualone, 250 mg, and diphenhydramine, 25 mg, in each pill.

(3 mg) and diazepam (10 mg). Amnestic properties of benzodiazepines will be discussed in greater detail subsequently.

Several groups have studied physiologic and biochemical parameters following oral premedications. Johnstone[21] used the plethysmographic digital pulse volume as an indicator of fear, with vasoconstriction indicating apprehension. Since the benzodiazepines do not produce sympathetic blockade, increase in pulse volume amplitude (vasodilation) can be interpreted as reduced apprehension occurring on a central basis. Mandrax and diazepam (20 mg) were equally unsatisfactory and inferior to nitrazepam (10 mg) as vasodilators. The combination of nitrazepam and droperidol was best, producing a greater degree of drowsiness in addition to vasodilation. The observed synergism of nitrazepam and droperidol was not due to the alpha-adrenergic blocking property of droperidol, since the vasoconstrictive response to cold was not impaired. Two studies involve plasma cortisol levels measured on the morning before surgery. Oyama and associates[22] found that diazepam (0.2 mg/kg), nitrazepam (0.2 mg/kg), and hydroxyzine (2.5 mg/kg) given preoperatively and on the night before surgery reduced plasma cortisol levels on the day of operation. Nitrazepam and diazepam were slightly superior by subjective assessment. James and Fisher[23] compared nitrazepam (40 mg) to placebo; the active drug was the superior sedative. Patients receiving nitrazepam had a fall in plasma cortisol following the drug, whereas a rise was noted in the placebo recipients. These findings support the conclusion (Chapter 8) that benzodiazepines can attenuate physiological responses to stress.

When given orally, benzodiazepines are at least as effective preoperative medications as traditional sedatives. It should be remembered that when large doses of long-acting benzodiazepine derivatives (chlordiazepoxide, diazepam) are given on the night prior to surgery, residual sedation may be present on the following morning and potentiate sedative effects of drugs given just prior to surgery. Short-acting barbiturates given as hypnotics, however, are largely eliminated by the following morning.

Parenteral Premedication

Preoperative medications are usually given by intramuscular injection rather than by mouth. This practice arises from the presumed danger of aspiration of retained gastric contents during induction. The actual risk is probably overrated. The absorption of most oral sedative-hypnotics is rapid and complete, and the stomach contents at the time of induction are negligible. McCaughey and Dundee[24] compared 10-mg doses of diazepam given orally and by the intramuscular route as premedicants prior to minor surgery in healthy females. Sedation was equivalent by both routes 40 min after the dose. At 60 and 90 min after administration, however, 84 to 88% of oral diazepam recipients were adequately sedated as compared to 52 to 56% of those receiving the drug intramuscularly. The results suggest that the continuing practice of intramuscular injection of premedicant drugs may be based more on tradition than on sound evidence that this route is the more appropriate.

Intramuscular chlordiazepoxide has received only limited evaluation. Gibbs and associates[25] showed that chlordiazepoxide (100 mg) was clinically somewhat superior to placebo as a premedicant for cardiac surgery. Burchmann and co-workers[26] found that this same dose (100 mg) was largely ineffective prior to surgery, but when given the night before operation allowed a better night's sleep than placebo. Tornetta[27] used intramuscular chlordiazepoxide (50 to 100 mg) in geriatric patients and found it superior to no sedation in a study that was not truly blind. The dose-dependent effect of chlordiazepoxide was demonstrated in studies by Haslett.[28,29] When given in a 50-mg dose, chlordiazepoxide was no more effective than placebo; 100 mg, however, was better than placebo and as good as diazepam (10 to 20 mg) at producing drowsiness and reducing apprehension and excitement as judged by the physician.

The superiority of intramuscular diazepam (10 to 20 mg) over placebo as a premedicant has been established with some consistency.[28-33] The combination of this dose of diazepam with either atropine or scopolamine (0.4 mg) appeared not to influence the overall efficacy of diazepam one way or another in a study by Steen and Hahl.[33] Dundee and associates,[32] however, found that the scopolamine-diazepam mixture increased the sedative, antianxiety, and amnestic effects of diazepam, but also produced paradoxical excitement much more frequently than did diazepam alone. There appears to be no good evidence that the 20-mg dose of diazepam is any more effective than 10 mg.[28,29,33] Two studies disputing the efficacy of diazepam were reported by Dobkin and co-workers,[34,35] who compared diazepam (10 mg), secobarbital (100 mg), doxepin (25 mg), and placebo. There were no substantial differences among the four treatment groups, except that diazepam increased the incidence of amnesia and also prolonged the time for recovery from anesthesia. An injectable preparation of doxepin is not available in the United States at the present time.

Cormier and associates[36] demonstrated that diazepam (5 to 10 mg) was approximately equivalent to meperidine (50 to 100 mg) as a premedicant. In more extensive studies at the Queen's University of Belfast, the superiority of diazepam over opiates, including meperidine (100 mg) and morphine (10 mg), has been documented with respect to the reduction of preoperative anxiety, the ease of induction, and the frequency of postoperative emesis and other adverse reactions.[31,32,37,38] The combination of meperidine plus diazepam has also been compared to each component given alone.[32] Opiate-induced emesis is reduced by the addition of diazepam, but cardiovascular toxicity is not. The sedative effects of the combination are greater than either drug by itself. Roberts[39] reported a study comparing diazepam (20 mg) to meperidine (100 mg) plus promethazine (25 mg). The antiemetic agent appeared to reduce the frequency of nausea associated with the opiate; nausea was only slightly more common with the combination than with diazepam alone. Patient acceptance of the mixture was greater than that of diazepam, and respiratory tract secretions were less of a problem. In other respects, the premedications were equivalent. In a similar study, Dixon and associates[40] compared diazepam (10 mg) and pentazocine (30 mg) to a mixture of the two. The two drugs given alone produced equivalent sedation and were no different as judged by the anesthetist's evaluation, whereas the combination was more satisfactory than either drug by itself. Pentazocine produced clinically minor respiratory depression which was not potentiated by diazepam. No respiratory depression occurred after diazepam alone.

Morrison[38] studied intramuscular droperidol (5 to 10 mg) as a premedicant compared to diazepam (10 mg). Droperidol caused excitement or respiratory upset during induction in more than 50% of cases and was clearly inferior to diazepam. Marrubini and Tretola[41] compared a belladonna preparation (atropine, 0.25 mg, plus scopolamine, 0.25 mg) with a belladonna-diazepam mixture. The addition of diazepam enhanced sedation and the overall acceptability of premedication, but "ideal" results were more frequently obtained when belladonna was combined with hydroxyzine (200 mg).

The nature of the patient populations in these studies must be emphasized. In all of the reports from the Department of Anesthesia at the Queen's University of Belfast, headed by Dr. John W. Dundee, the subjects are healthy females undergoing minor gynecological procedures. Whether this population responds uniquely to preoperative medications unfortunately cannot be assessed. Yet the findings of this group are reasonably consistent with those of other authors studying different groups of patients. In adequate doses both chlordiazepoxide and diazepam seem to be satisfactory premedicants for general surgery. Diazepam is at least as effective and is less toxic than an opiate by itself. The combination of diazepam plus an opiate or pentazocine is reasonable when sedation plus analgesia is desired; in addition, diazepam seems to reduce emetic sequelae associated with morphine or meperidine.

INDUCTION

The use of diazepam as an intravenous psychosedative prior to electroconvulsive therapy (Chapter 6) and cardioversion or endoscopy (Chapter 7) has been discussed previously. Many of the conclusions regarding the safety and efficacy of this drug are applicable to its use as an induction agent for general anesthesia. Since the use of placebo-controlled trials clearly is not feasible, conclusions must be based upon either uncontrolled open series or comparative trials with thiopental or methohexital.

Published reports dealing with nearly 2,500 patients are now available.[8,42-52] For purposes of induction, diazepam is given intravenously until dysarthria and sedation occur. Necessary dosage varies tremendously from patient to patient, ranging from only 5 mg to 60 mg or more. It has been suggested that patients chronically treated with other sedative-hypnotics require higher doses of diazepam,[51] but this has not been proven. Among those receiving premedication with opiates, scopolamine, or tranquilizers, smaller quantities of diazepam are required.[42] Effective total doses usually fall in the range of 10 to 30 mg; a total dose of 0.8 mg/kg will almost always be satisfactory. Some authors prefer to give a "loading" dose as a bolus of 15 to 35 mg, whereas others titrate the clinical effect using smaller increments of 5 to 10 mg.

Once sedation and dysarthria are achieved, nearly all patients will accept the face mask with no excitement or combativeness. Unlike those induced with barbiturates, diazepam-treated patients are rousable although they are drowsy and tranquil. A disadvantage of diazepam, however, is that second-to-second titration of the state of consciousness cannot be achieved. Whereas the depressant effects of thiopental or methohexital occur within one arm-brain circulation time, the sedation produced by diazepam is delayed from 30 to 120 sec after injection.

Adverse effects of diazepam induction are minimal and are less frequent than with barbiturate induction in the impression of most authors. Significant cardiovascular or respiratory depression rarely occurs, confirming the conclusions from studies cited in Chapter 7. Occasionally hiccoughs or yawning are associated with induction, but rarely restlessness or excitement. A non-life-threatening but significant problem associated with intravenous diazepam is pain on injection, occurring in up to 25% of cases depending upon dose, speed of injection, and size of the vein. In many cases local phlebitis is a sequel. It is unclear whether the drug itself or the propylene glycol solvent vehicle is responsible for this complication. Injection-site complications from intravenous diazepam are discussed in Chapters 4, 6, 7, and 12. Because diazepam is a highly lipid-soluble and slowly metabolized molecule, recovery from general anesthesia is prolonged when this drug is used for induction in place of short-acting barbiturates.

Diazepam in itself produces no significant analgesia (see Chapters 3 and 8), but opiate analgesics may be given as intramuscular premedicants, or intravenously together with diazepam at the time of induction. Aldrete et al.[53] have successfully used a fixed combination of diazepam (0.12 mg/ml) and pentazocine (0.35 mg/ml) as an induction agent. Although diazepam can be considered a central muscle relaxant, neither potentiation of succinylcholine nor reduction of succinylcholine requirements has been observed, consistent with the conclusions in Chapter 5. Two groups of investigators[54,54a] have noted that intravenous diazepam (0.2 to 0.4 mg/kg) reduced the alveolar concentration of volatile anesthetic necessary to eliminate spontaneous or provoked muscle movement.

Comparative Studies

Only a few comparative trials of diazepam and short-acting barbiturates have been published. Stovner and Endresen[55,56] found that diazepam produced amnesia with greater frequency and of longer duration than thiopental. Wyant and Studney[57] compared diazepam (0.3 to 0.45 mg/kg) to thiopental (2.5 mg/kg) in females undergoing gynecological procedures. Adequate anesthesia was reported in more than 90% of high-dose diazepam recipients, as opposed to less than 80% of those receiving thiopental. Recovery was significantly delayed in the diazepam group. Hellewell,[58] however, did not find that diazepam (0.16 to 0.32 mg/kg) significantly prolonged recovery time when compared to methohexital (1.6 mg/kg). Both medications were satisfactory induction agents, but apneic episodes occurred in 36% of barbiturate recipients versus only 7% of those receiving diazepam. Apnea was also more frequent after thiopental (average dose 4.1 mg/kg) than after diazepam (average dose 0.33 mg/kg) in a study reported by Fox and associates.[59] Induction was considered smooth in 70 to 80% of patients in both groups, while emergence from anesthesia was more rapid after thiopental induction. Hollis[60] reported that neither diazepam (0.32 mg/kg) nor thiopental (3.2 mg/kg) produced important alterations in systolic blood pressure. The barbiturate, however, reduced alveolar minute ventilation (V_A) by 40%, while diazepam reduced $\dot{V}_A$ by only 6%. Striking differences between these two drugs were reported by Dechene and Desrosiers.[61] After diazepam, mean arterial blood pressure fell from 89 to 87 mm Hg, and tidal volume fell slightly; after thiopental, mean blood pressure was reduced from 93 to 78 mm Hg, and tidal volume decreased more than 10-fold. Subjective impressions strongly favored diazepam over thiopental.

Diazepam has not fulfilled all the requirements as the ideal preanesthetic induction agent. Instantaneous control of consciousness cannot be achieved using this drug; in addition, diazepam appears to delay recovery from general anesthesia in many instances. Overall comparison with short-acting barbiturates, however, consistently suggests that diazepam is at least as effective and certainly is less toxic.

Amnesia

A significant advantage of diazepam is its ability to produce what is most accurately termed anterograde amnesia from the time of injection onward. This property is mentioned in many of the previously cited controlled and uncontrolled studies, and has also been noted by most authors using the drug for endoscopy and cardioversion (Chapter 7). Although patients are conscious following diazepam infusion, up to 100% of individuals recall nothing of the events occurring after receiving the drug. Anterograde amnesia appears to be much more frequent when the drug is given intravenously than after oral or intramuscular administration.

This property has been studied in more detail by several investigators. The route of administration is crucial. Pandit and Dundee[62] found that only 4% of patients had anterograde amnesia after intramuscular diazepam alone (10 mg). The incidence with intramuscular scopolamine alone (0.4 mg) was 14%. Scopolamine and diazepam combined produced anterograde amnesia in 26% of patients. By contrast, Turner and Wilson [63] found that intramuscular diazepam not only failed to suppress recall in most patients but also seemed to enhance unpleasant recall. After intravenous diazepam, however, 50% of patients had anterograde amnesia in a systematic test.[64] The combination of scopolamine, meperidine, and diazepam increased the incidence to 80%. Retrograde amnesia—lack of recall of events *prior* to intravenous drug infusion—was much less frequent. Dundee and Pandit[65] studied the time course of diazepam amnesia, and showed that the effect is immediate but short-lived. For 10 min following a 10-mg intravenous bolus of diazepam, there was essentially complete anterograde amnesia in 100% of subjects. After 10 min, the amnestic effect rapidly decayed. A 5-mg dose had a similar time course of action but was less effective. The effects of scopolamine (0.4 to 0.6 mg) were much slower in onset and longer in duration. Similar results were reported by Clarke and associates[66] using intravenous diazepam in doses of 0.25 mg/kg. There was no evidence of retrograde amnesia. Grove-White and Kelman[67] used much smaller doses of diazepam (0.05 mg/kg) in normal volunteers. Five min after the drug, recall of a six-digit number given 20 sec previously was impaired. At 15 min, impairment could no longer be demonstrated.

The short duration of diazepam-induced anterograde amnesia probably explains why the frequency of amnesia varies so widely from study to study. The degree of recall is critically dependent upon when the events took place relative to drug administration. It also is clear that when intravenous diazepam is to be used prior to cardioversion, endoscopy, electroconvulsive therapy, or general anesthesia, procedures are best performed immediately after the injection to insure minimal patient recall. The possibility that lorazepam also produces anterograde amnesia[20a,20b] deserves further investigation.

AFTER SURGERY

The benzodiazepines are of value as postoperative psychosedatives.[7] Derrick and associates[68] administered chlordiazepoxide (100 mg) or placebo to patients in a recovery room. Further sedatives or analgesics were not required in 72% of chlordiazepoxide recipients as opposed to only 16% of those treated with placebo. In a nonblind study, Bruce[69,70] administered diazepam (10 mg) or morphine (10 mg) to alternate patients requiring postoperative analgesia.

Adequate pain relief was reported nearly as often with diazepam (70% of patients) as with morphine (77% of patients). Vomiting was much less frequent after diazepam. McClish and associates[71] found that routine postoperative administration of diazepam (2.5 to 5.0 mg intravenously every 3 to 4 hr) to patients undergoing open-heart surgery considerably reduced the frequency of adverse psychiatric sequelae. Abel and Reis[72] reported that intravenous diazepam produced adequate sedation of agitated patients following cardiac surgery, with no evidence of cardiovascular depression.

Emergence Delirium

Intravenous ethanol has been tried as an induction agent for general anesthesia. Although the drug is an effective short-acting sedative-hypnotic, its use is limited by the high frequency of emergence delirium, estimated to occur in 50% of patients or more.[73] Reactions may be controlled by intravenous benzodiazepines or barbiturates at the time they occur, but recovery from anesthesia is thereby prolonged. Dundee and associates[74,75] have studied the influence of various premedications upon the incidence of emergence delirium with induction using 8% ethanol. Neither diazepam (10 to 30 mg) nor chlordiazepoxide (50 to 140 mg) as intramuscular premedications significantly influenced ethanol sequelae, nor increased the frequency of retrograde amnesia. In a second study from the same group,[76] intravenous diazepam or methohexital were combined with ethanol for induction. Methohexital was no help: hyperactivity or respiratory difficulties occurred in 50% of patients, and emergence delirium in 48%. With the diazepam-ethanol combination, the incidence of induction problems was reduced to 15%, and emergence delirium occurred in 25 to 30%. Recovery was markedly delayed when ethanol was combined with diazepam. The authors conclude that the complications associated with ethanol remain unacceptably common despite combination with diazepam.

An interesting alcohol-benzodiazepine interaction has been described by Dundee and associates.[74,77,78] They noted that following premedication with intramuscular chlordiazepoxide (100 to 140 mg), ethanol induction was more difficult, and patients more frequently required supplemental methohexital. Further investigation revealed that the dose of ethanol required to produce sleep was significantly increased, and the blood ethanol level at which sleep occurred was significantly elevated in patients premedicated with chlordiazepoxide. Meperidine (50 to 100 mg), diazepam (10 to 30 mg), and promethazine (50 mg) as intramuscular premedicants produced no such interaction. Pentobarbital (100 to 120 mg) produced slight ethanol potentiation. The results suggest that chlordiazepoxide antagonizes the central depressant effects of ethanol by acutely producing central tolerance. The basis for this interaction is unclear, but two groups of investigators[79,80] have made observations in animal studies which are consistent with these clinical findings of ethanol-chlordiazepoxide antagonism. The problem is further discussed in Chapter 11.

Emergence sequelae following ketamine anesthesia are a significant clinical problem. Two reports[81,82] have suggested that postoperative psychotomimetic reactions after ketamine may be reduced if diazepam supplementation is used. Systematic study has yielded conflicting results. A study by Collier[83] showed that routine postoperative diazepam increased patient acceptance of ketamine anesthesia. Erbguth and associates[84] also found that unpleasant recall and patient satisfaction following ketamine were favorably influenced by intravenous diazepam given after surgery. Chlorpromazine given prior to induction was equally useful, and in addition reduced the incidence of postoperative vomiting to less than 2%. Loh and associates,[85] however, were unable to demonstrate that intravenous diazepam (2 mg) after surgery reduced ketamine emergence delirium. Preoperative diazepam appears to be of no benefit.[86] Diazepam apparently does not influence the pattern of amnesia associated with ketamine.[84,87]

PREMEDICATION IN CHILDREN

The pediatric patient obviously presents a special problem to the anesthesiologist. The importance of premedication is considerable, since a fully alert child is likely to object violently to the events prior to surgery. At the same time, parenteral premedications seldom are quietly tolerated. Most studies deal with oral premedications in children undergoing tonsillectomy.

Uncontrolled observations by Dowell[88,89] suggest that oral diazepam is a satisfactory premedicant for children. The usual dose was 0.18 mg/kg given prior to surgery and on the previous night. Patients were conscious but cooperative during induction and seldom needed analgesics postoperatively. Several trials compare diazepam to trimeprazine, a phenothiazine derivative. Dowell[89] found that the two agents were equally satisfactory. Gordon and Turner[90] compared diazepam (0.22 mg/kg), trimeprazine (3.3 mg/kg), and phenobarbital (4.4 mg/kg) as oral premedicants in combination with scopolamine (0.4 to 0.6 mg). Preoperative behavior and response to induction were significantly more satisfactory with diazepam; in postoperative evaluations, the three drugs were equivalent. Haq and Dundee[91] found that overall patient acceptance of diazepam and trimeprazine was approximately the same, but trimeprazine was superior by most other evaluations. In both of these studies, trimeprazine was much more effective than diazepam in suppressing salivary secretions. Wilson and associates[92] reported that operative blood loss during tonsillectomy did not differ between children receiving diazepam (0.17 mg/kg), trimeprazine (3.3 mg/kg), or phenobarbital (4.4 mg/kg) as premedicants.

A nonblind trial reported by Bush[93] suggested that intramuscular meperidine was a more satisfactory premedication than oral diazepam.

McGarry[94] compared oral diazepam (0.4 mg/kg), meperidine (1.1 mg/kg), droperidol (0.05 mg/kg), and placebo. Diazepam proved to be the most satisfactory premedicant by a number of measures, whereas droperidol and placebo were the least. Romagnoli et al.[95] studied various combinations of diazepam, meperidine, anticholinergics, and pentobarbital, finding no consistent differences between the combinations. Boyd and Manford[95a] found that oral trichloroethyl phosphate (71 mg/kg) was a significantly more effective pediatric premedicant than diazepam (0.2 mg/kg).

The utility of diazepam as a pediatric premedicant has not been established. Since most surgical procedures in children are otolaryngological, diazepam by itself would, in general, be inadequate since it possesses no antisecretory properties. Yet even when diazepam is combined with an anticholinergic it has no consistent superiority over phenothiazines or opiates. More controlled study of this subject is required.

OTHER USES

Various reports have described the use of diazepam as a psychosedative adjunct for cystoscopy,[96,97] pneumoencephalography,[98] radiologic procedures in agitated or uncooperative patients,[99] or regional anesthesia.[100–102] In all of these publications, the results with diazepam are favorable. Cinotti and associates[103] found that intravenous chlordiazepoxide (20 to 40 mg) was superior to placebo as an adjunct to local anesthesia in patients undergoing cataract extraction. Further study is needed to establish the superiority of benzodiazepines over other psychosedatives in these situations.

DENTISTRY

The benzodiazepines appear to have a potentially important place in dental medicine and surgery. As discussed previously, the mere thought of dental manipulation for many individuals is sufficient to evoke severe symptomatic anxiety. Some, in fact, are so apprehensive that they refuse to submit to dental treatment despite its logical necessity. Several reports suggest that oral or parenteral premedication with chlordiazepoxide or diazepam may be effective in allaying apprehension in dental patients.[104–110] The need for adjuvants to local anesthesia in many dental procedures has been alluded to. Intravenous diazepam has received praise as a highly suitable adjunct.[111–126] The drug is used in much the same way as in cardioversion, with corresponding safety and efficacy in uncontrolled trials. The usual effective dose falls in the range of 10 to 20 mg. Adequate sedation, once achieved, lasts 30 to 60 min. Procedures may be carried out under local anesthesia, with many patients having no recollection of the events. Occasionally, small doses of supplemental methohexital are required. The patient usually is able to ambulate within 2 hr after termination of the procedure. Significant cardiovascular or pulmonary complications are extremely rare. The only consistent problem is injection pain and phlebitis.

In a controlled study of oral premedicants, Fisher and associates[127] compared diazepam (15 mg per day for 1 week) and placebo in a crossover trial in four patients undergoing multiple dental treatments. Diazepam did not significantly differ from placebo in antianxiety effects. In a much larger study using 50 patients per group, Baird and Curson[128] gave a total of 15 mg of oral diazepam in the 18 hr prior to dental treatment. Diazepam recipients were much less frightened prior to dental work than those receiving placebo. Two studies involve oxazepam and placebo given on the day preceding and again just prior to treatment. One group[129] reported that oxazepam was significantly superior to placebo in the patient's subjective evaluation. Norton,[130] however, found no significant drug-placebo differences. Chambrias[131] studied four tranquilizers (chlordiazepoxide, chlorpromazine, hydroxyzine, meprobamate) alone and in combination with secobarbital as oral premedicants in children. The combinations of secobarbital plus chlordiazepoxide and secobarbital plus chlorpromazine were superior to other mixtures and to the drugs given alone.

Intravenous diazepam has been compared in controlled trials to hydroxyzine,[132] pentazocine,[133] meperidine plus scopolamine,[134] and meperidine plus promethazine.[135] In each of the studies, diazepam is equally or more satisfactory than the comparison drug and produces fewer adverse reactions. Dixon and co-workers[136,137] reported that intravenous diazepam (0.12 to 0.32 mg/kg) was an effective sedative adjunct to local anesthesia and produced minimal cardiovascular depression. Postoperative tests of intellectual performance, however, showed significant impairment among diazepam recipients when compared to those receiving local anesthesia alone.[138]

COMMENT

The replacement of traditional sedative-hypnotics by benzodiazepine derivatives in anesthetic practice has both benefits and disadvantages. A consistent finding is that chlordiazepoxide and diazepam have minimal cardiovascular and respiratory depressant effects when compared to barbiturates. The importance of this property becomes greater among patients with obstructive pulmonary disease, advanced cardiac disease, or otherwise increased sensitivity to depressant drugs. In such cases, diazepam is probably preferable to short-acting barbiturates as premedicants or induction agents. Suppression of recall is another important property of diazepam. An intravenous bolus of this drug is followed by a short period of dense anterograde amnesia without unconsciousness. This may considerably enhance patient tolerance and acceptance of surgical or dental procedures, particularly among those who are severely apprehensive or who must undergo multiple procedures. When benzodiazepines are used in place of barbiturates, overall sedative and antianxiety effects are at least as satisfactory if not more so. In many of the cited controlled studies on which these conclusions are based, the authors make multiple statistical comparisons with single mean values. It is not obvious whether the appropriate adjustments of confidence limits have been made (see Chapter 9, under "Comment"), nor whether correct statistical treatment of incorrectly handled results would invalidate the reported conclusions.

For reasons which are uncertain, the central depressant effects of intravenous diazepam are less rapid in onset than those of methohexital or thiopental. When essentially instantaneous titration of the level of consciousness is required, diazepam by itself is not suitable. Some authors administer intravenous diazepam as the initial basal psychosedative, with small incremental doses of a barbiturate added as necessary. When diazepam is used as a premedicant or as an induction agent, a statistically significant delay in emergence from general anesthesia is frequently reported. Whether this delay is of clinical significance is uncertain. The data suggest, however, that ambulatory recipients of intravenous diazepam be advised against operation of automobiles or dangerous machinery for 24 hr following administration of the drug.

Other reviewers[139-143] support the conclusion that the availability of the benzodiazepines constitutes a significant advance in the psychopharmacology of anesthetic and dental practice.

REFERENCES

1. Norris W: The quantitative assessment of premedication. Brit J Anaesth 41:778-784, 1969
2. Coppolino CA, Wallace G: Evaluation of Librium® as a preanesthetic medication. Postgrad Med 29:619-621, 1961
2a. Elia JC: Pre-operative and postoperative otolaryngology. EENT Monthly 40:344-348, 1961
3. Inglis JM, Barrow MEH: Premedication—a reassessment. Proc Roy Soc Med 58:29, 1965
4. Corey PJ, Deaver JM, Haupt GJ: The use of Librium for surgical patients. Penn Med J 65:1053-1058, 1962
5. Robinson MM: The use of chlordiazepoxide to allay preoperative apprehension in abrasive surgery. Med Ann DC 30:719-721, 1961
6. Manku MS: Diazepam premedication in ophthalmic surgery. Brit J Ophthal 54:273-275, 1970
7. Lamphier TA, Chin S, Crooker L, Arthurs A, Goldberg RI: Chlordiazepoxide as a preoperative and postoperative medication. Clin Med 69:2466-2469, 1962
8. Kyles JR: Observations on the use of diazepam in anaesthesia. In, *Diazepam in Anaesthesia.* Edited by PF Knight, CG Burgess. Bristol, John Wright and Sons, 1968, pp 66-69
9. Apte NK: Chlordiazepoxide in otorhinolaryngological practice. J Indian Med Assoc 45:317-318, 1965
10. Bodi S: Observations with Seduxen in oto-rhino-laryngology. Therapia Hungarica 18:85-90, 1970

11. Somers K: Intravenous Librium as a supplement to local anesthesia in intraocular surgery. Ann Ophthalmol 4:847-850, 1972

12. Brandt AL, Lui SCY, Briggs BD: Trial of chlordiazepoxide as preanesthetic medication. Anesth Analg 41:557-564, 1962

13. Brandt AL, Oakes FD: Preanesthesia medication: double-blind study of a new drug, diazepam. Anesth Analg 44:125-129, 1965

14. Wordsworth VP: Oral use of diazepam. In, *Diazepam in Anaesthesia.* Edited by PF Knight, CG Burgess. Bristol, John Wright and Sons, 1968, pp 16-18

15. Powell WF, Comer WH: Controlled comparison of lorazepam and pentobarbital as hypnotics for presurgical patients. Anesth Analg 52:267-271, 1973

15a. Powell WF, Comer WH: Double-blind controlled comparison of lorazepam and glutethimide as night-before-operation hypnotics. Anesth Analg 52:313-316, 1973

16. Hare SA: Oral pre-anaesthetic medication with a new benzodiazepine hypnotic. South Afr Med J 47:109-111, 1973

17. Murray WJ, Bechtoldt AA, Berman L: Efficacy of oral psychosedative drugs for preanesthetic medication. JAMA 203:327-332, 1968

18. Moore PH, Hollis DA: Oral premedication with diazepam. Brit Med J 2:49, 1968

19. Norris W, Telfer ABM: Nitrazepam in premedication. Brit J Anaesth 41:877-879, 1969

20. Norris W, Wallace PGM: Wy 4036 (lorazepam): a study of its use in premedication. Brit J Anaesth 43:785-789, 1971

20a. Wilson J: Lorazepam as a premedicant for general anaesthesia. Curr Med Res Opin 1:308-316, 1973

20b. Turner DJ: Lorazepam as a premedicant in anaesthesia: a pilot study. Curr Med Res Opin 1:302-307, 1973

21. Johnstone M: The effects of oral sedatives on the vasoconstrictive reaction to fear. Brit J Anaesth 43:380-384, 1971

22. Oyama T, Kimura K, Takazawa T, Takiguchi H: An objective evaluation of tranquillizers as preanaesthetic medication: effect on adrenocortical function. Canad Anaesth Soc J 16:209-216, 1969

23. James M, Fisher A: Nitrazepam as a premedicant in minor surgery. An assessment. Anaesthesia 25:364-367, 1970

24. McCaughey W, Dundee JW: Comparison of the sedative effects of diazepam given by the oral and intramuscular routes (Abstract). Brit J Anaesth 44:901-902, 1972

25. Gibbs L, Svigals RE, Riklan M: A double-blind study of chlordiazepoxide as a preanesthetic agent in cardiac surgery. Anesth Analg 50:17-22, 1971

26. Buchmann G, Johansen SH, Schioler K: Chlordiazepoxide (Librium) used as premedication in operations for varicose veins. Acta Anaesth Scand 8:227-232, 1964

27. Tornetta FJ: Clinical evaluation of injectable Librium® in preanesthetic medication. Anesth Analg 42:463-469, 1963

28. Haslett WHK: A controlled study of diazepam and chlordiazepoxide as a premedicant for a standard operation. In, *Diazepam in Anesthesia.* Edited by PF Knight, CG Burgess. Bristol, John Wright and Sons, 1968, pp 19-24

29. Haslett WHK, Dundee JW: Studies of drugs given before anaesthesia. XIV: Two benzodiazepine derivatives—chlordiazepoxide and diazepam. Brit J Anaesth 40:250-258, 1968

30. Tornetta FJ: Diazepam as preanesthetic medication: a double-blind study. Anesth Analg 44:449-452, 1965

31. Dundee JW, Loan WB, Morrison JD: Studies of drugs given before anaesthesia. XIX: The opiates. Brit J Anaesth 42:54-58, 1970

32. Dundee JW, Haslett WHK, Keilty SR, Pandit SK: Studies of drugs given before anaesthesia. XX: Diazepam-containing mixtures. Brit J Anaesth 42:143-150, 1970

33. Steen SN, Hahl D: Controlled evaluation of parenteral diazepam as preanesthetic medication. Anesth Analg 48:549-554, 1969
34. Dobkin AB, Israel JS, Evers W, Bisset CM: Double-blind evaluation of diazepam for premedication. Canad Anaesth Soc J 17:52-60, 1970
35. Dobkin AB, Desai AA: Double-blind evaluation of doxepin hydrochloride (Sinequan®) for preanaesthetic medication. Canad Anaesth Soc J 19:129-137, 1972
36. Cormier A, Goyette M, Keeri-Szanto M, Rheault J: A comparison of the action of meperidine and diazepam in anaesthetic premedication. Canad Anaesth Soc J 13:368-373, 1966
37. Clarke RSJ, Dundee JW, Loan WB: The use of post-operative vomiting as a means of evaluating anti-emetics. Brit J Pharmacol 40:568P-569P, 1970
38. Morrison JD, Clarke RSJ, Dundee JW: Studies on drugs given before anaesthesia. XXI: Droperidol. Brit J Anaesth 42:730-735, 1970
39. Roberts JC: A double blind study comparing promethazine-pethidine with diazepam. In, *Diazepam in Anaesthesia*. Edited by PF Knight, CG Burgess. Bristol, John Wright and Sons, 1968, pp 9-15
40. Dixon HR, Tilton BE, Briggs BD: A comparison of the sedative and cardiorespiratory properties of diazepam and pentazocine for premedication. Anesth Analg 49:546-550, 1970
41. Marrubini MB, Tretola L: Diazepam as a pre-operative tranquillizer in neuroanaesthesia: a preliminary note. Brit J Anaesth 37:934-946, 1965
42. Brown SS, Dundee JW: Clinical studies of induction agents. XXV: Diazepam. Brit J Anaesth 40:108-112, 1968
42a. Urban BJ, Amaha K, Steen SN: Investigation of 1,4-benzodiazepine derivatives as basal anesthetic agents. Anesth Analg 45:733-736, 1966
43. Baker AB: Induction of anaesthesia with diazepam. Anaesthesia 24:388-394, 1969
44. Kurland P: Dissociative analgesia with diazepam and hyoscine. Anesthesia Progr 17:36-37, 1970
45. Goldman JA, Ovadia J, Eckerling B: Intravenous diazepam and pethidine-promethazine analgesia for minor gynaecological operations. Brit J Anaesth 44:381-382, 1972
46. McClish A: Diazepam as an intravenous induction agent for general anaesthesia. Canad Anaesth Soc J 13:562-575, 1966
47. McTigue JW, Urweider HA: The use of diazepam in ophthalmic surgery. Trans Amer Acad Ophthal Otolar 73:78-84, 1969
48. Eryasa Y: The use of diazepam in surgery. Southern Med J 64:27-29, 1971
49. Rollason WN: Diazepam as an intravenous induction agent for general anaesthesia. In, *Diazepam in Anaesthesia*. Edited by PF Knight, CG Burgess. Bristol, John Wright and Sons, 1968, pp 70-73
50. Brown SS: Studies of diazepam: an intravenous anaesthetic. In, *Diazepam in Anaesthesia*. Edited by PF Knight, CG Burgess. Bristol, John Wright and Sons, 1968, pp 52-55
51. Eisenberg L, Kwan AM: Neuroleptanaesthesia with diazepam-morphine in poor-risk surgical patients. Canad Anaesth Soc J 18:465-472, 1971
52. Beaulieu D, Goyette M, Keeri-Szanto M: Anaesthetic time/dose curves: VI. Experiences with diazepam. Canad Anaesth Soc J 14:326-332, 1967
53. Aldrete JA, Clapp HW, Fishman J, O'Higgins JW: "Pentazepam": a supplementary agent. Anesth Analg 50:498-504, 1971
54. Perisho JA, Buechel DR, Miller RD: The effect of diazepam (Valium®) on minimum alveolar anaesthetic requirement (MAC) in man. Canad Anaesth Soc J 18:536-540, 1971
54a. Tsunoda Y, Hattori Y, Takatsuka E, Sawa T, Hori T, Ikezono E: Effects of hydroxyzine, diazepam, and pentazocine on halothane minimum alveolar anesthetic concentration. Anesth Analg 52:390-394, 1973

55. Stovner J, Endresen R: Intravenous anaesthesia with diazepam. Acta Anaesth Scand supp 24:223-227, 1966
56. Stovner I, Endresen R: Diazepam as an induction agent. Der Anaesthetist 18:242-243, 1969
57. Wyant GM, Studney LJ: A study of diazepam (Valium®) for induction of anaesthesia. Canad Anaesth Soc J 17:166-171, 1970
58. Hellewell J: Induction of anaesthesia with diazepam. In, *Diazepam in Anaesthesia.* Edited by PF Knight, CG Burgess. Bristol, John Wright and Sons, 1968, pp 47-51
59. Fox GS, Wynands JE, Bhambhami M: A clinical comparison of diazepam and thiopentone as induction agents to general anaesthesia. Canad Anaesth Soc J 15:281-290, 1968
60. Hollis DA: Diazepam as an induction agent, II. In, *Diazepam in Anaesthesia.* Edited by PF Knight, CG Burgess. Bristol, John Wright and Sons, 1968, pp 60-65
61. Dechene J-P, Desrosiers R: Diazepam in pulmonary surgery. Canad Anaesth Soc J 16:162-166, 1969
62. Pandit SK, Dundee JW: Pre-operative amnesia. The incidence following the intramuscular injection of commonly used premedicants. Anaesthesia 25:493-499, 1970
63. Turner DJ, Wilson J: Effect of diazepam on awareness during caesarean section under general anaesthesia. Brit Med J 2:736-737, 1969
64. Pandit SK, Dundee JW, Keilty SR: Amnesia studies with intravenous premedication. Anaesthesia 26:421-428, 1971
65. Dundee JW, Pandit SK: Anterograde amnestic effects of pethidine, hyoscine, and diazepam in adults. Brit J Pharmacol 44:140-144, 1972
66. Clarke PRF, Eccersley PS, Frisby JP, Thornton JA: The amnesic effect of diazepam (Valium). Brit J Anaesth 42:690-697, 1970
67. Grove-White IG, Kelman GR: Effect of methohexitone, diazepam, and sodium 4-hydroxybutyrate on short-term memory. Brit J Anaesth 43:113-116, 1971
68. Derrick WS, Wette R, Hill DB: Librium® in the recovery room. Anesth Analg 46:171-175, 1967
69. Bruce IS: Diazepam in intravenous anaesthesia. Lancet 1:151, 1966
70. Bruce IS: Postoperative use of diazepam. In, *Diazepam in Anaesthesia.* Edited by PF Knight, CG Burgess. Bristol, John Wright and Sons, 1968, pp 89-91
71. McClish A, Andrew D, Tetreault L: Intravenous diazepam for psychiatric reactions following open-heart surgery. Canad Anaesth Soc J 15:63-79, 1968
72. Abel RM, Reis RL: Intravenous diazepam for sedation following cardiac operations: clinical and hemodynamic assessments. Anesth Analg 50:244-248, 1971
73. Dundee JW, Isaac M: Clinical studies of induction agents. XXIX: Ethanol. Brit J Anaesth 41:1063-1069, 1969
74. Dundee JW, Isaac M, Pandit SK, McDowell SA: Clinical studies of induction agents. XXXIV: Further investigations with ethanol. Brit J Anaesth 42:300-310, 1970
75. Isaac M, Pandit SK, Dundee JW, Galway JE: Intravenous ethanol anaesthesia. A study of sequelae and their implications. Acta Anaesth Scand 15:141-155,1971
76. Isaac M, Bovill JG, Dundee JW, Pandit SK: Clinical studies of induction agents. XXXV: Studies on combination of ethanol with methohexitone and diazepam. Brit J Anaesth 42:521-523, 1970
77. Dundee JW, Isaac M: Interaction between intravenous ethanol and some sedatives and tranquillizers. Brit J Pharmacol 39:199P-200P, 1970
78. Dundee JW, Howard AJ, Isaac M: Alcohol and the benzodiazepines. The interaction between intravenous ethanol and chlordiazepoxide and diazepam. Quart J Stud Alcohol 32:960-968, 1971
79. Hughes FW, Rountree CB, Forney RB: Suppression of learned avoidance and discriminative responses in the rat by chlordiazepoxide (Librium) and ethanol-chlordiazepoxide combinations. J Genetic Psychol 103:139-145, 1963

80. Hernandez-Peon R, Goldberg L, Rojas-Ramirez JA: Physiology and psychosomatic medicine: neurophysiological models of emotional behavior and of action of psychotropic drugs. In, *Psychotropic Drugs in Internal Medicine*. Edited by A Pletscher, A Marino, P Pinkerton. Amsterdam, Excerpta Medica Foundation, 1969, pp 16-46

81. Lowson AJ: Ketamine and diazepam in the adult patient. Med J Aust 2:448-449, 1971

82. McLean AG: Ketamine and diazepam in the adult patient. Med J Aust 2:338, 1971

83. Collier BB: Ketamine and the conscious mind. Anaesthesia 27:120-134, 1972

84. Erbguth PH, Reiman B, Klein RL: The influence of chlorpromazine, diazepam, and droperidol on emergence from ketamine. Anesth Analg 51:693-700, 1972

85. Loh L, Singer L, Morgan M, Moore PH: Influence of diazepam on the emergence reactions following ketamine anaesthesia. Canad Anaesth Soc J 19:421-425, 1972

86. Bovill JG, Clarke RSJ, Dundee JW, Pandit SK, Moore J: Clinical studies of induction agents. XXXVIII: Effect of premedicants and supplements on ketamine anaesthesia. Brit J Anaesth 43:600-608, 1971

87. Pandit SK, Dundee JW, Bovill JG: Clinical studies on induction agents. XXXVII: Amnestic action of ketamine. Brit J Anaesth 43:362-364, 1971

88. Dowell T: Diazepam in intravenous anaesthesia. Lancet 1:369-370, 1966

89. Dowell T: Diazepam premedication in paediatric patients. In, *Diazepam in Anaesthesia.* Edited by PF Knight, CG Burgess. Bristol, John Wright and Sons, 1968, pp 25-32

90. Gordon NH, Turner DJ: Oral paediatric premedication. A comparative trial of either phenobarbitone, trimeprazine, or diazepam with hyoscine, prior to guillotine tonsillectomy. Brit J Anaesth 41:136-142, 1969

91. Haq IU, Dundee JW: Studies of drugs given before anaesthesia. XVI: Oral diazepam and trimeprazine for adenotonsillectomy. Brit J Anaesth 40:972-978, 1968

92. Wilson SM, Owen M, Duff TB, Malcolm-Smith NA: Operative blood loss in guillotine tonsillectomy and adenoidectomy in children: a comparison of three premedicant drugs. Brit J Anaesth 45:86-89, 1973

93. Bush GH: Diazepam as a premedication in children. In, *Diazepam in Anaesthesia.* Edited by PF Knight, CG Burgess. Bristol, John Wright and Sons, 1968, pp 33-38

94. McGarry PMF: A double-blind study of diazepam, droperidol, and meperidine as premedication in children. Canad Anaesth Soc J 17:157-165, 1970

95. Romagnoli A, Cuison S, Cohen M: The use of diazepam in paediatric premedication. Canad Anaesth Soc J 15:603-609, 1968

95a. Boyd JD, Manford MLM: Premedication in children. A controlled clinical trial of oral triclofos and diazepam. Brit J Anaesth 45:501-506, 1973

96. Emmett JAJ: The use of intravenous diazepam (Valium®) as a sedative and relaxant in urological endoscopic procedures. Canad Anaesth Soc J 17:242-249, 1970

97. Blackard CE, McBride AM, Wedge JJ, Mellinger GT: Valium as an adjunct to cystoscopy. Minnesota Med 53:11-13, 1970

98. Edwards JC, Flowerdew GD: Diazepam and local analgesia for lumbar air encephalography. Brit J Anaesth 42:999-1004, 1970

99. Finby N, Kanick V: Radiological special procedures and the difficult patient. Intravenous Valium to salvage diagnostic studies. Radiology 94:101-103, 1970

100. Drolet H, Boisvert M: Diazepam as an adjuvant agent in regional anaesthesia. Canad Anaesth Soc J 19:283-289, 1972

101. Thompson GE, Moore DC: Ketamine, diazepam, and Innovar®: a computerized comparative study. Anesth Analg 50:458-463, 1971

102. Adamson JE, Cohen BI, Horton CE, Mladick RA, Gwyn PP: Intravenous diazepam: a helpful adjunct in plastic surgery. Plastic Reconstr Surg 45:145-149, 1971

103. Cinotti AA, Siliquini JJ, Long DL: Reinforcing anesthesia in cataract surgery. Report on a new technique. Arch Ophthal 74:360-364, 1965

104. Collopy FJ: The use of chlordiazepoxide in general dental practice. Aust Dent J 10:431-432, 1965
105. Black A: Diazepam. Brit Dent J 125:244, 1968
106. Ahlin JH, Steinberg AI: Chlordiazepoxide HCl (Librium®) as a premedicant for dental patients: a preliminary report. J Oral Med 24:39-41, 1969
107. Lipkin KM: The reduction of anxiety: the dentist, the psychiatrist, and diazepam. Oral Surg Oral Med Oral Pathol 25:131-133, 1968
108. Grant GH: Chlordiazepoxide used for apprehensive dental patients: preliminary observations. J Amer Dent Assoc 66:182-185, 1963
109. Peabody JB: Premedicating periodontic patients. Texas Dent J 83:12-14. (Oct) 1965
110. Goffen BS: Patient acceptance of the anesthetic process II: Diazepam (Valium®) premedication. J Amer Soc Psychosom Dent Med 16:108-119, 1969
111. Healy TEJ, Lautch H, Hall N, Tomlin PJ, Vickers MD: Interdisciplinary study of diazepam sedation for outpatient dentistry. Brit Med J 3:13-17, 1970
112. Rattray IJ: Observations on the use of diazepam in general dental practice. Brit Dent J 125:495-498, 1968
113. Harris D: Intravenous diazepam. Brit Dent J 129:57, 1970
114. Shepherd PR, Aust JH: Diazepam. Brit Dent J 125:184, 1968
115. Hall W: Diazepam. Brit Dent J 125:244, 1968
116. Brown PRH, Main DMG, Lawson JIM: Diazepam in dentistry. Report on 108 cases. Brit Dent J 125:498-501, 1968
117. Litchfield NB, Gerard P: Diazepam intravenous sedation in dentistry. A report of 1,557 cases. Aust Dent J 16:25-33, 1971
118. Poswillo D: Intravenous amnesia for dental and oral surgery. New Zealand Dent J 63:265-270, 1967
119. O'Neil R, Verrill P: Intravenous diazepam in minor oral surgery. Brit J Oral Surg 7:12-14, 1969
120. O'Neil R, Verrill PJ, Aellig WH, Laurence DR: Intravenous diazepam in minor oral surgery. Further studies. Brit Dent J 128:15-18, 1970
121. Schofield IDFS: Investigation into the use of diazepam as an intravenous premedicant in minor oral surgery. J Ontario Dent Assoc 47:306-310, 1970
122. Driscoll EJ, Smilack ZH, Lightbody PM, Fiorucci RD: Sedation with intravenous diazepam. J Oral Surg 30:332-343, 1972
123. Shane SM: Amnesia for brief exodontia procedures using small doses of diazepam and methohexital with local block anesthesia for ambulatory patients. J Oral Surg 29:191-193, 1971
124. Main DMG: The use of diazepam in dental anaesthesia. In, Diazepam in Anaesthesia. Edited by PF Knight, CG Burgess. Bristol, John Wright and Sons, 1968, pp 85-87
125. Foreman PA, Neels R, Willetts PW: Diazepam in dentistry. Clinical observations based on the treatment of 167 patients in general dental practice. Anesthesia Progr 15:253-259, 1968
126. Edmondson HD, Roscoe B, Vickers MD: Biochemical evidence of anxiety in dental patients. Brit Med J 4:7-9, 1972
127. Fisher S, Pillard RC, Yamada L: Hard-core anxiety in dental patients: implications for drug screening. In, The Present Status of Psychotropic Drugs. Pharmacological and Clinical Aspects. Edited by A Cerletti, FJ Bové. Amsterdam, Excerpta Medica Foundation, 1969, pp 381-382
128. Baird ES, Curson I: Orally administered diazepam in conservative dentistry. A double-blind trial. Brit Dent J 128:25-27, 1970
129. Dental Practitioner Research Unit: Oxazepam before dental treatment. Brit J Clin Prac 24:323-326, 1970

130. Norton GA: A clinical investigation of oxazepam as an adjunct for periodontal therapy. J Periodontol 40:485-489, 1969

131. Chambrias PG: Sedation for dentistry in children: selective medication. Aust Dent J 14:245-254, 1969

132. Schechter HO, Cosentino BJ: Combinations of psychotherapeutic drugs and local anesthesia for dental procedures. J Oral Surg 28:280-284, 1970

133. Brown PRH, Donaldson D, Gray IG, Main DMG: Intravenous sedation in dentistry: a comparative study of diazepam and pentazocine. Dent Prac Dent Rec 21:2-6, (Sept) 1970

134. Chambrias PG: Evaluation of sedatives in dental practice. Preliminary report. Aust Dent J 15:112-118, 1970

135. Khosla VM, Boren W: Diazepam (Valium) as preoperative medication in oral surgery. Oral Surg Oral Med Oral Pathol 28:671-679, 1969

136. Dixon RA, Day CD, Eccersley PS, Thornton JA: Intravenous diazepam in dentistry: monitoring results from a controlled trial. Brit J Anaesth 45:202-206, 1973

137. Dixon RA, Hatt SD, Rowse CW: Intravenous diazepam in dentistry: operating conditions in a controlled clinical trial. J Dent 1:2-6, 1972

138. Dixon RA, Thornton JA: Tests of recovery from anaesthesia and sedation: intravenous diazepam in dentistry. Brit J Anaesth 45:207-215, 1973

139. Hughes G: Diazepam in the dental surgery. Ann Royal Coll Surg Engl 48:38-39, 1971

140. Hollis DA: Diazepam: its scope in anaesthetic practice. Proc Roy Soc Med 62:806-807, 1969

141. Dundee JW, Haslett WHK: The benzodiazepines. A review of their actions and uses relative to anaesthetic practice. Brit J Anaesth 42:217-234, 1970

142. Dundee JW, Keilty SR: Diazepam. Int Anaesth Clin 7:91-121, 1969

143. Foreman PA: Intravenous diazepam in general dental practice. New Zealand Dent J 65:243-253, 1969

Chapter 11

The Treatment of Alcoholism and Other Drug-Dependent States

The use of sedatives and tranquilizers has long been an important aspect of the treatment of drug addiction. The problem has two quite distinct components. The first is the acute withdrawal syndrome. Withdrawal from an habituating drug is a medical problem, often requiring hospitalization. The efficacy of a sedative or tranquilizer in acute withdrawal syndromes is measured by the degree to which it reduces the severity and duration of the syndrome, the mortality and frequency of complications, and the subjectively unpleasant nature of withdrawal. It appears that almost any choice of "replacement drug"—barbiturates, paraldehyde, ethanol, benzodiazepines or phenothiazines—is better than placebo or no treatment in patients acutely withdrawing from alcohol, barbiturates, or opiates. Which of the available replacement drugs is most suitable, however, is unclear.

When the state of physiologic addiction is terminated, the issue becomes one of preventing relapse. The appropriate use of pharmacotherapy in this stage of the treatment of drug abuse is primarily a psychiatric problem. The efficacy of a psychotropic drug in this setting is measured by the patient's willingness to return for follow-up care, his return to work and functional citizenship, and the prevention of relapse to addiction to the original drug of abuse. As opposed to acute withdrawal, almost any choice of psychotropic drug in this situation is likely to fail. A large proportion of patients drop out of therapy and return to the original addiction with its associated social and medical consequences.

Aside from its apparent lack of efficacy, long-term pharmacotherapy of drug addiction has been questioned on other grounds. Critics point out that in the addiction-prone personality, sequential or concurrent abuse of multiple drugs—alcohol, barbiturates, opiates, hallucinogens, amphetamines—is common.[1,2] It has been claimed with some justification that simply transferring the state of addiction from one drug to another accomplishes very little in terms of treating the patient's underlying psychopathology.

Yet there is more to the problem than the issue of drug dependence alone. Prolonged use of certain drugs is associated with unacceptably grave medical sequelae. The association of alcoholism and cirrhosis is a classic example. With respect to opiate abuse, it is becoming clear that the eventual downfall of most addicts is related to the infectious disease consequences of repeated nonsterile intravenous injections. The effects of long-term chlordiazepoxide use in humans, for example, are not known at present, but it is likely that replacement of alcohol or opiates with chlordiazepoxide would reduce or eliminate serious medical hazards. Use of legal rather than illegal drugs also relieves the obligation to participate in counterproductive social behavior. It may well be, therefore, that addiction to ethanol or heroin should be terminated even if prolonged use of chlordiazepoxide or methadone is a possible consequence.

This chapter reviews the role of the benzodiazepines in the acute and chronic treatment of addiction to other drugs. Most published studies deal with alcoholism. A few reports describe the use of the benzodiazepines in states of dependence on barbiturates, opiates, and tobacco.

INTERACTION OF BENZODIAZEPINES AND ETHANOL

Some of the experimental and clinical studies cited in Chapter 10 (references 77-80) suggest that chlordiazepoxide and ethanol have opposing effects upon the central nervous system. Most other studies, however, demonstrate that ethanol and the benzodiazepines produce additive central depression. The effects are most obvious in laboratory animals. Combining either chlordiazepoxide or diazepam with ethanol increases the muscle-relaxant[3,4] and hypnotic[4-9] effects over those produced when the drugs are given alone. Norio et al.,[6] however, were unable to demonstrate significant potentiation of ethanol in rats by large doses of nitrazepam (10 to 100 mg/kg). Milner[8] found that diazepam did not enhance the lethal effects of alcohol in mice despite significant prolongation of sleeping time. Others have similarly reported that additive behavioral depression is more obvious than additive lethality.[10,11] In human studies, significant benzodiazepine-ethanol interactions are minimal or absent. Chlordiazepoxide, diazepam, and medazepam have been tested in controlled trials.[9,12-16] In these studies administration of drug or placebo is begun as early as several days before testing and continues up to several hours before the trial session. Psychomotor performance is then tested after a standard dose of ethanol. In all of the reports, significant impairment is produced by ethanol alone, but the impairment is not potentiated to any important degree in subjects also receiving benzodiazepines. Reggiani and associates[9] found that a single 10-mg dose of chlordiazepoxide did not potentiate the effects of ethanol on automobile operation by normal volunteers. Betts and co-workers[16a] administered 50 mg of chlordiazepoxide in divided doses to healthy individuals over the 36 hr prior to low-speed driving performance tests. Subjects who also received ethanol just before testing performed the same as those receiving chlordiazepoxide without ethanol. These two reports are the only ones describing study of realistic life situations. The interaction of ethanol with high doses of benzodiazepines also has received little attention. Until these areas are investigated more thoroughly, physicians are urged to counsel their patients conservatively regarding potentiation of ethanol depression by any tranquilizers, including benzodiazepines.

From limited investigation it appears that the benzodiazepines have little effect upon the metabolism of ethanol. Blood levels of ethanol in rats 1 hr after a standard dose were not influenced by concurrent administration of chlordiazepoxide (20 mg/kg).[17] Morselli and associates[18] studied the kinetics of ethanol disappearance in humans before and after 10 days of treatment with diazepam (15 mg per day). There was no alteration of ethanol half-life by diazepam treatment. Reggiani and associates[9] found that the pharmacokinetics of absorption, distribution, and metabolism of a single oral dose of ethanol in humans (700 mg/kg) was not changed when the ethanol was given together with chlordiazepoxide (20 mg).

ALCOHOL WITHDRAWAL

The benzodiazepines currently are the tranquilizing agents most commonly used in the treatment of acute alcohol withdrawal.[19] There is ample evidence for the efficacy of chlordiazepoxide and diazepam in this setting. Guerrero-Figueroa and associates[20] made cats ethanol-dependent by daily infusion through a gastric cannula for periods as long as 5 months. Cessation of alcohol administration was followed by clinical signs of withdrawal, epileptiform activity as measured by electroencephalography, and grand mal seizures in animals with implanted aluminum oxide seizure foci. Diazepam (1.5 mg/kg per day) produced immediate cessation of seizure activity and behavioral relaxation. A similar experiment in mice was reported by Goldstein who produced ethanol dependence after 3 days of administration.[21] Intraperitoneal chlordiazepoxide (20 to 100 mg/kg) or diazepam (5 to 50 mg/kg) given 5 hr after alcohol cessation clearly reduced the intensity of the withdrawal syndrome. Barbiturates were also effective, but only at doses which produced ataxia.

The clinical use of the benzodiazepines in alcohol withdrawal has been described in many reports[22–38] Intramuscular chlordiazepoxide has received the most attention, and in the majority of cases this drug produces satisfactory sedation by itself. In some reports, anticonvulsants (diphenylhydantoin, carbamazepine) are added as necessary.[36–38] High doses of intramuscular chlordiazepoxide are used initially—100 to 200 mg when the patient first comes under medical care, then repeated every few hours as often as necessary. Typically, 300 to 400 mg is required in the first 24 hr, but doses as high as 800 to 1,000 mg can be safely given. Other supportive measures are provided concurrently: parenteral thiamine and other vitamins, intravenous fluids, magnesium and potassium supplements, reassurance, and restraints as necessary.[39] Unless there is a preexisting seizure disorder, seizures associated with alcohol withdrawal when they occur are a self-limited phenomenon confined to the early stages of withdrawal and do not usually require anticonvulsant medication.[40] Occasionally harm is done when large doses of barbiturates or paraldehyde are given to treat seizure activity—not only are convulsions arrested, but the patient is made apneic and comatose. Antibiotics and corticosteroids are best withheld unless a specific indication exists.

The long duration of action of chlordiazepoxide (see Chapter 2) has both benefits and hazards. A few doses early in the course of withdrawal may be sufficient to suppress symptoms for a full 24 to 48 hr. Excessive doses given initially, or continued administration once adequate sedation is achieved, can produce central depression for much longer than is needed, with the associated hazards of infection of the respiratory tract and intravenous catheter sites. The need for dosage titration is crucial—chlordiazepoxide should be given in sufficient but not excessive dosage. After the acute phase of withdrawal, smaller doses (75 to 150 mg/day) can be given by mouth.

Controlled studies of sedatives and tranquilizers in alcohol withdrawal are difficult to perform. When paraldehyde is involved, for example, double-blindness is impossible for purely olfactory reasons. Brown and associates[41] attempted to compare intravenous diazepam and chlordiazepoxide in patients with delirium tremens. They were able to study only seven patients per treatment group and found no difference between the drugs. What impressed the authors most were the difficulties inherent in controlled study of this subject. Many of the trials subsequently discussed do not strictly adhere to the double-blind design.

Four trials compare chlordiazepoxide to a placebo. In the study by Kissen,[42] the results strongly favored chlordiazepoxide with respect to symptomatology and time for recovery. The dosage was 100 mg intravenously to start, followed by oral medication tapering from 80 to 30 mg daily. Rosenfield and Bizzoco[43] also reported a strong chlordiazepoxide-placebo difference in a study with dosage variable according to patient needs. Kaim and associates[44] gave intramuscular chlordiazepoxide parenterally (200 mg) on the first day of withdrawal, followed by oral therapy on a "p.r.n." basis for the next 9 days. Less than 1% of patients developed full-blown delirium tremens or seizures in the chlordiazepoxide-treated group as opposed to more than 5% of the placebo group. With respect to objective evaluations by nurse and physician, however, drug and placebo were largely indistinguishable.[45] Sereny and Kalant[46] found that chlordiazepoxide was only slightly better than placebo; the major difference was an enhancement of sleep by the active drug.

Most comparisons with phenothiazine tranquilizers involve either chlorpromazine or promazine, both of which have potent sedating properties. Ban and associates[47] and Muller[48] found that chlordiazepoxide and chlorpromazine were essentially equivalent, although neither of the studies was blind. In a well-controlled trial, Kaim et al.[44,45] showed that these two drugs were equivalent in efficacy, but chlorpromazine was much more toxic.

Seizures occurred in chlorpromazine-treated patients even more often than in those receiving placebo. Similar findings are reported in three comparisons with promazine.[46,49,50] Hypotension, seizures, and other serious or fatal complications were invariably more frequent among promazine-treated patients. In a comparison of chlordiazepoxide and perphenazine, however, Kaim and Klett[51] found the two drugs approximately equivalent in efficacy and toxicity. Chambers and Shultz[49] found that diazepam was inferior in efficacy to either chlordiazepoxide or promazine.

Two studies compare chlordiazepoxide to the traditional combination of paraldehyde and chloral hydrate. Muller[48] reported that chlordiazepoxide was more frequently associated wtih complications (ataxia, delirium tremens, relapse to drinking, fever, prolonged obtundation), but no statistics are presented because the number of cases treated was small. Golbert and associates[50] also found more complications in chlordiazepoxide-treated patients, but no subjects with delirium tremens were included in the study. Comparing chlordiazepoxide with paraldehyde alone and with pentobarbital, Kaim and Klett[51] found no significant difference between the three treatments. Kissen[52] compared chlordiazepoxide to a "control" treatment consisting of barbiturates, other tranquilizers, or placebo. Disability was more rapidly reduced in the chlordiazepoxide group, but patients who developed complications were eliminated from the study. Hekimian et al.[53] administered a single dose of chlordiazepoxide (100 mg), nicotinamide adenine dinucleotide (NAD, 100 mg), or placebo at the beginning of alcohol withdrawal with no subsequent treatment. Global improvement with chlordiazepoxide and placebo was equivalent, and superior to NAD. Prozine® (meprobamate plus promazine) was the comparison preparation in a study by Wegner and Fink.[54] All patients initially received promethazine and promazine to control agitation; they were then assigned to chlordiazepoxide, Prozine®, or placebo treatment groups. Recipients of Prozine® appeared to do better than patients treated with either chlordiazepoxide or placebo. The results of this study, however, are hardly conclusive, since all patients who failed to respond to placebo were switched to Prozine® treatment.

Bliding [540] compared oxazepam (120 to 240 mg/day), chlorprothixene (60 to 120 mg/day), and placebo in patients with "alcohol post-intoxication symptoms." Individuals with severe symptoms and/or delirium tremens were excluded. Oxazepam was significantly superior to both chlorprothixene and placebo according to ratings by patient, physician, and hospital personnel. Oxazepam-treated patients had fewer side effects than those receiving either of the other two treatments.

These studies in general support the concept that patients in the acute phase of alcohol withdrawal benefit from treatment with sedatives or tranquilizers. Chlordiazepoxide is as effective as any. The phenothiazines, on the other hand, appear to be hazardous with respect to enhancement of seizure activity and impairment of postural blood pressure regulation.

Many authors have interpreted the study by Golbert and associates[50] as demonstrating that chloral hydrate plus paraldehyde is the preferable drug therapy for alcohol withdrawal. It must be remembered, however, that no comparison with chlordiazepoxide was made in the most severely ill patients—those with delirium tremens. In many such patients, parenteral drug therapy is necessary, which is unavailable with chloral hydrate and undesirable in the case of paraldehyde because of the large volume required.

CHRONIC ALCOHOLISM

Viamontes[55] has reviewed drug studies in the treatment of chronic alcoholism. By his evaluation the results are poor with all drugs, including benzodiazepines. Although 14 of 16 uncontrolled trials show the benzodiazepines to be of value, all nine reported controlled trials reveal failure. Unfortunately, Viamontes does not define criteria for "success" or "failure," and no bibliography is available.

Our own survey of the literature reveals that, relative to the lifelong nature of chronic alcoholism, most studies are "short-term," lasting 6 weeks or less. Some trials deal only with hospitalized patients. In these studies, criteria for success are similar to those described in Chapter 4—global symptomatic improvement or relief of anxiety or depression. Uncontrolled short-term trials usually demonstrate improvement associated with benzodiazepine therapy,[56-59] while the results of controlled trials are less impressive. Two groups were unable to demonstrate significant drug-placebo differences with chlordiazepoxide[60] or diazepam.[61] Malmgren[62] found chlordiazepoxide (75 mg/day) superior to placebo by patient preference in a crossover trial. Shaffer and associates[63] found no overall difference between chlordiazepoxide (30 to 60 mg/day) and placebo in 1 month of study, although a significant increase in the acquiescent set response subgroup of the Minnesota Multiphasic Personality Inventory could be demonstrated in association with the active drug.[64] In a later study, the same investigators showed a weak superiority of chlordiazepoxide and prazepam over placebo.[65] Bowman and Thiman[66] compared chlordiazepoxide, oxazepam, promazine, and placebo in a 6-week trial in convalescing alcoholics. All three active drugs were essentially equivalent and significantly better than placebo with respect to symptomatic improvement and the physician's global rating. In two studies of doxepin and diazepam, the two drugs were equivalent in one study,[61] with doxepin superior in the other.[67] Ditman and associates[68] tested single doses of chlordiazepoxide (75 mg), methylphenidate (75 mg), and LSD (200 μg) given intravenously to rehabilitating alcoholics. Unlike the other two drugs, chlordiazepoxide calmed the subjects without arousing sensory or perceptual distortions.

None of these studies provides data on the crucial question of whether drug therapy prevents relapse to drinking among chronic alcoholics in remission. Ditman and associates[69,70] examined the incidence of drop-out from outpatient therapy over a 6-week period. Chlordiazepoxide was compared to several other treatments, including thioridazine, methocarbamol, and placebo. The return-to-clinic rate with chlordiazepoxide was significantly better than with all other treatments, but still was only about 50% after 6 weeks. In other studies, Kissin and associates[71,72] continued the investigations for up to 1 year, with correspondingly dismal results. One-third of patients failed to keep even three early follow-up visits. After 1 year, no more than 10% of patients had improvement in drinking habits, regardless of chlordiazepoxide or placebo. There is a suggestion that the combination of imipramine and chlordiazepoxide may be associated with more sustained improvement than placebo or either drug alone,[72] but this requires further confirmation.

Our review, in general, supports the conclusion of Viamontes[55] that the results of drug therapy in chronic alcoholism are disappointing.

OTHER DRUG-RELATED DISEASES

Norton[73] used chlordiazepoxide to treat barbiturate-withdrawal convulsions in the rat. Dependence upon barbital was produced by daily administration of 400 mg/kg for 5 weeks. Seizures appeared upon cessation of treatment but could be prevented by chlordiazepoxide (200 mg/kg per day). Reports of benzodiazepine treatment of barbiturate dependence and withdrawal in humans are anecdotal,[22,74] and the problem has not yet been systematically studied.

Diazepam appears to be suitable for the treatment of opiate withdrawal. In experimental studies, the withdrawal syndrome in morphine-dependent mice is completely suppressed by administration of diazepam (7.5 to 50 mg/kg).[75] Litt and associates[75] at Montefiore Hospital in New York City used diazepam (40 mg per day) as the only therapy for detoxifying 85 adolescent heroin addicts. The results were uniformly successful. The same workers also used diazepam, up to 6 mg per day, to suppress opiate withdrawal in 18 infants born to heroin-dependent mothers.[76] Full control was achieved in 17 of 18 infants with diazepam alone. Sugerman and associates[77] compared prazepam and placebo in male narcotic addicts who had completed the withdrawal process. Prazepam tended to produce more symptomatic improvement early in the trial, but the differences had largely disappeared by the end of the 3-week study. The frequency of relapse was not investigated.

The possible use of chlordiazepoxide and diazepam as smoking deterrents was investigated in two studies.[78,79] Only a few subjects were involved, and the results were not encouraging. Epidemiologic data from the Boston Collaborative Drug Surveillance Program[80] has suggested that cigarette smokers are less sensitive to the central depressant effects of benzodiazepines than nonsmokers. The basis for this finding is unclear. It may simply reflect the fact that smokers are more anxious, tense, or agitated than nonsmokers.

Alternatively, it may reflect the enzyme-inducing effects of chronic cigarette smoking, with consequent enhancement of metabolic degradation of benzodiazepines.

Agitation, delirium, or panic can be associated with the ingestion of hallucinogenic drugs. Although these symptoms are not manifestations of addiction or withdrawal, they may be severe enough to require pharmacologic treatment. Phenothiazines are hazardous because of their autonomic side effects. Debilitating postural hypotension may occur after small doses of chlorpromazine or promazine. Phenothiazines may actually potentiate and prolong delirium in anticholinergic overdosage.[81] Recent reports have suggested that diazepam is an appropriate drug for treating hallucinogenic drug crises. Solursh and Clement[82] used diazepam successfully in 67 of 69 such cases. Levy[83] has suggested that diazepam behaves as a specific antidote in "bad trips" following LSD. No comparisons with chlordiazepoxide have been reported, but there is no reason to expect that chlordiazepoxide would be any less effective. Adverse reactions to hallucinogenic drugs are best treated without sedatives or tranquilizers whenever possible. When attention and reassurance by themselves are insufficient, however, diazepam and chlordiazepoxide are probably among the most reasonable choices of tranquilizing agents.

COMMENT

The use of tranquilizers in the management of alcohol withdrawal is sound, but the proper choice of drug is not so obvious. Many physicians favor chlordiazepoxide,[19,39,84,85] although its superiority is not overwhelmingly clear. Certainly chlordiazepoxide is the least toxic of tranquilizers, and is easily administered by mouth or parenterally. Diazepam has not been studied as extensively, but it is probably equally safe and effective. Sleep disturbance may be an important aspect of alcohol withdrawal.[85] Prolonged suppression of dreaming by ethanol leads to rebound upon withdrawal, and this may underlie many of the unpleasant subjective symptoms. The noninterference of chlordiazepoxide and other benzodiazepines with rapid eye movement sleep (see Chapter 9) is a theoretical advantage of this group of drugs, inasmuch as rapid eye movement recovery may be important in the escape from alcohol dependence. Barbiturates and high doses of chloral hydrate also suppress dreaming and would appear to have the potential to prolong the withdrawal syndrome and delay recovery. Respiratory depression is another objectionable property of the barbiturates, since most chronic alcoholics are heavy cigarette smokers with a high incidence of obstructive pulmonary disease. Respiratory failure may easily be precipitated by high doses of barbiturates in such patients. The phenothiazine tranquilizers, particularly chlorpromazine and promazine, are potent sedatives, but in many trials are associated with serious complications—hypotension and shock, exacerbation of seizure activity, and disturbance of temperature regulation. Paraldehyde, particularly by intramuscular injection, is more painful than therapeutic; without reservation, we discourage the use of this drug.

Alcoholism is among the most destructive of chronic diseases. The prognosis is the worst in patients served by city and municipal hospitals for whom the environment is the least supportive. Except for unusually motivated individuals who are candidates for aversive drug therapy or group psychotherapy, physicians have very little to offer the chronic alcoholic outside of availability for reassurance during remission and for acute medical care during exacerbations. Psychiatrists and internists frequently prescribe sedatives or tranquilizers for alcoholics, yet there is no convincing evidence that such drugs favorably influence the drinking patterns of these patients. The benzodiazepines, at least, seldom do harm. Addiction does not often occur, and overdosage is rarely if ever fatal (see Chapter 12).

Acute adverse reactions to hallucinogenic drugs are often encountered by physicians staffing the emergency facilities of general hospitals. The majority of such patients do not require drug therapy: they will calm down if simply reassured by a physician that they are only suffering a temporary drug effect and are not "losing their mind." Many unnecessary iatrogenic hospital admissions have been precipitated by adverse reactions to phenothiazines: seizures, intractable postural hypotension, persistent obtundation, or acute dystonic reactions. Although benzodiazepines are the most reasonable drugs to use in these situations, patients may still become so sedated that they are unable to leave the hospital. The hallucinogenic drug crisis may exemplify a situation in which the physician does best by giving as little additional medication as possible.

REFERENCES

1. Devenyi P, Wilson M: Abuse of barbiturates in an alcoholic population. Canad Med Assoc J 104:219-221, 1971

2. Freed EX: Drug abuse by alcoholics: a review. Int J Addictions 8:451-473, 1973

3. Danechmand L, Casier H, Hebbelinck M, DeSchaepdryver A: Combined effects of ethanol and psychotropic drugs on muscular tone in mice. Quart J Stud Alcohol 28:424-429, 1967

4. Gebhart GF, Plaa GL, Mitchell CL: The effects of ethanol alone and in combination with phenobarbital, chlorpromazine, or chlordiazepoxide. Toxicol Appl Pharmacol 15:405-414, 1969

5. Madan BR, Sharma JD, Vyas DS: Some neuropharmacological actions of Librium. Ann Biochem Exp Med 12:221-224, 1962

6. Norio M, Isoaho R, Idänpään-Heikkilä J: Interaction of benzodiazepines and ethanol on sleeping time in rats. Scand J Clin Lab Invest 27(supp 116):76, 1971

7. Milner G: Interaction between barbiturates, alcohol, and some psychotropic drugs. Med J Aust 1:1204-1207, 1970

8. Milner G: The effect of antidepressants and "tranquillizers" on the response of mice to ethanol. Brit J Pharmacol 34:370-376, 1968

9. Reggiani G, Hurlimann A, Theiss E: Some aspects of the experimental and clinical toxicology of chlordiazepoxide. In, *Proceedings of the European Society for the Study of Drug Toxicity. Vol 9. Toxicity and Side-Effects of Psychotropic Drugs.* Edited by SBD Baker, JR Boissier, W Koll. Amsterdam, Excerpta Medica Foundation, 1968, pp 79-97

10. Votava Z, Vojtechovsky M: An experimental and clinical contribution to interaction of alcohol and diazepam. Activ Nerv Sup 13:197-198, 1971

11. Vapoatalo H, Karppanen H: Combined toxicity of ethanol with chlorpromazine, diazepam, chlormethiazole, or pentobarbital in mice. Agents and Actions 1:43-45, 1969

12. Hoffer A: Lack of potentiation by chlordiazepoxide (Librium) of depression or excitation due to alcohol. Canad Med Assoc J 87:920-921, 1962

13. Miller AI, D'Agostino A, Minsky R: Effects of combined chlordiazepoxide and alcohol in man. Quart J Stud Alcohol 24:9-13, 1963

14. Lawton MP, Cahn B: The effects of diazepam (Valium®) and alcohol on psychomotor performance. J Nerv Ment Dis 136:550-554, 1963

15. Bernstein ME, Hughes FW, Forney RB: The influence of a new chlordiazepoxide analogue on human mental and motor performance. J Clin Pharmacol 7:330-335, 1967

16. Hughes FW, Forney RB, Richards AB: Comparative effect in human subjects of chlordiazepoxide, diazepam, and placebo on mental and physical performance. Clin Pharmacol Ther 6:139-145, 1965

16a. Betts TA, Clayton AB, MacKay GM: Effects of four commonly-used tranquillizers on low-speed driving performance tests. Brit Med J 4:580-584, 1972

17. Khan AU, Forney RB, Hughes FW: Effect of tranquilizers on the metabolism of ethanol. Arch Int Pharmacodyn 150:171-176, 1964

18. Morselli PL, Veneroni E, Zaccala M, Bizzi A: Further observation on the interaction between ethanol and psychotropic drugs. Arzneim-Forsch 21:20-23, 1971

19. Jones RW, Helrich AR: Treatment of alcoholism by physicians in private practice. A national survey. Quart J Stud Alcohol 33:117-131, 1972

20. Guerrero-Figueroa R, Rye MM, Gallant DM, Bishop MP: Electrographic and behavioral effects of diazepam during alcohol withdrawal stage in cats. Neuropharmacology 9:143-150, 1970

21. Goldstein DB: An animal model for testing effects of drugs on alcohol withdrawal reactions. J Pharmacol Exp Ther 183:14-22, 1972

22. Armour PS: Management of acute alcohol and barbiturate withdrawal states. Western Med 4:369-384, 1963

23. Lawrence FE: The outpatient management of the alcoholic. Quart J Stud Alcohol 22(supp 1):117-128, (Nov) 1961

24. Schultz JD: Treatment of alcoholism in a general hospital. Quart J Stud Alcohol 22(supp 1):85-92, (Nov) 1961

25. D'Agostino A, Schultz JD: Clinical experience with chlordiazepoxide in acute alcoholism. Psychosomatics 2:362-365, 1961

26. Rummele W: Prophylaxis and therapy of delirium tremens. In, *Proceedings of the Fourth World Congress of Psychiatry.* Edited by JJL Ibor. Amsterdam, Excerpta Medica Foundation, 1968, pp 1404-1411

27. Short MJ, Moore WJ: Treatment of alcoholic withdrawal states with chlordiazepoxide. Military Med 130:1203-1206, 1965

28. Floyd JB, Collins MC: Management of alcohol withdrawal. J South Carolina Med Assoc 59:229-233, 1963

29. Baroody NB, Baroody WG, Mead WR: Management of alcohol withdrawal. Observation using chlordiazepoxide as chief tranquilizing agent. J South Carolina Med Assoc 58:439-440, 1962

30. Karolus HE: Chlordiazepoxide in the treatment of acute alcoholism: a preliminary report. Illinois Med J 120:96-99, 1961

31. Salzberger GJ: Treatment of acute alcohol poisoning in a state mental hospital. Dis Nerv Syst 25:293-297, 1964

32. Morrison JM: Treatment of chronic alcoholism. Dis Nerv Syst 24:430-443, 1963

33. Ziporyn M: Effective management of delirium tremens. Appl Ther 5:137-138, 1963

34. Koutsky CD, Sletten IW: Chlordiazepoxide in alcohol withdrawal. Minnesota Med 46:354-357, 1963

35. Spenader WF, Schwamberger BV: The treatment of acute alcoholism in a small rural hospital. Illinois Med J 140:508,530-531, 1971

36. McCurdy RL, Kane FJ: Orthostatic hypotension associated with high dosage of Librium. Amer J Psychiat 120:601-602, 1963

37. Brune F, Busch H: Anticonvulsive-sedative treatment of delirium alcoholicum. Quart J Stud Alcohol 32:334-342, 1971

38. Doeff JW, Pendleton JL: Wernicke's syndrome treated with parenteral and oral chlordiazepoxide. Amer J Psychiat 121:183, 1964

39. Becker CE, Scott R: The treatment of alcoholism. Rational Drug Ther 6: Oct, 1972

40. Victor M, Brausch C: The role of abstinence in the genesis of alcoholic epilepsy. Epilepsia 8:1-20, 1967

41. Brown JH, Moggey DE, Shane FH: Delirium tremens: a comparison of intravenous treatment with diazepam and chlordiazepoxide. Scottish Med J 17:9-12, 1972

42. Kissen MD: Management of psychomotor agitation in acute alcoholism. A double-blind study using chlordiazepoxide. Dis Nerv Syst 26:364-368, 1965

43. Rosenfeld JE, Bizzoco DH: A controlled study of alcohol withdrawal. Quart J Stud Alcohol 22(supp 1):77-84, (Nov) 1961

44. Kaim SC, Klett CJ, Rothfeld B: Treatment of the acute alcohol withdrawal state: a comparison of four drugs. Amer J Psychiat 125:1640-1646, 1969

45. Klett CJ, Hollister LE, Caffey EM, Kaim SC: Evaluating changes in symptoms during acute alcohol withdrawal. Arch Gen Psychiat 24:174-178, 1971

46. Sereny G, Kalant H: Comparative clinical evaluation of chlordiazepoxide and promazine in treatment of alcohol-withdrawal syndrome. Brit Med J 1:92-97, 1965

47. Ban TA, Lehmann HE, Matthews V, Donald M: Comparative study of chlorpromazine and chlordiazepoxide in the prevention and treatment of alcohol withdrawal symptoms. Clin Med 72:59-67, 1965

48. Muller DJ: A comparison of three approaches to alcohol-withdrawal states. Southern Med J 62:495-496, 1969

49. Chambers JF, Schultz JD: Double-blind study of three drugs in the treatment of acute alcoholic states. Quart J Stud Alcohol 26:10-18, 1965

50. Golbert TM, Sanz CJ, Rose HD, Leitschuh TH: Comparative evaluation of treatments of alcohol withdrawal syndromes. JAMA 201:99-102, 1967

51. Kaim SC, Klett CJ: Treatment of delirium tremens. A comparative evaluation of four drugs. Quart J Stud Alcohol 33:1065-1072, 1972

52. Kissen MD: The treatment of alcoholics. Quart J Stud Alcohol 22(supp 1): 101-106, (Nov) 1961

53. Hekimian LJ, Friedhoff AJ, Alpert M: Treatment of acute brain syndrome from alcohol with nicotinamide adenine dinucleotide and methaminodiazepoxide. Quart J Stud Alcohol 27:214-220, 1966

54. Wegner ME, Fink DW: Chlordiazepoxide (Librium) compared with meprobamate and promazine (Prozine) for the withdrawal symptoms of acute alcoholism. Wisconsin Med J 64:436-440, 1965

54a. Bliding A: Efficacy of antianxiety drug therapy in alcohol post-intoxication symptoms.

A double-blind study of chlorprothixen, oxazepam, and placebo. Brit J Psychiat 122:465-468, 1973

55. Viamontes JA: Review of drug effectiveness in the treatment of alcoholism. Amer J Psychiat 128:1570-1571, 1972

56. Mitchell EH: Rehabilitation of the alcoholic. Quart J Stud Alcohol 22(supp 1):93-100, (Nov) 1961

57. Chesrow EJ, Kaplitz SE, Levine JM, Musci JP, Sabatini R: The use of chlordiazepoxide (Librium) in the alcoholic patient: a clinical study of forty cases. J Amer Geriat Soc 10:264-269, 1962

58. Hoff EC: The use of pharmacological adjuncts in the psychotherapy of alcoholics. Quart J Stud Alcohol 22(supp 1):138-150, (Nov) 1961

59. Ota KY, Kurland AA, Turek I: A clinical trial of SCH-12041 with chronic alcoholic patients. Curr Ther Res 13:463-468, 1971

60. Bartholomew AA, Guile LA: A controlled evaluation of "Librium" in the treatment of alcoholics. Med J Aust 2:578-581, 1961

61. Gallant DM, Bishop MP, Guerrero-Figueroa R, Selby M, Phillips R: Doxepin versus diazepam: a controlled evaluation in 100 chronic alcoholic patients. J Clin Pharmacol 9:57-65, 1969

62. Malmgren G: Comparative investigation of the effects of dixyrazine, placebo and chlordiazepoxide on alcoholics during hospital care. Int J Neuropsychiat 3:413-417, 1967

63. Shaffer JW, Freinek WR, Wolf S, Foxwell NH, Kurland AA: A controlled evaluation of chlordiazepoxide (Librium) in the treatment of convalescing alcoholics. J Nerv Ment Dis 137:494-507, 1963

64. Shaffer JW: Chlordiazepoxide (Librium) and acquiescent response set. Psychol Rep 13:463-465, 1963

65. Shaffer JW, Yeganeh ML, Foxwell NH, Kurland AA: A comparison of the effects of prazepam, chlordiazepoxide, and placebo in the short-term treatment of convalescing alcoholics. J Clin Pharmacol 8:392-399, 1968

66. Bowman EH, Thimann J: Treatment of alcoholism in the subacute stage. (A study of three active agents). Dis Nerv Syst 27:342-346, 1966

67. Butterworth AT, Watts RD: Treatment of hospitalized alcoholics with doxepin and diazepam. A controlled study. Quart J Stud Alcohol 32:78-81, 1971

68. Ditman KS, Moss T, Forgy EW, Zunin LM, Lynch RD, Funk WA: Dimensions of the LSD, methylphenidate, and chlordiazepoxide experiences. Psychopharmacologia 14:1-11, 1969

69. Ditman KS: Evaluation of drugs in the treatment of alcoholics. Quart J Stud Alcohol 22(supp 1):107-116, (Nov) 1961

70. Mooney HB, Ditman KS, Cohen S: Chlordiazepoxide in the treatment of alcoholics. Dis Nerv Syst 22(July supp):44-51, 1961

71. Charnoff SM, Kissin B, Reed JI: An evaluation of various psychotherapeutic agents in the long-term treatment of chronic alcoholism. Results of a double-blind study. Amer J Med Sci 246:172-179, 1963

72. Kissin B, Gross MM: Drug therapy in alcoholism. Amer J Psychiat 125:31-41, 1968

73. Norton PRE: The effects of drugs on barbiturate withdrawal convulsions in the rat. J Pharm Pharmacol 22:763-766, 1970

74. Remington FB: The use of chlordiazepoxide (Librium) in the barbiturate abstinence syndrome. Amer J Psychiat 120:402-403, 1963

75. Litt IF, Colli AS, Cohen MI: Diazepam in the management of heroin withdrawal in adolescents: preliminary report. J Pediat 78:692-696, 1971

76. Nathenson G, Golden GS, Litt IF: Diazepam in the management of the neonatal narcotic withdrawal syndrome. Pediatrics 48:523-527, 1971

77. Sugerman AA, Miksztal MW, Freymuth HW: Comparison of prazepam and placebo in

the treatment of convalescing narcotic addicts. J Clin Pharmacol 11:383-387, 1971

78. Whitehead RW, Davies JM: A study of methylphenidate and diazepam as possible smoking deterrents. Curr Ther Res 6:363-367, 1964

79. Graff H, Hammett VBO, Bash N, Fackler W, Yanovski A, Goldman A: Results of four antismoking therapy methods. Penn Med J 69:39-43, (Feb) 1966

80. Boston Collaborative Drug Surveillance Program: Clinical depression of the central nervous system due to diazepam and chlordiazepoxide in relation to cigarette smoking and age. New Eng J Med 288:277-280, 1973

81. Shader RI, Greenblatt DJ: Belladonna alkaloids and synthetic anticholinergics: uses and toxicity. In, *Psychiatric Complications of Medical Drugs.* Edited by RI Shader. New York, Raven Press, 1972, pp 103-147

82. Solursh LP, Clement WR: Use of diazepam in hallucinogenic drug crises. JAMA 205:644-645, 1968

83. Levy RM: Diazepam for L.S.D. intoxication. Lancet 1:1297, 1971

84. Benor D, Ditman KS: Tranquilizers in the management of alcoholics: a review of the literature to 1964. Part I. J New Drugs 6:319-337, 1966

85. Greenblatt DJ, Greenblatt M: Which drug for alcohol withdrawal? J Clin Pharmacol 12:429-431, 1972

Chapter 12
Unwanted Effects

Chlordiazepoxide and diazepam share with other widely used pharmacologic agents the questionable distinction of implication in almost every conceivable drug-induced disease. Any symptom or syndrome which develops while a patient is taking a drug, and subsequently disappears when the drug is discontinued, may be attributed to the drug by patient and/or physician. When a drug-associated event is commonly observed or is related to intrinsic pharmacologic properties, such as drowsiness after chlordiazepoxide, assignment of a causal relationship is reasonable. When events are rare or unrelated to the drug's primary action, causality seldom can be established conclusively. Chance associations with many such events occur when drugs are used by millions of patients, and the cases often appear as isolated reports in the literature. Since many unusual drug reactions are serious ones, confirmatory techniques such as rechallenge are ethically precluded. The medical community is then left with drug-associated reactions for which the causal role of the drug cannot be confirmed.

Unfortunately, much of the data on unwanted effects of the benzodiazepines is of this anecdotal type. Larger epidemiologic studies do exist, but even these do not clarify the possible association of the benzodiazepines with events such as hepatic toxicity or fetal malformations. For this reason, many of the conclusions presented in this chapter must be regarded as tentative or equivocal.

CENTRAL NERVOUS SYSTEM TOXICITY

The most common adverse effects of the benzodiazepines involve depression of the central nervous system (CNS). Whether "drowsiness" is an unwanted effect depends on the therapeutic indication. When the drug is given as a nighttime hypnotic, drowsiness and sleep are desired effects; central depression persisting into the next day is, of course, unwanted. Benzodiazepines given during the daytime as antianxiety agents are meant to reduce anxiety without producing generalized sedation. Excess CNS depression may take many forms, including muscle weakness, ataxia, dysarthria, incoordination, diplopia, blurring of vision, confusion, apathy, vertigo, dizziness, or somnolence.[1-9] The symptom complex may resemble alcoholic intoxication or a Korsakoff-like syndrome.[10] Enuresis[11] and failure of ejaculation[12] are less common manifestations. In clinical trials of the benzodiazepines in psychiatry (Chapter 4), drowsiness invariably occurs in some of the patients, usually with an incidence that exceeds drowsiness associated with placebo. Nearly always, central depression is dose-dependent, occurring more often in patients receiving high doses and remitting when dosage is lowered. It also appears that drowsiness is more common in elderly patients, and that individuals with a recent history of abuse of ethanol or barbiturates have a reduced susceptibility to the central depressant effects of benzodiazepines. Bartholomew and Bruce[13] have reported that combining amiphenazole with chlordiazepoxide significantly reduces the incidence of drowsiness associated with chlordiazepoxide. The influence of the stimulant upon the therapeutic effect of chlordiazepoxide, however, was not reported.

A realistic estimation of the frequency of unwanted CNS depression produced by chlordiazepoxide and diazepam cannot be made on the basis of small series, since doses and patient populations vary widely within and between studies. More reliable estimates are available from larger epidemiologic surveys, to be discussed subsequently.

Other central effects of benzodiazepines are less frequent and more unpredictable. In some individuals, benzodiazepines produce stimulation instead of sedation. A number of manifestations have been observed. Occasionally, a reduced threshold for grand mal seizures is seen in patients receiving benzodiazepines for anticonvulsant therapy (see Chapter 6). Excitement, rage, and hostility associated with chlordiazepoxide[14,15] are discussed in Chapters 1 and 4. Maguire and associates[16] reported a patient with a syndrome of hyperkinesis and agitation apparently induced by chlordiazepoxide. The authors state that paradoxical stimulation by chlordiazepoxide is most likely to occur in patients with mild anxiety receiving high doses of the drug. Similar paradoxical reactions have been attributed to diazepam (Chapter 4). It is not clear whether all benzodiazepines have the potential to produce such effects, but reports are not limited to chlordiazepoxide and diazepam. Bladin[17] reported that clonazepam caused behavioral and motor stimulation in 10 of 27 children receiving the drug as an anticonvulsant. Increased irritability, irrational antisocial behavior, and outbursts of aggressive temper were observed in these patients, and necessitated discontinuation of the drug in some cases. Zucker[18] has made observations of "strange behavior" in patients receiving oxazepam. One patient noted unusual bodily sensations; another was arrested for disrobing in public; a third woman became uncommonly argumentative with her husband.

Viscott[19] described seven patients receiving chlordiazepoxide who developed hypnagogic hallucinations. They usually occurred during induction of sleep, and terminated rapidly with reality testing. Anecdotal reports in the British literature have suggested a causal association of nitrazepam with increased dreaming[20] and nightmares[21,22] (see also Chapter 9). Taylor[22] states that the nightmares are intense during the first few nights of nitrazepam therapy, then become less intense as drug use continues. The dream content often involves episodes of personal stress in the patient's past. Goossens and associates[22a] suggest that the disinhibiting property of nitrazepam allows distressing subconscious processes to enter into the realm of dreams. Evans and Jarvis[23] have emphasized the hazards of nitrazepam use in the elderly, reporting the case of a 75-year-old woman who developed ataxia, incontinence, dysarthria, and confusion during nightly nitrazepam therapy. All of the symptoms disappeared when the drug was withdrawn. The syndrome resembles that reported by Glasgow[9] associated with chlordiazepoxide in three elderly patients. In another report,[24] nitrazepam appeared to induce a reversible motor and sensory impairment involving both hands in a 55-year-old woman.

Important changes in affect have been attributed to diazepam. Ryan and associates[25] described eight patients in whom exacerbation of depression and suicidal ideation occurred after diazepam therapy was begun. Affect changes developed insidiously after several days to several weeks of diazepam. Two patients committed suicide; the others improved when diazepam was discontinued. Hall and Joffee[26] characterized the syndrome more specifically in a study of six patients. All six were female, and all had other organic diseases (ischemic or hypertensive heart disease, seizure disorder, thyrotoxicosis, diabetes, glomerulonephritis). After 6 to 8 days of relatively high-dose diazepam therapy (40 mg per day or more), patients developed tremulousness, impaired concentration and memory, episodes of spontaneous crying, insomnia, nightmares, and in two cases nocturnal confusion. They became apprehensive and depressed with ego-alien suicidal ideation. The symptoms remitted within 10 days after discontinuation of the drug. Diazepam is known to be a potent inhibitor of Stage IV slow-wave sleep (see Chapter 9). Fisher and associates[27] reported the successful use of this drug in the treatment of non-REM (rapid eye movement) night terrors, a phenomenon associated with slow-wave sleep. One patient in this series experienced a "displacement" of night terrors to the daytime hours ("daymares" or "day terrors") while on diazepam. The patient reported spontaneous episodes of panic as well as persistent, highly disturbing, intrusive thoughts of a self-destructive nature. The symptoms described by this individual bear some resemblance to those reported in the series of Hall and Joffe.[26] It may be that impairment of Stage IV sleep underlies the enhancement or production of self-destructive ideation attributed to diazepam therapy.

The problem of adverse reactions to parenteral benzodiazepines is an important one. The data surveyed in Chapters 6, 7, and 10 would suggest that cardiovascular and respiratory depression rarely occur after intravenous diazepam. Those who do develop hypotension or apnea appear to be those with serious underlying disease or who received other central depressant drugs concurrently. Case reports of apnea following intravenous diazepam continue to be published,[28-30] but the frequency of such reactions cannot be assessed without epidemiologic data. Greenblatt and Koch-Weser[31] reported that 173 of almost 15,000 hospitalized medical patients monitored by the Boston Collaborative Drug Surveillance Program received intravenous diazepam during one or more hospital admissions. Most patients received the drug for the management of severe anxiety or agitation or for the control of seizure activity. Patients receiving intravenous diazepam were among a seriously ill group, including many respirator cases. The eventual hospital mortality was 24%. Only six patients experienced adverse reactions attributable to diazepam. The three reactions that were considered serious or life-threatening occurred in patients with advanced or terminal organic disease, one of whom received numerous other parenteral sedatives and tranquilizers concurrently with diazepam. No adverse reactions occurred among 32 patients who received intravenous diazepam as premedication for endoscopy or cardioversion.

No injection-site complications were attributed to intravenous diazepam in this series. However, injection pain and/or subsequent local phlebitis are not infrequently reported in other series cited in this volume (see Chapters 4, 6, 7, and 10). Langdon and associates[32] noted that phlebitis was a complication of intravenous diazepam in approximately 3.5% of 1,500 patients receiving the drug as premedication for endoscopy. In a subsequent study,[32a] phlebitis occurred in 23 (7%) of 328 patients premedicated with intravenous diazepam. The incidence was not significantly reduced by "flushing" the vein with hydrocortisone or heparin. However, flushing with 150 to 250 ml of saline significantly reduced the incidence of phlebitis to 2.2%. Wehlage[33] reported that the repeated use of an antecubital vein for injection of diazepam as a premedicant for sequential daily electroconvulsive treatments invariably leads to induration and tenderness of the vein. Precipitation occurs when the parenteral diazepam preparation is mixed with aqueous solutions.[33a] It may be that precipitated particles of drug are responsible for local irritation. The propylene glycol solvent alone has also been suggested as the cause of phlebitis.[33b]

Intramuscular diazepam produces an elevation in the serum creatine phosphokinase (CPK) activity. Kuster[34] found that intramuscular diazepam (10 mg) given to 15 volunteers produced nearly a fourfold rise in mean serum CPK 12 hr after the dose. No changes in CPK were observed after intramuscular saline or oral diazepam. The propylene glycol solvent could be responsible for local muscle irritation leading to the rise in CPK. Greenblatt and associates[35] noted a similar CPK elevation in a subject receiving an intramuscular injection of the propylene glycol solvent alone. The findings suggest that intramuscular diazepam should be avoided whenever serum CPK levels are of diagnostic importance.

Although serious adverse reactions to parenteral benzodiazepines appear to be uncommon, intravenous administration of these drugs as well as other sedatives and tranquilizers should be undertaken with caution.

HEPATOXICITY

The clinical studies reviewed in Chapter 4 provide no substantial evidence that the benzodiazepines have an hepatotoxic potential. Two groups[36,37] specifically investigated changes in liver function tests occurring with chlordiazepoxide, both alone and in combination with other psychotropic drugs. No significant changes were attributable to chlordiazepoxide.

Six case reports describe hepatic disease associated with chlordiazepoxide or diazepam. In the report of Abbruzzeze and Swanson,[38] acute hepatitis developed 6 weeks after chlordiazepoxide therapy was begun; the patient was also receiving sulfisoxazole, and had antecedent symptoms suggestive of a viral infection. A 64-year-old woman described by Pickering[39] developed jaundice after 12 days of chlordiazepoxide therapy, with liver biopsy findings consistent with acute hepatocellular disease and necrosis. The nature of the association was not further elucidated. Cacioppo and Merlis[40] reported the case of a male patient on long-term therapy with diphenylhydantoin and phenobarbital who became jaundiced after 5 days of chlordiazepoxide. In the case reported by Lo and associates,[41] jaundice was noted in a 26-year-old female following 2 weeks of chlordiazepoxide, 30 mg per day. Three days prior to beginning chlordiazepoxide, she gave birth to a normal male infant; she received no blood during labor or delivery. Two days after beginning chlordiazepoxide, symptoms of a flu-like illness appeared for which she was treated with penicillin. A liver biopsy on the 19th day of jaundice showed cholestasis but no parenchymal damage. An intravenous cholangiogram performed after resolution of jaundice revealed that the common bile duct was patent. A 54-year-old woman reported by Cunningham[42] was hospitalized following nearly 5 months of therapy with diazepam and amitriptyline. She became comatose and died 2 weeks later. Post-mortem examination revealed a small, shrunken liver and acute hepatic necrosis. Finally, Winkelmayer[43] described a 35-year-old man who became jaundiced following 5 days of chlordiazepoxide (75 mg per day) and 1 day of thioridazine (300 mg per day). In the previous 4 months he had received chlorpromazine and fluphenazine. After resolution of jaundice and laboratory abnormalities, rechallenge with chlordiazepoxide alone was followed by reappearance of jaundice. Rechallenge with thioridazine alone had no effect.

In the final case, a causal role of chlordiazepoxide is suggested. In all other cases, however, chance association with viral hepatitis, hepatic toxicity from other drugs, or other causes of jaundice cannot be ruled out. At present, the evidence substantiating benzodiazepine-induced hepatic damage is very weak.

HEMATOLOGIC EFFECTS

Adverse hematologic effects of the benzodiazepines, if they occur, are probably as rare as hepatotoxicity.[36,37,44] Litvak and Kaebling[45] surveyed hematologic laboratory tests in 5,993 patients taking psychotropic drugs. There were 111 instances in which white blood cell (WBC) counts below 3,700 per cubic mm were noted. In 27 cases, leukopenia had a non-drug etiology, and in 30 the depressed white count occurred for no apparent reason while the patients were not taking drugs. Of the remaining 54 drug-associated episodes, phenothiazines were being taken in 50 cases; in none of the remaining four cases could a benzodiazepine be implicated.

Again, case reports require cautious interpretation. Menon[46] described two instances of pancytopenia associated with chlordiazepoxide. The first occurred in a 30-year-old female who had taken chlordiazepoxide continuously for 2 years prior to the event. Two days before admission, tetracycline, 1.0 g/day, was begun. She was admitted with purpura, a facial abscess, and pancytopenia (hemoglobin 7.6 g/100 ml; WBC 2,000 per cubic mm; platelets 24,000 per cubic mm). She recovered following treatment with antibiotics and corticosteroids. The second case was also a woman, aged 42, who received chlordiazepoxide for 9 months prior to the event. She entered with petichiae and severe pancytopenia. No other drugs were implicated. Wilcox[47] reported agranulocytosis in a 43-year-old woman after 3 months of chlordiazepoxide therapy. Other medications included aspirin, triflupromazine, and ethchlorvynol. She was febrile and had a total white count of 558 per cubic mm, but recovered with corticosteriod therapy. The 23-year-old woman reported by Kaebling and Conrad[48] had manifested cutaneous sensitivity to chlorpromazine prior to chlordiazepoxide treatment. After receiving chlordiazepoxide for 1 month, she developed pharyngitis, fever, and a white blood cell count as low as 1,600 per cubic mm with no granulocytes noted. She recovered with antibiotics and corticosteroids. Bitnun[49] noted persistent granulocytopenia (total WBC 3,500 per cubic mm, 28% granulocytes) in an infant born to a woman who had taken chlordiazepoxide during pregnancy. In none of these cases could chlordiazepoxide be established as the causative agent.

A final unexplained observation was reported by Dhawan and associates[50] who administered intramuscular chlordiazepoxide (15 mg/kg) to rabbits. Twenty-four hr after the injection, the prothrombin time had dropped from 7.6 to 6.5 sec. There was no change in bleeding or coagulation times. The meaning of this finding is unclear.

ALLERGIC REACTIONS

Almeyda[51] has reviewed cutaneous reactions to benzodiazepines. He states that allergic dermatitides following chlordiazepoxide have been reported to take the form of urticaria, angioneurotic edema, or maculopapular eruptions. Mackie and Mackie,[52] in a review of 179 drug eruptions, stated that five nonurticarial reactions were due to chlordiazepoxide alone, and one due to the combination of chlordiazepoxide and diazepam. Luton and Finchum[53] described a photosensitivity reaction to chlordiazepoxide in a 53-year-old man. The patient received chlordiazepoxide for approximately 1 week prior to the onset of a diffuse severe eczematous reaction over sun-exposed areas. The reaction was reproduced by rechallenge with chlordiazepoxide plus ultraviolet light. Fixed drug eruptions have been reported as well.[54] Gaul[55] verified by rechallenge that chlordiazepoxide was the etiologic agent in a 66-year-old female. Copperman[56] described a 65-year-old woman who developed a generalized purpuric rash after receiving chlordiazepoxide for 1 year. Her platelet count was normal, but the tourniquet test was positive. Abnormalities resolved after chlordiazepoxide was discontinued. Rechallenge with chlordiazepoxide at a later date was rapidly followed by reappearance of the nonthrombocytopenic purpuric eruption. Swelling of the tongue following flurazepam use was reported by Rapp.[57] The patient was a 65-year-old man who had previously taken both chlordiazepoxide and diazepam with no adverse effects. Two days after beginning flurazepam, 30 mg nightly, tongue swelling appeared. The drug was discontinued after four doses, and the swelling resolved.

An anaphylactic reaction to chlordiazepoxide is implied in the report of O'Grady and Pokorny.[58] The patient, an asthmatic, received parenteral aminophylline (500 mg) and ACTH (40 units), as well as oral chlordiazepoxide (30 mg). Thirty min later the patient became comatose and cyanotic, and required resuscitation. In view of the nature of the underlying disease and the properties of the concurrently administered drugs, allergy to chlordiazepoxide seems to be an extremely unlikely explanation for the event.

Salzman and associates[59] have described a collagen disease-like syndrome following administration of isoquinazepon, an experimental drug having an eight-membered 1,4-benzodiazepine structure. Two healthy male subjects developed polyarthralgia and pruritis during treament with the drug. One subject also experienced a macular, erythematous skin rash together with malaise, anorexia, leukocytosis, elevation of the sedimentation rate, and trace albuminuria. Symptomatic relief was obtained with diphenhydramine, and the syndrome resolved completely within a few weeks of drug discontinuation. Isoquinazepon was subsequently withdrawn from clinical testing.

CYTOGENETIC EFFECTS

A number of studies have investigated the influence of benzodiazepines upon chromosomal abnormalities. In no case is the clinical relevance of the experimental results obvious. Human fibroblast cells grown in tissue culture show no increase in chromosomal abnormalities when chlordiazepoxide is added in concentrations as high as a 100 μg/ml,[60,61] although at high concentrations the growth rate is reduced.[61] Lymphocytes incubated with these concentrations of chlordiazepoxide also show no abnormalities.[62] No aberrations were seen in marrow cells of hamsters treated with chlordiazepoxide, 150 mg/kg per day for 10 days.[63] Human lymphocytes of subjects treated with chlordiazepoxide are indistinguishable from those of untreated controls when chromosomal patterns are studied.[61,64] Diazepam in similar concentrations is likewise innocent in studies of fibroblast tissue cultures[60,62] and hamsters under chronic treatment[63] and in lymphocytes of human subjects receiving the drug.[64,65] Stenchever and associates[62] noted that chromosomal breaks in human lymphocytes were significantly more frequent after incubation with diazepam in concentrations exceeding 10 $\mu g/ml$. Staiger,[66] however, found no significant changes with concentrations as high as 50 $\mu g/ml$. Breen and Stenchever[67] noted striking ultrastructural electron micrographic changes in human fibroblasts incubated with diazepam at 10 to 20 $\mu g/ml$.

Istvan[68] reported a female infant born with complete absence of the first digits bilaterally, and a congenital dislocation of the head of the right radius. The mother had taken diazepam early in the first trimester. Experimental studies, however, have uniformly failed to reveal a teratogenic potential of the benzodiazepines (see Chapter 1 and references 69 and 69a of this chapter).

ADVERSE REACTIONS TO BENZODIAZEPINES: EPIDEMIOLOGIC STUDIES

Reliable data on the frequency of unwanted side effects of benzodiazepines can be obtained only through surveys of large numbers of patients. Unfortunately, only two such studies are currently available.

Svenson and Hamilton[70] reviewed 287 clinical studies of chlordiazepoxide published through 1965. A total of 17,935 patients were involved. Most were outpatients receiving chlordiazepoxide for anxiety, but a wide variety of

TABLE 12-1. *Side effects of chlordiazepoxide among 17,935 patients**

Drowsiness	3.90%
Ataxia	1.70%
Paradoxical excitement	0.70%
Dizziness or vertigo	0.64%
Constipation	0.40%
Appetite stimulation	0.36%
Nausea or vomiting	0.34%
Muscular weakness	0.30%
Gas pain, dysphagia, or diarrhea	0.26%
Decrease in libido	0.26%
Irritability	0.24%
Weight gain	0.20%
Dysarthria	0.20%
Skin reactions	0.20%

*Svenson SE, Hamilton RG: Curr Ther Res 8:455-464, 1966

diagnoses, indications for therapy, and dosages are represented, all of which were massed together for the purpose of the survey. Adverse *events*, rather than *patients* with adverse reactions, are tabulated, so that some individuals are undoubtedly represented more than once. Table 12-1 shows the frequency of side effects which occurred with an overall rate of at least 2 per 1,000 patients. Drowsiness was the most frequent side effect, reported in 3.9% of patients at an average daily dose of 75 mg per day. Ataxia occurred in 1.7% of chlordiazepoxide recipients at an average dose of 96 mg per day. The authors emphasize that 75% of all symptoms were reported as being dose-related.

The limitations of the survey are numerous. Reports arise from many different investigators, each with a different approach to documenting adverse reactions. The frequency of events elicited by physician interview, for example, may differ widely from that derived from statements volunteered by the patient. Most of the studies were uncontrolled, and it cannot be said how often the infrequent events were actually due to the drug. A significant proportion of patients receiving placebo experience side effects which they attribute to the pill they are taking. The survey does not consider *differences* in frequencies of drug-attributed events between active-drug and placebo groups. Yet this review does provide confirmation that the most common side effects of chlordiazepoxide involve central depression (drowsiness, ataxia) and that these effects seem to be dose-related.

The Boston Collaborative Drug Surveillance Program[71] utilizes trained nurse monitors to record data on hospitalized medical patients in nine hospitals in the United States, Canada, Israel, and New Zealand. Information is collected on patient characteristics, diagnoses, the therapeutic effects of all drugs administered, and full details of dosage and duration of therapy. When drug treatment is instituted, the prescribing physician is interviewed

TABLE 12-2. *Epidemiology of benzodiazepine usage in the Boston Collaborative Drug Surveillance Program*

Chlordiazepoxide		Diazepam
2,086	Number of recipients	2,623
15.6%	% of total patients surveyed	19.8%
51 years	Mean age	54 years
68.6%	% of male patients	55.6%
10.8%	Hospital mortality (coincidental)	8.8%
	Indications for Therapy	
79.9%	Anxiety	71.8%
8.5%	Psychiatric disturbance	2.9%
2.4%	Insomnia	8.8%
0.0%	Seizures	1.5%
0.0%	Depression	0.7%
0.6%	Preoperative	8.7%
8.6%	Other	5.6%

TABLE 12-3. *Adverse reactions to benzodiazepines*
in the Boston Collaborative Drug Surveillance Program

Chlordiazepoxide			Diazepam	
2,086		Total number of recipients	2,623	
		Number with adverse reactions (%)		
181	(8.7%)	Drowsiness	151	(5.7%)
14	(0.7%)	Confusion, excitement, agitation, hallucinations, or nightmares	9	(0.3%)
10	(0.5%)	Hypotension, respiratory depression, or coma	15	(0.6%)
7	(0.3%)	Rash or drug fever	10	(0.4%)
7	(0.3%)	Vertigo or ataxia	5	(0.2%)
0		Gastrointestinal disturbance	8	(0.3%)
2		Other	4	
221	(10.6%)	Total patients with adverse reactions	202	(7.7%)
183	(8.8%)	Drug discontinued or dosage changed due to adverse reaction	174	(6.6%)
3		Drug-attributed deaths	3	

to determine the therapeutic indications. Reasons for termination of therapy and descriptions of suspected adverse reactions are recorded as well. Between 1966 and 1972, a total of 13,349 patients were studied of whom 2,086 (15.6%) received chlordiazepoxide and 2,623 (19.8%) received diazepam during one or more hospitalizations. Approximately 10 to 15% of patients in each group received both drugs. Other benzodiazepines were infrequently used; nitrazepam was prescribed to 333 patients, flurazepam to 146, and oxazepam to only 16. Table 12-2 shows pertinent data for recipients of chlordiazepoxide and diazepam. Patients treated with chlordiazepoxide were more often male, were younger, and had a higher hospital mortality. The common use of this drug for the treatment of alcohol withdrawal in municipal and veterans' hospitals accounts for these differences as well as the more frequent occurrence of "psychiatric disturbance" as an indication for therapy. Anxiety was the most common therapeutic indication for both drugs, but diazepam was used more often than chlordiazepoxide for insomnia, seizures, and as preoperative medication for endoscopy, cardioversion, and prior to transfer to a surgical service.

Table 12-3 shows adverse reactions reported by physicians and attributed to the drugs. For each patient the major manifestation of toxicity is tabulated, so that each patient is represented only once. Adverse reactions were reported in 10.6% of chlordiazepoxide recipients and in 7.7% of those receiving diazepam. In most cases the adverse reaction precipitated drug discontinuation or alteration of dosage. Drowsiness was the most common event; some patients in this group were also confused or disoriented. Other reactions are infrequently reported, including the serious ones (hypotension, respiratory depression, or coma). A total of six hospital deaths, occurring in patients with advanced or terminal disease, were attributed in part to the drugs.

In a subsequent study,[72] the dependence of drowsiness upon dose and age was examined in a subgroup of patients who received chlordiazepoxide or diazepam for the treatment of anxiety. Table 12-4 shows that drowsiness attributed to both drugs becomes more common at higher daily doses. The frequency of drowsiness is also greater in older patients, even though this group did not receive higher doses. Another finding described in this publication is an inverse relationship of drowsiness to cigarette smoking—patients with a history of heavy smoking developed drowsiness less frequently than nonsmokers.

The epidemiologic studies of Svenson and Hamilton and of the Boston Collaborative Drug Surveillance Program differ in important ways. One is a retrospective survey of published reports dealing mainly with anxious neurotic outpatients, whereas the other is a monitoring program dealing with hospitalized medical patients. For obvious reasons ataxia is more common in the former study, while drowsiness is more common in the latter. Other adverse reactions occur in less than 1% of patients surveyed in both studies. For those relatively rare events which are not plausible dose-related manifestations of CNS depression, prospective studies on large numbers of patients will be needed to clarify the possible causal role of the benzodiazepines.

TABLE 12-4. *Relation of dose and age to drowsiness attributed to benzodiazepines**

Daily dosage	% of patients with drowsiness
Chlordiazepoxide	
less than 40 mg	4.9
40-79 mg	6.5
80 mg or more	10.4
Diazepam	
less than 10 mg	4.1
10-19 mg	8.6
20 mg or more	11.2

Patient age	% of patients with drowsiness attributed to either drug
40 years or younger	4.4
41-50 years	4.2
51-60 years	7.6
61-70 years	8.6
older than 70 years	10.9

*Boston Collaborative Drug Surveillance Program: New Eng J Med 288:277-280, 1973

TOLERANCE AND HABITUATION

Animal studies have suggested that the benzodiazpines can produce both acute and chronic tolerance. Some of these effects are evident in behavioral investigations cited in Chapter 3. Margules and Stein[73] noted that early in the course of high-dose oxazepam treatment in rats, generalized behavioral depression was much more prominent than disinhibition. After several days of drug therapy, tolerance to depressant effects developed, and disinhibition was unmasked. A similar pattern was noted with lorazepam treatment.[74] Cannizzarro and associates[75] reported that acute treatment of rats with flurazepam (5 to 10 mg/kg) resulted in reduced spontaneous activity, with no potentiation of behavior suppressed by punishment. After 8 days of alternate-day treatment, depressant effects were much less prominent and punishment-suppressed behavior was enhanced. Tolerance to chlordiazepoxide has been reported by several groups.[76–78] Hoogland and associates[78] studied paralysis times and plasma half-times of chlordiazepoxide (100 mg/kg) in rats. In non-pretreated rats, the paralysis time was 115 min and the plasma half-time 6.3 hr; in animals receiving five consecutive daily doses of chlordiazepoxide prior to testing, the results were 65 min and 3.1 hr, respectively.

Barnett and Fiore[79–81] have described acute tolerance to diazepam in an experimental model. The linguomandibular reflex (LMR) was measured in anesthetized cats. Diazepam (2 mg/kg) produced 79% inhibition of the LMR in unpretreated animals; in those receiving the same dose of diazepam 2 hr prior to the test, 2 mg/kg intravenously produced only 23% inhibition. Tolerance was greater when diazepam was given intraduodenally rather than intravenously. A similar pattern of tolerance was observed in these animals using the anterior tibial flexor reflex or the EEG amplitude as the test response.[81] The authors provide evidence to suggest that one of the less active metabolites of diazepam (desmethyldiazepam, temazepam, or oxazepam) may antagonize the action of diazepam itself.

The addicting properties of benzodiazepines in animals have received limited investigation. Findley and associates[82] studied monkeys with indwelling devices for intravenous administration of drugs. Addiction to chlordiazepoxide could be produced by doses of 1 mg/kg given every 3 hr. When the animals were then given a choice of intravenous self-administration of chlordiazepoxide (1 mg/kg) or secobarbital (9 mg/kg), they gradually evolved to secobarbital dependence over a period of 60 days. Stolerman et al.[83] noted that when chlordiazepoxide was made available to rats in an aqueous solution of 0.5 mg/ml, no animals developed dependence upon the drug. Harris and associates[84] forced rats to drink such a solution by depriving them of other liquid. The animals simply reduced their liquid intake. When allowed to choose between drugged and undrugged liquid, they all returned to pure liquid with no evidence of addiction or tolerance. In a further study,[84] food was withheld, except when administered on a fixed-ratio schedule contingent upon drinking of chlordiazepoxide-containing water. After 25 days of conditioning, the rats were then allowed a choice between drugged and undrugged liquid, and they continued to choose the solution containing chlordiazepoxide. Gotesdam[85] devised a system by which rats could self-administer intragastric medazepam contingent upon a lever-pressing response. Rates of response in food-deprived animals receiving medazepam contingently were significantly higher than in animals receiving placebo. Yanagita and Takahashi[85a] reported that daily intravenous administration of chlordiazepoxide (75 to 113 mg/kg), diazepam (8 to 10 mg/kg), or oxazolam (20 to 60 mg/kg) to monkeys resulted in addiction after 1 month. Habituation could also be produced if the animals were allowed to self-administer the drugs intravenously. These studies suggest that benzodiazepines may produce a relatively weak state of habituation or addiction in animals.

The issue of the abuse potential of benzodiazepines in humans obviously is of great importance. British and Australian authors have stated that habituation or addiction to chlordiazepoxide, diazepam, and nitrazepam does occur but seems to be unusual.[86,87] Reggiani and associates[88] claim that addiction to chlordiazepoxide cannot occur with ordinary therapeutic doses; the drug must be taken in 10 to 20 times the usual doses over a period of months, and produces a dependent state of only moderate intensity. They estimate the frequency of dependence at less than one per one million users. Smith and Wesson[89] state that addicting doses are large—300 to 600 mg per day of chlordiazepoxide, or 80 to 120 mg per day of diazepam—and must be taken for at least 40 to 60 days before habituation occurs. Others suggest that chlordiazepoxide dependence may be much more common in certain populations, notably in chronic alcoholics. Finer[90] states that many alcoholics become addicted to chlordiazepoxide, exhibiting typical pleading and cajoling behavior to obtain the drug. The withdrawal syndrome resembles that associated with barbiturate abstinence. The author claims that he has not seen a similar type of addiction to diazepam. Ewing and Bakewell[91] surveyed 128 hospital admissions due to drug abuse or addiction, finding that chlordiazepoxide was involved in at least 10 cases. Swanson and associates[91a] retrospectively studied the records of 225 patients hospitalized between 1966 and 1972 because of prescription drug abuse. Meprobamate was implicated in 29 cases (13%), diazepam in 22 (9.8%), chlordiazepoxide in 17 (7.6%), oxazepam in 7 (3.1%), and flurazepam in one. Bowes[92] reported that overt dependence occurred in 1% of 500 outpatients receiving diazepam for various emotional disorders.

Unfortunately, few reliable data are available, and our understanding is based on case reports and anecdotal evidence. Much has been made of the study by Hollister and associates,[93] who gave chlordiazepoxide, 100 to 600 mg daily, to 36 hospitalized psychiatric patients for periods of 1 to 7 months. Eleven patients were abruptly changed to placebo on a single-blind basis.

TABLE 12-5. *Habituation to benzodiazepines: Case reports*

Ref.	Author	Patient characteristics (age, sex)	Drug	Dose (mg/day)	Duration	Result
95	Barten, 1965	52, female	Diazepam	40-60	3 mos	Acute delirium tremens-like syndrome upon discontinuation of drug
96	Clare, 1971	39, female, history of barbiturate & alcohol abuse	Diazepam	Max. of 500	wks	Diazepam withdrawal syndrome suppressed by ethanol
97	Darcy, 1972	51, male	Nitrazepam	20 mg nightly	yrs	Acute delirium tremens-like syndrome upon discontinuation of drug
98	Gordon, 1967	23, female	Diazepam	60	1 yr	Tremulous, diaphoretic, and agitated upon discontinuation of drug
99	Guile, 1963	44, female	Chlordiazepoxide	160	dosage increased over 2 mos	Withdrawal syndrome prevented by trifluoperazine
100	Hanna, 1972	29, male	Oxazepam	90	18 mos	Severe agitation and depression upon discontinuation of drug
101	Relkin, 1966	20, male, with dystonia musculorum deformans	Diazepam	40-60	11 days	Severe withdrawal syndrome and death 3 days after drug discontinuation
102	Selig, 1966	29, female	Oxazepam	400-600	6 wks	Acute toxic delirium 5 days after discontinuation of drug
103	Slater, 1966	37, female	Chlordiazepoxide	50-140	yrs	Abdominal pain, diaphoresis, hallucinations upon discontinuation; symptoms suppressed by reinstituting drug

Ten of the 11 patients developed objective or subjective signs of withdrawal, including depression in six, aggravation of psychosis in five, insomnia and agitation in five, decreased appetite in four, seizures in three, and twitching in one. Most symptoms appeared 4 to 8 days after drug discontinuation, and had largely subsided by the 10th day. The authors calculated the plasma half-life of chlordiazepoxide to be 48 hr. Burke and Anderson[94] performed a similar study on 25 hospitalized male chronic alcoholics, administering 75 to 150 mg of chlordiazepoxide per day for 2 weeks. There was no sign of withdrawal in any of the patients when the drug was abruptly discontinued. Covi and associates[94a] compared the effects of sudden discontinuation of chlordiazepoxide after continuous administration of 45 mg per day to anxious neurotic outpatients for either 10 or 20 weeks. Symptomatic distress (tenseness, trembling, dizziness, loss of appetite) after drug termination was worse in those who had received it for 20 weeks. The authors state that it is not clear whether symptoms were due to a withdrawal syndrome or only to recurrence of pretreatment anxiety. However, they suggest that chlordiazepoxide should not be abruptly discontinued if patients have been taking the drug continuously for 16 weeks or more.

Case reports of benzodiazepine abuse or addiction are listed in Table 12-5. Chlordiazepoxide, diazepam, oxazepam, and nitrazepam have all been inplicated. The reports do suggest that addiction to any of the benzodiazepines is indeed possible, but the frequency of addiction among all users of the drugs remains unknown. Certainly many individuals take large doses over long periods of time with no evidence of dependence. Ditman and Benor,[104] for example, reported a 53-year-old alcoholic patient who took up to 200 mg per day of diazepam for many years, with no evidence of a withdrawal syndrome when the drug was discontinued.

At one time or another, most psychoactive drugs are abused by the intravenous or "mainline" route. Richman and Harris[105] describe a 32-year-old male who prepared three chlordiazepoxide capsules for intravenous injection. Shortly after the infusion, the patient developed acute pulmonary edema, fever, leukocytosis, and acidosis. The heart was not enlarged by X-ray. The patient recovered without sequelae. The syndrome has been reported in association with intravenous opiate abuse,[106] and probably represents a sensitivity phenomenon either to the drug, the preservatives, or the vehicle used for injection.

DRUG INTERACTIONS

Interactions of benzodiazepines with other drugs are of two general types. The most straightforward are the acute interactions. Potentiation of the depressant effect of ethyl alcohol is discussed in Chapter 11. In animal studies, the benzodiazepines also potentiate the central depressant properties of barbiturates and other hypnotic agents.[88,107-110] Chlordiazepoxide has also been shown to enhance the lethal effects of cholinesterase inhibitors[111] and amphetamines.[112] Stahnke[113] demonstrated that diazepam (5 to 10 mg/kg) lowered the lethal dose of scorpion venom in mice. In a study by Frommel and associates,[114] chlordiazepoxide-induced sleeping time was prolonged by concurrent administration of morphine but shortened by nalorphine. Nicotine has been shown to antagonize the sedative effects of chlordiazepoxide.[115]

The influence of the propylene glycol solvent vehicle (Table 2-4) upon the pharmacologic activity of the benzodiazepines has been discussed previously (see Chapters 5-7). Propylene glycol is not inert: it possesses weak but significant central depressant and anticonvulsant effects.[116] The sedative effects of water-insoluble benzodiazepines (diazepam, nitrazepam, medazepam) are enhanced when the drugs are administered in the propylene glycol solvent as opposed to a suspension in carboxymethyl cellulose plus polysorbate-80.[117] The potency of chlordiazepoxide, a water-soluble drug, is not influenced. Bradshaw and Pleuvry[118] showed that the 50% lethal dose (LD_{50}) of intraperitoneal nitrazepam in mice was reduced from 640 to 38 mg/kg when the drug was given in propylene glycol rather than as a suspension; the LD_{50} of diazepam was also reduced, from 120 to 87 mg/kg. Schiff and associates[119] demonstrated that the commercially available preparation of injectable diazepam displaced bilirubin from albumin binding sites in an *in vitro* system. The effect was reproduced using the solvent alone without diazepam. This interaction appears not to be of clinical significance.[119a] It is clear, however, that physicians should bear in mind the possibility of drug interactions involving the propylene glycol solvent system. This vehicle is used for injectable preparations of diphenylhydantoin and digoxin as well as diazepam.

Benzodiazepine interactions with drugs other than ethanol in humans have not been investigated in depth. In a non-blind trial, Tammisto and associates[120] studied the effect of various preoperative medications upon the depressant properties of a standard dose of thiopental. Oral chlordiazepoxide pretreatment significantly prolonged thiopental-induced obtundation from an average of 58 sec to 86 sec. The apneic period, however, was not lengthened. Meperidine plus promethazine premedication prolonged obtundation to 142 sec and also lengthened the apneic period. Vajda and associates[121] noted that average plasma diphenylhydantoin levels in patients receiving benzodiazepines concurrently were nearly twice as high as those in patients not receiving benzodiazepines. The explanation is unclear, but the authors suggest that benzodiazepine therapy may precipitate diphenylhydantoin toxicity in patients receiving this drug. Taylor[122] made a similar observation in a patient on stable anticoagulant therapy with bishydroxycoumarin for more than 2 years. Initiation of diazepam therapy (20 mg per day) was followed in 2 weeks by excessive hypoprothrombinemia (prothrombin time 52 sec) and spontaneous ecchymoses. At a later date, it was demonstrated that the hypoprothrombinemic effect of a single oral dose of bishydroxycoumarin was potentiated by concurrent diazepam. Mackie[123] reported a case of a parkinsonian patient receiving L-DOPA, 2 g per day. Addition of chlordiazepoxide (30 mg per day) was followed by nearly complete recrudescense of parkinsonian symptoms despite continuation of L-DOPA. After chlordiazepoxide was discontinued, the symptoms again disappeared. These anecdotal observations are of interest, but require further confirmation and explanation.

Enzyme Induction

Chronic pretreatment of animals or humans with any of a number of sedative-hypnotic agents, most notably barbiturates, is known to enhance the subsequent metabolism of other drugs.[124] The enzyme-inducing properties of the benzodiazepines have been investigated in some detail. In general, effects can be demonstrated in animals but appear to be of little consequence in humans.

Animal studies are summarized in Table 12-6. Most of these investigations are performed in rats, and most demonstrate some degree of enzyme induction. The results, however, are not completely consistent. Orme and associates[131] found a strong effect of chlordiazepoxide pretreatment (40 mg/kg per day), but neither diazepam nor nitrazepam produced any changes at the same dosage. In several of the other reports, however, enzyme induction was evident following pretreatment with similar doses of diazepam.[110,125,132,133] These inconsistencies may in part be explained by differences in the testing parameters as well as age-, sex-, and strain-dependent variations in drug-metabolizing function in laboratory animals.

A number of studies have been performed in humans. Stevenson and associates[135] and O'Malley[136] investigated the plasma half-life of phenyl-butazone and antipyrine following 3 weeks of nightly hypnotic medication. Amobarbital (200 mg nightly) significantly enhanced antipyrine disappearance; nitrazepam (5 to 10 mg nightly) had no effect upon either parameter. Casier et al.[137] found that ethanol metabolism was unaltered in subjects chronically pretreated with diazepam (10 mg per day). Whitfield and co-workers[138] used plasma gamma-glutamyl transpeptidase (GGT) activity as an indicator of hepatic drug-metabolizing activity. Treatment of subjects with barbiturates increased plasma GGT activity, whereas benzodiazepine treatment produced no change. Vesell and associates[134] found that 7 days of prazepam administration (30 mg per day) to healthy males did not produce enhanced metabolism of either prazepam or antipyrine.

All other studies involve coumarin anticoagulants, known to be metabolized by hepatic microsomes.[139] The barbiturates and glutethimide produce clinically important stimulation of oral anticoagulant metabolism in man.[140–142] The benzodiazepines have been studied by two approaches. In the first, the plasma half-life and hypoprothrombinemic effect of a single dose of an oral

TABLE 12-6. Enzyme induction by benzodiazepines: Animal studies*

Ref.	Author	Drug	Daily dose (mg/kg)	Duration of pretreatment	Result
125	Albanus et al., 1971	Diazepam** / Oxazepam**	35 / 150	13 days	Antipyrine half-time shortened by diazepam, prolonged by oxazepam
126	Ballinger et al., 1971	Chlordiazepoxide / Nitrazepam	10-100 / 10-200	4 wks / 4 wks	In vitro barbiturate oxidation enhanced by both drugs
127	Berte el al., 1969	Oxazepam	20	14-30 days	No effect upon oxazepam metabolism by homogenates of placental tissue
78	Hoogland et al., 1966	Chlordiazepoxide	100	5 days	Barbiturate sleeping time shortened; ascorbic acid excretion enhanced; liver weight increased
110	Jori et al., 1969	Chlordiazepoxide / Diazepam	100 / 50-100	3 days / 3 days	Barbiturate sleeping time shortened; enhanced in vitro metabolism of para-nitrophenol, para-aminophenol, 4-aminoantipyrine
128	Kato & Chiesara, 1962	Chlordiazepoxide	50	Single dose 48 hr before test	No effect upon barbiturate metabolism or sleeping time
129	Kato & Vassanelli, 1962	Chlordiazepoxide	50	Single dose 48 hr before test	No effect upon meprobamate metabolism or sleeping time
130	Manzo et al., 1969	Oxazepam	20	4 days	Enhanced oxazepam metabolism by homogenates of tissue (liver, kidney, lung, brain) taken from mother and fetus.
131	Orme et al., 1972	Chlordiazepoxide / Diazepam / Nitrazepam	40 / 40 / 40	4 days / 4 days / 4 days	Chlordiazepoxide shortened pentobarbital sleeping time, enhanced pentobarbital metabolism in vivo; enhanced ethylmorphine N-demethylase activity of hepatic microsomes in vitro. Diazepam and nitrazepam had no effect
132	Ristola et al., 1971	Diazepam / Diazepam***	10 / 2	7 days / 7 days	Enhancement of warfarin metabolism / Shortening of warfarin half-life
133	Szeberenyi et al., 1969	Diazepam	100	5 days	Shortening of metyrapone half-life
134	Vesell et al., 1972	Prazepam	100	4-7 days	Enhanced activity of microsomal ethylmorphine N-demethylase and aniline hydroxylase

anticoagulant are determined in the same subject before and after a course of therapy with a benzodiazepine derivative. In all published studies of chlordiazepoxide,[131,143-145] diazepam,[131,132,145] nitrazepam,[131] and flurazepam,[146] both of these parameters remain unaffected. The second approach involves addition of benzodiazepine therapy to the regimen of a patient on stable oral anticoagulation. The patient is then closely monitored for a decrease in hypoprothrombinemic response or an increase in the anticoagulant dose required to maintain the prothrombin time in a therapeutic range. Chlordiazepoxide,[131,147,148] diazepam,[131] nitrazepam,[131,149,150] and flurazepam[146] all have been found to produce no change in anticoagulant control. At the present time, there is little evidence that any of the benzodiazepines cause clinically important enzyme induction in man.

THYROID FUNCTION

Concern that the benzodiazepines might interfere with thyroid function was precipitated by two reports[151,152] appearing in 1967. The authors presented anecdotal evidence that chlordiazepoxide and diazepam interfered with iodine uptake. They stated that in several clinically thyrotoxic patients taking these drugs, the uptake of radioactive iodine (I^{131}) by the thyroid gland was much lower than expected. These observations remain unexplained. Schindler and associates[153] studied the effects of chlordiazepoxide and diazepam upon the hypothalamic-pituitary-thyroid system in mice. Neither drug altered the thyroid uptake of I^{131} nor influenced the release of thyroid-stimulating hormone (TSH) caused by propylthiouracil. In humans, both drugs have been thoroughly investigated in controlled trials involving normal subjects[154-159] as well as patients with thyrotoxicosis.[157-161] Parameters of thyroid function under study included protein-bound iodine, I^{131} uptake, total thyroxine, free thyroxine, *in vitro* triiodothyronine uptake, plasma TSH, thyroid-binding globulin, antithyroid antibodies, and cholesterol. In no case did the benzodiazepines significantly alter any of these parameters.

In vitro studies by Schussler[162] have revealed that very high concentrations of diazepam (142 μg/ml) displace thyroxine and triiodothyronine from binding sites on thyroid-binding globulin. Tegeris and associates[163] found that addition of diazepam (100 μg/ml) to the serum of healthy subjects receiving no drugs increased the observed protein-bound iodine level by 150%. In clinically relevant concentrations, however, there is no evidence that the benzodiazepines alter any parameters of thyroid function, nor interfere with laboratory determinations thereof.

INFLUENCE UPON LABORATORY TESTS

Zileli and associates[164,165] reported the case of a 45-year-old man hospitalized with a large overdosage of oxazepam. No glycosuria, ketonuria, or acidosis was present, but the blood glucose value on admission was reported at 1,680 mg/100 ml. The authors concluded that oxazepam itself produces a false-positive reaction for glucose. They suspended a commercial 10-mg tablet of oxazepam in a small amount of water; the supernatant yielded glucose values of 590 mg/100 ml and higher using Somogyi and glucose oxidase techniques. Other authors[166-168] subsequently pointed out that the positive glucose reaction was due to the lactose "filler" used in packaging the drug. Pure oxazepam by itself did not test positively.

In an early publication[169] it was stated that chlordiazepoxide interferes with the laboratory determinations of 17-ketosteroids and 17-hydroxycorticosteroids. This claim has been widely perpetuated in various review articles but appears not to be true.[170]

OVERDOSE

The problem of poisoning with psychotropic agents has been reviewed in several publications.[171-173] As tranquilizing agents become more widely used, overdosage becomes more common. Minor tranquilizers are involved in 10 to 25% of cases of intentional self-poisoning according to several recent surveys.[174-176] Ingestion of multiple drugs is common; poisoning with barbiturates, glutethimide, or methaqualone remains the most important problem, both numerically and with respect to the gravity of the medical syndrome. Lawson and Mitchell[177] reviewed nearly 1,000 cases of drug ingestion seen since 1960. About 12% involved benzodiazepines, and none of these patients died. In another review of almost 1,200 cases, Sharman and associates[178] also found that benzodiazepines were involved in 12%. Barbiturate overdosage accounted for most of the total cases and most of the deaths in both of these series.

It is generally accepted that the benzodiazepines are the most benign of all psychotropic drugs with respect to the danger of overdosage. A total of 5,849 deaths due to drug ingestion are on file at the General Registrar's Office in London for the period 1968 through 1969. In only 16 cases was a benzodiazepine by itself implicated (nitrazepam, eight times; chlordiazepoxide and diazepam, each four times).[179,180] In the medical literature there are no reported cases of fatal overdosage due to benzodiazepines alone.

Nitrazepam poisoning has been studied in detail at the Regional Poisoning Treatment Center of the Edinburgh Royal Infirmary.[181] Out of 1,176 hypnotic drug overdosages, 102 involved nitrazepam.[182] Only six patients were deeply comatose and none was obtunded for more than 12 hr. No patients required intubation, and only one was hypotensive. Among 706 barbiturate overdosages, however, 35% were deeply comatose, 15% remained comatose for more than 12 hr, 12% required intubation, and 24% were hypotensive. Poisoning with methaqualone and glutethimide was of equal gravity.

Electroencephalographic studies[183] were consistent with deep coma in many barbiturate ingestions, but revealed predominantly beta and theta activity in nitrazepam overdosage. Tomsett[184] performed blood level studies in 10 cases of overdosage. Concentrations of unchanged nitrazepam ranged from 0.1 to 7.0 µg/ml. Metabolites formed by reduction of the 7-amino group (see Chapter 2) were present in concentrations of 0.7 to 12.0 µg/ml. Unfortunately, details of the quantities of drug ingested are not available.

In three series of chlordiazepoxide overdosage, a total of 148 cases were reported.[185–187] Doses ranged from 60 to 2,250 mg or as high as 50 mg/kg. Patients' ages ranged from 15 months to 65 years. There was no deep coma, respiratory depression, or hypotension in any of the cases, and all recovered without sequelae. Patients had symptoms of somnolence and drowsiness, but generally were rousable. Symptoms usually disappeared within 48 hr of ingestion. Jatlow[188] analyzed blood samples of 60 patients after large overdoses of chlordiazepoxide. Blood concentrations ranged from 2 to 66 µg/ml. Levels greater than 20 µg/ml were associated with drowsiness; patients with blood concentrations of 40 µg/ml were asleep but rousable. True coma was extremely rare, even in patients with levels exceeding 60 µg/ml.

Further documentation of benzodiazepine overdosage exists as case reports, summarized in Table 12-7. These include chlordiazepoxide in 11 cases, diazepam in five, and oxazepam in three. Brief reports of overdosage appearing in the clinical studies reviewed in Chapter 4 are not included. In this series, the largest diazepam ingestion was 1.4 g together with 40 Mandrax pills.[192] Hypothermia was noted in one episode of diazepam poisoning, but this patient also took 7.5 g of glutethimide.[195] Death from coma and hypothermia in an 84-year-old male following therapeutic doses of diazepam has been mentioned previously;[207] in this case, the patient was probably myxedematous and thus predisposed to develop hypothermia. Cruz and associates[194] reported a fatal case of multiple drug ingestion. The blood level of chlordiazepoxide was 24 µg/ml, and elimination appeared to be hastened by dialysis. The drug was not detectable in the dialysate, however. Both chlordiazepoxide and diazepam are strongly protein-bound, and dialysis would not be expected to be of great help. Fortunately, dialysis is seldom required. Decker et al.[208] found that in vitro dialysis of plasma containing chlordiazepoxide and diazepam caused very little drug removal. Dialysis against activated charcoal, however, enchanced drug removal considerably. Rice et al.[209] showed that forced diuresis was of little value in experimental chlordiazepoxide poisoning. Bullous skin lesions, thought to be characteristic of barbiturate overdosage, have been observed in at least one case of nitrazepam poisoning.[210]

The available evidence supports the contention that the benzodiazepines are the least hazardous of available sedative or psychotropic drugs. At the present time flurazepam is the only benzodiazepine hypnotic available in the United States, and there is little or no experience with flurazepam

TABLE 12-7. *Case reports of benzodiazepine overdosage*

Ref.	Author	Age, sex	Drug and dosage (mg)	Comment
189	Austin, 1966	42, F	CDX, 480	With amobarbital, 1 g, and phenelzine, 600 mg. Hypotensive, required tracheostomy
190	Bardhan, 1969	23, M	NTZ, 180	Predominant symptoms: ataxia, dysarthria, nystagmus
191	Burston, 1969	68, F	CDX, 400	With pentobarbital, 600 mg
192	Carroll, 1970	20, F	DZ, 1,400	With 10 g methaqualone and 1 g diphenhydramine
193	Clarke et al., 1961	44, F	CDX, 875	Benign course in both cases
		22, M	CDX, 1,630	
194	Cruz et al., 1967	43, F	CDX, ? dose	With ethchlorvynol, barbiturates, ethanol, propoxyphene; CDX level 24 μg/ml. Died despite dialysis.
195	Fell & Dendy, 1968	38, F	DZ, ? dose	With glutethimide, 7.5 g; developed severe hypothermia
196	Ganguli et al., 1970	16, M	OXZ, 900	Deep coma; rapid recovery
197	Gilbert, 1961	38, F	CDX, 1,250	With ethanol; deep coma
198	Hillyer, 1965	? age, M	DZ, 250	Benign course
199	Jenner & Parkin, 1961	23, F	CDX, 1,850	Benign course
200	Pennington & Synge, 1961	32, F	CDX, 600	Blood level 2 μg/ml
201	Schaeffer, 1962	11, M	CDX, 425	Blood level 9 μg/ml. Recovered in 3 days
202	Shimkin & Shaivitz, 1966	2, F	OXZ, 90	Blood level 5 μg/ml
203	Smith, 1961	47, F	CDX, 1,150	With ethanol
204	Spark & Goldman, 1965	2, M	DZ, 20-24	Rapid recovery
205	Tanner & Moorhead, 1968	2, F	DZ, 300	—
206	Thompson & Glen, 1961	?	CDX, 190	Not comatose
165	Zileli et al., 1972	45, M	OXZ, ? dose	Deep coma. Required tracheostomy & exchange transfusion

overdosage. Yet it is reasonable to extrapolate from studies of nitrazepam overdosage and assume that flurazepam is equally innocuous. If for this reason only, nitrazepam and flurazepam are clearly preferable to other hypnotic agents provided drug cost is not an overwhelming consideration.

COMMENT

Very few unequivocal statements can be made concerning unwanted effects of benzodiazepines. Chlordiazepoxide and diazepam appear to produce excess

CNS depression, manifested as drowsiness and/or ataxia, in 3 to 10% of users. The effects are dose-dependent and can be controlled by adjusting dosage downward. Clinically significant drug interactions do not appear to be a problem. The hazard of overdosage is minimal—very large doses produce obtundation and coma only rarely. On the other hand, the degree to which the benzodiazepines produce adverse effects such as addiction, bone marrow depression, or fetal malformations cannot be adequately estimated without further systematic epidemiologic investigation. It is important that the apparent innocuousness of the benzodiazepines not lead to the assumption that such investigation is unnecessary.

REFERENCES

1. Lemere F: Toxic reactions to chlordiazepoxide. JAMA 174:893, 1960
2. Fullerton AG, Bethell MS: Side-effects of Librium. Lancet 2:875, 1960
3. Bartholomew AA: A dramatic side effect of a new drug, "Librium." Med J Aust 2:436-438, 1961
4. Currie JP: Hypnotic effects of chlordiazepoxide. Lancet 1:724, 1961
5. Noack CH: An unfortunate effect from the ill-judged self-administration of chlordiazepoxide ("Librium"). Med J Aust 1:930-931, 1962
6. Kane FJ, Taylor TW: A toxic reaction to combined Elavil-Librium therapy. Amer J Psychiat 119:1179-1180, 1963
7. Abdou FA: Elavil-Librium combination. Amer J Psychiat 120:1204, 1964
8. Daly RJ, Kane FJ: Two severe reactions to benzodiazepine compounds. Amer J Psychiat 122:577-578, 1965
9. Glasgow JFT: A neurological disorder associated with chlordiazepoxide therapy. Clin Toxicol 2:5-11, 1969
10. Hallberg RJ, Lessler K, Kane FJ: Korsakoff-like syndrome associated with benzodiazepine overdosage. Amer J Psychiat 121:188-189, 1964
11. Ditman KS, Gottlieb L: Transient enuresis from chlordiazepoxide and diazepam. Amer J Psychiat 120:910-911, 1964
12. Hughes JM: Failure to ejaculate with chlordiazepoxide. Amer J Psychiat 121:610-611, 1964
13. Bartholomew AA, Bruce DW: The modification of a side effect (drowsiness) of chlordiazepoxide ("Librium") by amiphenazole: preliminary communication. Med J Aust 1:927-928, 1962
14. Murray N: Covert effects of chlordiazepoxide therapy. J Neuropsychiat 3:168-170, 1962
15. Ayd FJ: A critical appraisal of chlordiazepoxide. J Neuropsychiat 3:177-180, 1962
16. Maguire GP, Aitken RCB, Zealley AK: Hyperkinesis due to chlordiazepoxide. J Int Med Res 1:15-17, 1972
17. Bladin PF: The use of clonazepam as an anticonvulsant—clinical evaluation. Med J Aust 1:683-688, 1973
18. Zucker HS: Strange behavior with oxazepam. NY State J Med 72:974, 1972
19. Viscott DS: Chlordiazepoxide and hallucinations. Report of cases. Arch Gen Psychiat 19:370-376, 1968
20. Fraser AG, Shepherd FGG: Trial of a new hypnotic in general practice. Practitioner 196:829-833, 1966
21. Girdwood RH: Nitrazepam nightmares. Brit Med J 1:353, 1973
22. Taylor F: Nitrazepam in the elderly. Brit Med J 1:113-114, 1973

22a. Goossens T, Bulckaert M, Wakeling E: Nitrazepam and the subconscious. Brit Med J 2:488, 1973

23. Evans JG, Jarvis EH: Nitrazepam and the elderly. Brit Med J 4:487, 1972

24. MacLean H: Nitrazepam: another interesting syndrome. Brit Med J 1:488, 1973

25. Ryan HF, Merrill FB, Scott GE, Krebs R, Thompson BL: Increase in suicidal thoughts and tendencies. Association with diazepam therapy. JAMA 203:1137-1139, 1968

26. Hall RWC, Joffe JR: Aberrant response to diazepam: a new syndrome. Amer J Psychiat 126:738-742, 1972

27. Fisher C, Kahn E, Edwards A, Davis DM: A psychophysiological study of nightmares and night terrors. The suppression of stage 4 night terrors with diazepam. Arch Gen Psychiat 28:252-259, 1973

28. Doughty A: Unexpected danger of diazepam. Brit Med J 2:239, 1970

29. Buskop JJ, Price I, Molnar I: Untoward effect of diazepam. New Eng J Med 277:316, 1967

30. Clinical anesthesia conference. Unexpected responses following diazepam. NY State J Med 71:578-580, 1971

31. Greenblatt DJ, Koch-Weser J: Adverse reactions to intravenous diazepam: a report from the Boston Collaborative Drug Surveillance Program. Amer J Med Sci 266:261-266, 1973

32. Langdon DE, Harlan JR, Bailey RL: Thrombophlebitis with diazepam used intravenously. JAMA 223:184-185, 1973

32a. Langdon DE: Thrombophlebitis following diazepam. JAMA 225:1389, 1973

33. Wehlage DF: Diazepam phlebitis. JAMA 224:128-129, 1973

33a. Jusko WJ, Gretch M, Gassett R: Precipitation of diazepam from intravenous preparations. JAMA 225:176, 1973

33b. Keller MF: Intravenous diazepam administration. JAMA 225:750, 1973

34. Kuster J: Increased creatine-kinase concentrations after intramuscular injection of diazepam. German Med 2:154-155, 1972

35. Greenblatt DJ, Duhme DW, Koch-Weser J: Pain and CPK elevation after intramuscular digoxin. New Eng J Med 288:689, 1973

36. Holden JMC, Itil TM: Laboratory changes with chlordiazepoxide and thioridazine, alone and combined. Canad Psychiat Assoc J 14:299-301, 1969

37. Kurland AA, Bethon GD, Michaux MH, Agallianos DD: Chlorpromazine-chlordiazepoxide and chlorpromazine-imipramine treatment: side effects and clinical laboratory findings. J New Drugs 6:80-95, 1966

38. Abbruzzeze A, Swanson J: Jaundice after therapy with chlordiazepoxide hydrochloride. New Eng J Med 273:321-322, 1965

39. Pickering D: Hepatic necrosis after chlordiazepoxide therapy. New Eng J Med 274:1449, 1966

40. Cacioppo J, Merlis S: Chlordiazepoxide hydrochloride (Librium®) and jaundice: report of a case. Amer J Psychiat 117:1040-1041, 1961

41. Lo K-J, Eastwood IR, Eidelman S: Cholestatic jaundice associated with chlordiazepoxide hydrochloride (Librium) therapy. Report of a case and review of the literature. Amer J Dig Dis 12:845-849, 1967

42. Cunningham ML: Acute hepatic necrosis following treatment with amitriptyline and diazepam. Brit J Psychiat 111:1107-1109, 1965

43. Winkelmayer R: Subicterus following the administration of thioridazine and chlordiazepoxide. Delaware Med J 38:334-336, 1966

44. Ebert MH, Shader RI: Hematological effects. In, *Psychotropic Drug Side Effects. Clinical and Theoretical Perspectives.* By RI Shader, A DiMascio, and associates. Baltimore, Williams and Wilkins, 1970, pp 164-174

45. Litvak R, Kaebling R: Agranulocytosis, leukopenia, and psychotropic drugs. Arch Gen Psychiat 24:265-267, 1971

46. Menon GN: Hypoplastic anaemia—an unusual complication of chlordiazepoxide hydrochloride therapy. Postgrad Med J 41:282-283, 1965
47. Wilcox WW: A case of agranulocytosis. Alaska Med 4:31-32, (March) 1962
48. Kaebling R, Conrad FG: Agranulocytosis due to chlordiazepoxide hydrochloride. JAMA 174:1863-1865, 1960
49. Bitnun S: Possible effect of chlordiazepoxide on the fetus. Canad Med Assoc J 100:351, 1969
50. Dhawan BN, Mathur GB, Rajvanshi VS: Effects of some centrally acting drugs on blood coagulation. Jap J Pharmacol 18:445-453, 1968
51. Almeyda J: Cutaneous reactions to imipramine and chlordiazepoxide. Brit J Dermatol 84:298-300, 1971
52. Mackie BS, Mackie LE: Antihistamines in the treatment of drug eruptions. Med J Aust 2:1034-1037, 1966
53. Luton EF, Finchum RN: Photosensitivity reaction to chlordiazepoxide. Arch Dermatol 91:362-363, 1965
54. Savin JA: Current causes of fixed drug eruptions. Brit J Dermatol 83:546-549, 1970
55. Gaul LE: Fixed drug eruption from chlordiazepoxide. Arch Dermatol 83:1010-1011, 1961
56. Copperman IJ: Purpura in a patient taking chlordiazepoxide. Brit Med J 4:485-486, 1967
57. Rapp MS: Reaction to flurazepam. Canad Med Assoc J 105:1020-1021, 1971
58. O'Grady JA, Pokorny C: Drug allergy. Severe allergic reaction to Librium®: case report. J Kansas Med Soc 65:65-66, 1964
59. Salzman C, Shader RI, DiMascio A: Collagen disease-like syndrome following administration of a benzodiazepine derivative. Dis Nerv Syst 28:614-615, 1967
60. Staiger GR: Chlordiazepoxide and diazepam: absence of effects on the chromosomes of diploid human fibroblast cells. Mutation Res 7:109-115, 1969
61. Stenchever MA, Frankel RS, Jarvis JA, Veress K: Effect of chlordiazepoxide hydrochloride on human chromosomes. Amer J Obstet Gynecol 106:920-923, 1970
62. Stenchever MA, Frankel RS, Jarvis JA, Veress K: Some effects of diazepam in human cells in vitro. Amer J Obstet Gynecol 103:836-842, 1969
63. Schmid W, Staiger GR: Chromosome studies on bone marrow from Chinese hamsters treated with benzodiazepine tranquillizers and cyclophosphamide. Mutation Res 7:99-108, 1969
64. Cohen MM, Hirschhorn K, Frosch WA: Cytogenetic effects of tranquilizing drugs in vivo and in vitro. JAMA 207:2425-2426, 1969
65. Stenchever MA, Frankel RS, Jarvis JA: Effect of diazepam on chromosomes of human leukocytes in vivo. Amer J Obstet Gynecol 107:456-460, 1970
66. Staiger GR: Studies on the chromosomes of human lymphocytes treated with diazepam *in vitro*. Mutation Res 10:635-644, 1970
67. Breen PC, Stenchever MA: Some effects of diazepam on the fine structure of human fibroblasts in tissue culture. Amer J Obstet Gynecol 108:520-527, 1970
68. Istvan EJ: Drug-associated congenital abnormalities. Canad Med Assoc J 103:1394, 1970
69. Beall JR: Study of the teratogenic potential of diazepam and SCH 12041. Canad Med Assoc J 106:1061, 1972
69a. Owen G, Smith THF, Agersborg HPK: Toxicity of some benzodiazepine compounds with CNS activity. Toxicol Appl Pharmacol 16:556-570, 1970
70. Svenson SE, Hamilton RG: A critique of overemphasis on side effects with the psychotropic drugs: an analysis of 18,000 chlordiazepoxide-treated cases. Curr Ther Res 8:455-464, 1966
71. Miller RR: Drug surveillance utilizing epidemiologic methods: a report from the Boston Collaborative Drug Surveillance Program. Amer J Hosp Pharm 30:584-592, 1973
72. Boston Collaborative Drug Surveillance Program: Clinical depression of the central nervous system due to diazepam and chlordiazepoxide in relation to cigarette smoking and age. New Eng J Med 288:277-280, 1973

73. Margules DL, Stein L: Increase of "antianxiety" activity and tolerance of behavioral depression during chronic administration of oxazepam. Psychopharmacologia 13:74-80, 1968

74. Stein L, Berger BD: Psychopharmacology of 7-chloro-5-(o-chlorophenyl)-1,3-dihydro-3-hydroxy-2H-1,4-benzodiazepin-2-one (lorazepam) in squirrel monkey and rat. Arzneim-Forsch 21:1073-1078, 1971

75. Cannizzaro G, Nigito S, Provenzano PM, Vitikova T: Modification of depressant and disinhibitory action of flurazepam during short-term treatment in the rat. Psychopharmacologia 26:173-184, 1972

76. Goldberg ME, Manian AA, Efron DH: A comparative study of certain pharmacologic responses following acute and chronic administrations of chlordiazepoxide. Life Sci 6(Part I):481-491, 1967

77. Matsuki K, Iwamoto T: Development of tolerance to tranquillizers in the rat. Jap J Pharmacol 16:191-197, 1966

78. Hoogland DR, Miya TS, Bousquet WF: Metabolism and tolerance studies with chlordiazepoxide-2-^{14}C in the rat. Toxicol Appl Pharmacol 9:116-123, 1966

79. Barnett A, Fiore JW: Acute tolerance to diazepam in cats: lack of cross-tolerance to phenobarbital and methocarbamol. Eur J Pharmacol 14:301-302, 1971

80. Barnett A, Fiore JW: Acute tolerance to diazepam in cats and its possible relationship to diazepam metabolism. Eur J Pharmacol 13:239-243, 1971

81. Barnett A, Fiore JW: Acute tolerance to diazepam in cats. In, *The Benzodiazepines.* Edited by S Garattini, E Mussini, LO Randall. New York, Raven Press, 1973, pp 545-557

82. Findley JD, Robinson WW, Peregrino L: Addiction to secobarbital and chlordiazepoxide in the rhesus monkey by means of self-infusion preference procedure. Psychopharmacologia 26:93-114, 1972

83. Stolerman IP, Kumar R, Steinberg H: Development of morphine dependence in rats: lack of effect of previous ingestion of other drugs. Psychopharmacologia 20:321-336, 1971

84. Harris RT, Claghorn JL, Schoolar JC: Self-administration of minor tranquilizers as a function of conditioning. Psychopharmacologia 13:81-88, 1968

85. Gotesdam KG: Intragastric self-administration of medazepam. Psychopharmacologia 28:87-94, 1973

85a. Yanagita T, Takahashi S: Dependence liability of several sedative-hypnotic agents evaluated in monkeys. J Pharmacol Exp Ther 185:307-316, 1973

86. Edgley R: Diazepam, nitrazepam, and the N.H.S. Med J Aust 1:186-187, 1970

87. Glatt MM: Benzodiazepines. Brit Med J 2:444, 1967

88. Reggiani G, Hurlimann A, Theiss E: Some aspects of the experimental and clinical toxicology of chlordiazepoxide. In, *Proceedings of the European Society for the Study of Drug Toxicity. Vol. 9. Toxicity and Side-Effects of Psychotropic Drugs.* Edited by SBD Baker, JR Boissier, W Koll. Amsterdam, Excerpta Medica Foundation, 1968, pp 79-97

89. Smith DE, Wesson DR: A new method for treatment of barbiturate dependence. JAMA 213:294-295, 1970

90. Finer MJ: Habituation to chlordiazepoxide in an alcoholic population. JAMA 213:1342, 1970

91. Ewing JA, Bakewell WE: Diagnosis and management of depressant drug dependence. Amer J Psychiat 123:909-917, 1967

91a. Swanson DW, Weddige RL, Morse RM: Abuse of prescription drugs. Mayo Clin Proc 48:359-367, 1973

92. Bowes HA: The role of diazepam (Valium) in emotional illness. Psychosomatics 6:336-340, 1965

93. Hollister LE, Motzenbecker FP, Degan RO: Withdrawal reactions from chlordiazepoxide ("Librium"). Psychopharmacologia 2:63-68, 1961

94. Burke GW, Anderson CWG: Response to Librium in individuals with a propensity for addiction. A pilot study. J Louisiana State Med Soc 114:58-60, 1962

94a. Covi L, Lipman RS, Pattison JH, Derogatis LR, Uhlenhuth EH: Length of treatment with anxiolytic sedatives and response to their sudden withdrawal. Acta Psychiat Scand 49:51-64, 1973

95. Barten HH: Toxic psychosis with transient dysmnestic syndrome following withdrawal from Valium. Amer J Psychiat 121:1210-1211, 1965

96. Clare AW: Diazepam, alcohol, and barbiturate abuse. Brit Med J 4:340, 1971

97. Darcy L: Delirium tremens following withdrawal of nitrazepam. Med J Aust 2:450, 1972

98. Gordon EB: Addiction to diazepam (Valium). Brit Med J 1:112, 1967

99. Guile LA: Rapid habituation to chlordiazepoxide ("Librium"). Med J Aust 2:56-57, 1963

100. Hanna SM: A case of oxazepam (Serenid D) dependence. Brit J Psychiat 120:443-445, 1972

101. Relkin R: Death following withdrawal of diazepam. NY State J Med 66:1770-1772, 1966

102. Selig JW: A possible oxazepam abstinence syndrome. JAMA 198:951-952, 1966

103. Slater J: Suspected dependence on chlordiazepoxide hydrochloride (Librium). Canad Med Assoc J 95:416, 1966

104. Ditman KS, Benor D: Diazepam (Valium) very high dosage: longitudinal and single case study. Western Med 7:109-110, 1966

105. Richman S, Harris RD: Acute pulmonary edema associated with Librium abuse. Radiology 103:57-58, 1972

106. Duberstein JL, Kaufman DM: A clinical study of an epidemic of heroin intoxication and heroin-induced pulmonary edema. Amer J Med 51:704-714, 1971

107. Fujimori H: Potentiation of barbital hypnosis as an evaluation method for central nervous system depressants. Psychopharmacologia 7:374-378, 1965

108. Frank GB, Jhamandas K: Effects of drugs acting alone and in combination on the motor activity of intact mice. Brit J Pharmacol 39:696-706, 1970

109. Macko E, Wilfon G, Greene L, Bender AD, Tedeschi RE: Pharmacological properties of the isopropyl ester of *o*-sulfamoyl-benzoic acid. Arch Int Pharmacodyn 168:220-234, 1967

110. Jori A, Prestini PE, Pugliatti C: Effect of diazepam and chlordiazepoxide on the metabolism of other drugs. J Pharm Pharmacol 21:387-390, 1969

111. Weiss LR, Orzel RA: Enhancement of toxicity of cholinesterases by central depressant drugs in rats. Toxicol Appl Pharmacol 10:334-339, 1967

112. Gardocki JF, Schuler ME, Goldstein L: Reconsideration of the central nervous system pharmacology of amphetamine. II. Influence of pharmacologic agents on cumulative and total lethality in grouped and isolated mice. Toxicol Appl Pharmacol 9:536-554, 1966

113. Stahnke HL: Effect of Thorazine and Valium on scorpion venom toxicity. Arizona Med 29:424, 1972

114. Frommel E, von Ledebur I, Seydoux J: Study of the effects of morphine and nalorphine. Arch Int Pharmacodyn 152:144-155, 1964

115. Bhattacharya IC, Goldstein L, Pfeiffer CC: Influence of acute and chronic nicotine administration on EEG reactivity to drugs in rabbits. 2. Psychoactive agents. Res Comm Chem Pathol Pharmacol 1:109-114, 1970

116. Zaroslinski JF, Browne RK, Possley LH: Propylene glycol as a drug solvent in pharmacologic studies. Toxicol Appl Pharmacol 19:573-578, 1971

117. Crankshaw DP, Raper C: The effect of solvents on the potency of chlordiazepoxide, diazepam, medazepam, and nitrazepam. J Pharm Pharmacol 23:313-321, 1971

118. Bradshaw EG, Pleuvry BJ: Respiratory and hypnotic effects of nitrazepam, diazepam, and pentobarbitone and their solvents in the rabbit and the mouse. Brit J Anaesth 43:637-643, 1971

119. Schiff D, Chan G, Stern L: Fixed drug combinations and the displacement of bilirubin from albumin. Pediatrics 48:139-141, 1971

119a. Adoni A, Kapitulnik J, Kaufmann NA, Ron M, Blondheim SH: Effect of maternal administration of diazepam on the bilirubin-binding capacity of cord blood serum. Amer J Obstet Gynecol 115:577-579, 1973

120. Tammisto T, Elfving G, Saikku K, Titinen P: The effect of reserpine, chlordiazepoxide, and imipramine treatment on the potency of thiopental in man. Ann Chir Gynaecol Fenn 56:323-326, 1967

121. Vajda FJE, Prineas RJ, Lovell RRH: Interaction between phenytoin and the benzodiazepines. Brit Med J 1:346, 1971

122. Taylor PJ: Hemorrhage while on anticoagulant therapy precipitated by drug interaction. Arizona Med 24:697-699, 1967

123. Mackie L: Drug antagonism. Brit Med J 2:651, 1971

124. Conney AH: Pharmacological implications of microsomal enzyme induction. Pharmacol Rev 19:317-366, 1967

125. Albanus L, Jonsson M, Sparf B, Vessman J: A study of the induction effect of phenobarbital, diazepam, and oxazepam in the dog (Abstract). Acta Pharmacol Toxicol 29(supp 4):55, 1971

126. Ballinger B, O'Malley K, Stevenson IH, Turnbull MJ: Stimulation of drug metabolism by centrally active drugs. Brit J Pharmacol 41:383P, 1971

127. Berte F, Manzo L, DeBernardi M, Benzi G: Ability of the placenta to metabolize oxazepam and aminopyrine before and after drug stimulation. Arch Int Pharmacodyn 182:182-185, 1969

128. Kato R, Chiesara E: Increase of pentobarbitone metabolism induced in rats pretreated with some centrally acting compounds. Brit J Pharmacol Chemother 18:29-38, 1962

129. Kato R, Vassanelli P: Induction of increased meprobamate metabolism in rats pretreated with some neurotropic drugs. Biochem Pharmacol 11:779-794, 1962

130. Manzo L, Berte F, DeBernardi M: Oxazepam glucuronidation "in vitro" in some maternal and fetal tissues of the rat. Effects of pretreatment with oxazepam and phenobarbital. Estratto Boll Chim Farm 108:19-24, 1969

131. Orme M, Breckenridge A, Brooks RV: Interactions of benzodiazepines with warfarin. Brit Med J 3:611-614, 1972

132. Ristola P, Pyorala K, Jalonen K, Suhonen O: The effect of diazepam on the rate of warfarin metabolism in man, rabbit, and rat. Scand J Clin Lab Invest 27(supp 116):18, 1971

133. Szeberenyi S, Szalay KS, Garrattini S: Removal of plasma metyrapone in rats submitted to previous pharmacological treatment. J Pharm Pharmacol 21:201-202, 1969

134. Vesell ES, Passananti GT, Viau J-P, Epps JE, DiCarlo FJ: Effects of chronic prazepam administration on drug metabolism in man and rat. Pharmacology 7:197-206, 1972

135. Stevenson IH, Browning M, Crooks J, O'Malley K: Changes in human drug metabolism after long-term exposure to hypnotics. Brit Med J 4:322-324, 1972

136. O'Malley K: Safety of hypnotics. Brit Med J 1:729, 1971

137. Casier H, Danechmand L, DeSchaepdryver A, Hermans W, Piette Y: Blood alcohol levels and psychotropic drugs. Arzneim-Forsch 16:1505-1507, 1966

138. Whitfield JB, Moss DW, Neale G, Orme M, Breckenridge A: Changes in plasma γ-glutamyl transpeptidase activity associated with alterations in drug metabolism in man. Brit Med J 1:316-318, 1973

139. Coon WW, Willis PW: Some aspects of the pharmacology of oral anticoagulants. Clin Pharmacol Ther 11:312-336, 1970

140. O'Reilly RA, Aggeler PM: Determinants of the response to oral anticoagulant drugs in man. Pharmacol Rev 22:35-96, 1970

141. Koch-Weser J, Sellers EM: Drug interactions with coumarin anticoagulants. New Eng J Med 285:487-498, 547-558, 1971

142. Greenblatt DJ, Shader RI: The clinical choice of sedative-hypnotics. Ann Intern Med 77:91-100, 1972

143. Robinson DS, Sylwester D: Interaction of commonly prescribed drugs with warfarin. Ann Intern Med 72:853-856, 1970

144. van Dam FE, Gribnau-Overkamp MJH: The effect of some sedatives (phenobarbital, gluthetimide [sic], chlordiazepoxide, chloral hydrate) on the rate of disappearance of ethyl biscoumacetate from the plasma. Folia Med Neerl 10:141-145, 1967

145. Solomon HM, Barakat MJ, Ashley CJ: Mechanisms of drug interaction. JAMA 216:1997-1999, 1971

146. Robinson DS, Amidon EL: Interaction of benzodiazepines with warfarin in man. In, *The Benzodiazepines*. Edited by S Garattini, E Mussini, LO Randall. New York, Raven Press, 1973, pp 641-646

147. Lackner H, Hunt VE: The effect of Librium on hemostasis. Amer J Med Sci 256:368-372, 1968

148. Bibawi E, Girgis B, Abu-Khatwa H: Effect of hypnotics and psychotropic drugs on prothrombin level. J Egyptian Med Assoc 46:933-936, 1963

149. Breckenridge A, Orme M: Clinical implications of enzyme induction. Ann NY Acad Sci 179:421-431, 1971

150. Bieger R, de Jonge H, Loeliger EA: Influence of nitrazepam on oral anticoagulation with phenprocoumon. Clin Pharmacol Ther 13:361-365, 1972

151. Baron JM: Chlordiazepoxide (Librium) and thyroid-function tests. Brit Med J 1:699, 1967

152. Harvey RF: Drugs and thyroid-function tests. Brit Med J 2:52, 1967

153. Schindler WJ, Matthews MG, McHorse TS: Influence of centrally acting drugs on pituitary TSH release and thyroid activity in the mouse. Fed Proc 25:380, 1966

154. Oberman H, Buse J, Herbert EG, Ellison HS, Buse MG: Effect of chlordiazepoxide on thyroid function. JAMA 184:342, 1963

155. Saldanha VF, Bird R, Havard CWH: Effect of diazepam (Valium) on dialysable thyroxine. Postgrad Med J 47:326-328, 1971

156. Mazzaferri EL, Skillman TG: Diazepam (Valium®) and thyroid function: a double-blind, placebo controlled study in normal volunteers showing no effect. Amer J Med Sci 257:388-394, 1969

157. Clark F, Hall R: Chlordiazepoxide (Librium) and tests of thyroid function. Brit Med J 2:266-268, 1970

158. Clark F, Hall R, Ormston BJ: Diazepam and tests of thyroid function. Brit Med J 1:585-586, 1971

159. Slater SD: The effect of chlordiazepoxide and amylobarbitone upon thyroid function test. Brit J Clin Prac 26:463-465, 1972

160. Greenberg AH, Czernichow P, Blizzard RM: Diazepam (Valium®) in thyrotoxicosis. Negative results. Johns Hopkins Med J 126:134-138, 1970

161. Barnes HV, Greenberg AH, Owings J, Blizzard RM: The effect of chlordiazepoxide (Librium) on thyroid function in thyrotoxicosis. Johns Hopkins Med J 131:298-302, 1972

162. Schussler GC: Diazepam competes for thyroxine binding sites. J Pharmacol Exp Ther 178:204-209, 1971

163. Tegeris AS, Cottrell JC, Cruz EA: The in vitro effect of some commonly prescribed drugs on routine laboratory tests (Abstract). Toxicol Appl Pharmacol 14:618, 1969

164. Zileli MS, Teletar F, Deniz S, Ilter E, Adalar N: Oxazepam intoxication simulating non-ketoacidotic diabetic coma. JAMA 215:1986, 1971

165. Zileli MS, Telatar F, Deniz S, Ilter E, Adalar N: Pseudohyperosmolar nonketoacitotic coma due to oxazepam intoxication. Clin Toxicol 5:337-341, 1972

166. Frings CS: Absence of interference of oxazepam with glucose determination. JAMA 217:1244, 1971

167. Spiegel HE, Enthoven D: Autoanalyzer glucose problems. JAMA 220:1499, 1972
168. Teller JD: False glucose values with use of oxazepam. JAMA 222:209, 1972
169. Borushek S, Gold JJ: Commonly used medications that interfere with routine endocrine laboratory procedures. Clin Chem 10:41-52, 1964
170. Cryer PE, Sode J: Drug interferences with measurement of adrenal hormones in urine: analgesics and tranquilizer-sedatives. Ann Intern Med 75:697-702, 1971
171. Brophy JJ: Suicide attempts with psychotherapeutic drugs. Arch Gen Psychiat 17:652-657, 1967
172. Greenblatt DJ, Shader RI: Acute poisoning with psychotropic drugs. In, *Psychotropic Drug Side Effects: Clinical and Theoretical Perspectives.* By RI Shader, A DiMascio, and associates. Baltimore, Williams and Wilkins, 1970, pp 214-234
173. Davis JM, Bartlett E, Termini BA: Overdosage of psychotropic drugs: a review. Dis Nerv Syst 29:157-164, 246-256, 1968
174. Smith AJ: Self-poisoning with drugs: a worsening situation. Brit Med J 4:157-159, 1972
175. Ianzito BM: Attempted suicide by drug ingestion. Dis Nerv Syst 31:453-458, 1970
176. Birtchnell J, Alarcon J: Depression and attempted suicide: a study of 91 cases seen in a casualty department. Brit J Psychiat 118:289-296, 1971
177. Lawson AAH, Mitchell I: Patients with acute poisoning seen in a general medical unit (1960-1971). Brit Med J 4:153-156, 1972
178. Sharman JR, Taylor HW, Scott RD: Drug overdosages and poisonings in Christchurch during 1971. New Zealand Med J 76:402-404, 1972
179. Poisoning cases in 1968. Pharmaceut J 204:703-707, 1970
180. Poisoning cases in 1969. Pharmaceut J 206:422-426, 1971
181. Matthew H, Proudfoot AT, Aitken RCB, Raeburn JA, Wright N: Nitrazepam—a safe hypnotic. Brit Med J 3:23-25, 1969
182. Matthew H, Roscoe P, Wright N: Acute poisoning. A comparison of hypnotic drugs. Practitioner 208:254-258, 1972
183. Haider I, Matthew H, Oswald I: Electroencephalographic changes in acute drug poisoning. Electroenceph Clin Neurophysiol 30:23-31, 1971
184. Tompsett SL: Nitrazepam (Mogadon) in blood serum and urine and Librium in urine. J Clin Pathol 21:366-371, 1968
185. Malizia E, Bertolini G, Venturi VM: Comparison between experimental responses and clinical intoxications caused by central nervous system depressants and by antihistaminic drugs. In, *Proceedings of the European Society for the Study of Drug Toxicity. Vol. 6. Experimental Studies and Clinical Experience—The Assessment of Risk.* Amsterdam, Excerpta Medica Foundation, 1965, pp 179-184.
186. Zbinden G, Bagdon RE, Keith EF, Phillips RD, Randall LO: Experimental and clinical toxicology of chlordiazepoxide (Librium®). Toxicol Appl Pharmacol 3:619-637, 1961
187. Gjerris F: Poisoning with chlordiazepoxide (Librium®). Danish Med Bull 13:170-172, 1966
188. Jatlow P: Ultraviolet spectrophotometric measurement of chlordiazepoxide in plasma. Clin Chem 18:516-518, 1972
189. Austin TR: Mixed drug overdosage with phenelzine, amytal, and chlordiazepoxide. A case report. Anaesthesia 21:249-252, 1966
190. Bardhan KD: Cerebellar syndrome after nitrazepam overdosage. Lancet 1:1319-1320, 1969
191. Burston GR: Self-poisoning in elderly patients. Gerontol Clin 11:279-289, 1969
192. Carroll BJ: Attempted suicide: hypnotics and sedatives. Med J Aust 2:806, 1970
193. Clarke TP, Simpson TR, Wise SP: Two unsuccessful suicidal attempts with a new drug: methaminodiazepoxide (Librium). Texas State J Med 57:24-26, 1961
194. Cruz IA, Cramer NC, Parrish AE: Hemodialysis in chlordiazepoxide toxicity. JAMA 202:438-440, 1967
195. Fell RH, Dendy PR: Severe hypothermia and respiratory arrest in diazepam and glutethimide intoxication. Anaesthesia 23:636-640, 1968

196. Ganguli LK, Sen D, Chatterjee P, Mandal JN: Oxazepam overdosage. J Indian Med Assoc 54:424-425, 1970

197. Gilbert JE: Ingestion of a massive dose of Librium. South Dakota J Med Pharm 14:307-309, 1961

198. Hillyer DM: An overdosage of "Valium." Med J Aust 1:565, 1965

199. Jenner FA, Parkin D: A large overdose of chlordiazepoxide. Lancet 2:322-323, 1961

200. Pennington GW, Synge VM: Chloridazepoxide ("Librium") overdosage. J Irish Med Assoc 49:187-188, 1961

201. Schaeffer S: Toxicity from drug overdosage in an eleven-year-old boy. Case report. Clin Pediat 1:103-104, 1962

202. Shimkin PM, Shaivitz SA: Oxazepam poisoning in a child. JAMA 196:662-663, 1966

203. Smith ME: Suicidal attempt by oral ingestion of chlordiazepoxide (Librium). Clin Med 68:72-74, 1961

204. Spark H, Goldman AS: Diazepam intoxication in a child. Amer J Dis Child 109:128-129, 1965

205. Tanner TB, Moorhead SH: High dose poisoning with diazepam (Valium) and survival in a two-year-old child. J Med Assoc Georgia 57:534-536, 1968

206. Thomson J, Glen AIM: A large overdosage of chlordiazepoxide. Lancet 2:722-723, 1961

207. Irvine RE: Hypothermia due to diazepam. Brit Med J 2:1007, 1966

208. Decker WJ, Combs HF, Treuting JJ, Banez RJ: Dialysis of drugs against activated charcoal. Toxicol Appl Pharmacol 18:573-578, 1971

209. Rice AJ, Gruhn SW, Gibson TP, Delle M, DiBona GF: Effect of saline infusion on the renal excretion of secobarbital, meprobamate, and chlordiazepoxide. J Lab Clin Med 80:56-62, 1972

210. Ridley CM: Bullous lesions in nitrazepam overdosage. Brit Med J 3:28, 1971

Chapter 13
The Price We Pay

Elsewhere in this volume reference has been made to the relatively high dollar cost of benzodiazepine tranquilizers and hypnotics in the United States. We suggested that the price of benzodiazepines might be a significant drawback to their use. To put these concepts in perspective, this chapter presents more specific data on the cost and extent of use of tranquilizers and hypnotics in the United States.

WHOLESALE PRICE

Table 13-1 shows wholesale prices of antianxiety agents as taken from a common reference source.[1] The cost per 100 comparable dose units of oral benzodiazepine preparations is similar. Intermediate-strength dosages are most commonly prescribed; their prices range from $7.23 to $9.00 per 100 units. Meprobamate is somewhat less expensive when prescribed by trade name and much less expensive when prescribed by generic name. Phenobarbital can be obtained for only $0.35 per 100 dose units—less expensive even than placebo.

Table 13-2 shows wholesale prices of commonly prescribed hypnotic drugs. Barbiturates and chloral hydrate are the least expensive agents, particularly when prescribed by generic name. In all cases, the cost to the consumer is higher than the quoted price because of the pharmacist's dispensing fee. The usual mark-up is $1.00 to $3.00 per prescription.

EXTENT OF USE

Figure 13-1 shows the number of prescriptions for various types of psychotropic drugs filled in American retail pharmacies during the last 3 years. The data are based upon the ongoing survey of retail pharmacy transactions performed by R. A. Gosselin and Co., Inc.,[2] and are quoted with permission. Antianxiety agents accounted for nearly 95 million prescriptions in 1972. They are the most commonly used psychotropic drugs, and the number of prescriptions is increasing yearly.

Table 13-3 shows the extent of use of selected antianxiety agents. All quoted figures are in *millions*. Given in parentheses are the percentages of all prescriptions which were *new* as opposed to *refills*. The total dollar cost

TABLE 13-1. *Average wholesale prices of antianxiety agents*

Generic name	Trade name	Manufacturer	Unit dose size (mg) (tablet or capsule)	Wholesale price per 100 dose units
Chlordiazepoxide	Librium, Libritabs	Roche	5	$ 5.64
			10	7.32
			25	10.50
Diazepam	Valium	Roche	2	7.20
			5	8.70
			10	11.94
Oxazepam	Serax	Wyeth	10	5.82
			15	7.23
			30	10.05
Chlorazepate	Tranxene	Abbott	3.75	6.00
			7.5	9.00
			15	15.00
Meprobamate	Miltown	Wallace	400	6.50
Meprobamate	Equanil	Wyeth	400	7.06
Meprobamate	—	(many)	400	1.11*
Phenobarbital	—	(many)	15	0.35*
			30	0.35*
Placebo	—	(many)	tablet	0.75*
			capsule	1.30*

*Indicates the lowest price when many are quoted.

(in millions) is also shown. As intimated in Chapter 4, benzodiazepines are the most commonly prescribed antianxiety agents. More than 200 million dollars was spent on outpatient prescriptions for benzodiazepines in 1972. If drug use in hospitals were also accounted for, the figure would be about 25% higher.[3] About two-thirds of prescriptions were for diazepam. Usage of benzodiazepines—particularly diazepam—is increasing at a rapid pace. European observers note that "at this rate the arrival of the millennium would coincide with the total tranquillisation of America."[4]

Flurazepam, available only since June 1970, has rapidly become a popular hypnotic agent. Prescriptions for flurazepam accounted for more than 10% of all hypnotic drug prescriptions in 1972. Only short-acting barbiturates, glutethimide, and methaqualone were used more frequently.

COMMENT

These data raise three issues of medical and political importance.

1. Are anxiety and insomnia so prevalent and severe in the population as to justify the extent of tranquilizer and hypnotic use?
2. Are benzodiazepine derivatives so much more effective and safe as

to justify the increased cost to society when these drugs are used rather than less expensive sedative-hypnotics?

3. Are pharmaceutical manufacturers justified in reaping huge profits from the sales of patent-protected benzodiazepine tranquilizers and hypnotics?

Implicit in the first question is the therapeutic dilemma, described in Chapters 4 and 9, that plagues all practicing physicians. Undoubtedly, many sedative-hypnotic prescriptions are unnecessary and therefore constitute a kind of drug misuse. One possible remedy to the situation is "tighter" tranquilizer control. By classifying benzodiazepines as Schedule IV substances, the Drug Enforcement Administration would take steps to ensure their proper distribution and use. Under the new classification, prescriptions could be refilled for no longer than 6 months after the initial prescription is written, with no more than five refills allowed for that prescription per 6 months. Physician education can potentially lead to voluntary tranquilizer control. Small-scale studies[5] have demonstrated that programs which intensively indoctrinate the principles of rational sedative-hypnotic use result in less prevalent prescription of these drugs. It is not clear, however, that the trend toward more rational drug use produced by such programs would be anything more than a transient one. The present health care system itself is as much at fault for sedative-hypnotic misuse as is the collective pharmacologic unsophistication of practicing physicians. Primary care physicians—doctors who do most of the nation's "doctoring"—are so pressured by too many patients and too few

TABLE 13-2. *Average wholesale prices of hypnotic drugs*

Generic name	Trade name	Manufacturer	Unit dose size (mg) (tablet or capsule)	Wholesale price per 100 dose units
Secobarbital	Seconal	Lilly	100	$2.16
Secobarbital	—	(many)	100	1.05*
Pentobarbital	Nembutal	Abbott	100	2.59
Pentobarbital	—	(many)	100	1.00*
Methyprylon	Noludar	Roche	200	5.16
			300	6.12
Glutethimide	Doriden	USV	250	3.30
			500	5.51
Ethchlorvynol	Placidyl	Abbott	100	2.53
			200	3.93
			500	6.66
			750	9.18
Chloral hydrate	—	(many)	500	1.20*
Flurazepam	Dalmane	Roche	15	5.10
			30	6.12

*Indicates the lowest price when many are quoted.

hours that a pharmacologic "crutch" is the answer to many medical complaints arising from anxiety rather than organic disease. Neither educational programs nor strict controls can relieve these burdens on the nation's primary physicians. Tranquilizer misuse and overuse is inherent in a health care system which does not allow the practitioner time for interpersonal therapy of his patients with insomnia, anxiety, and psychosomatic complaints.

The complexity of the second question is attested by the length of this volume alone. Physicians are increasingly forced to choose between several or many drugs available for use in a given clinical situation. Each drug has its benefits and drawbacks, which the clinician must evaluate before making a choice. His choice must be rational not only to himself and his

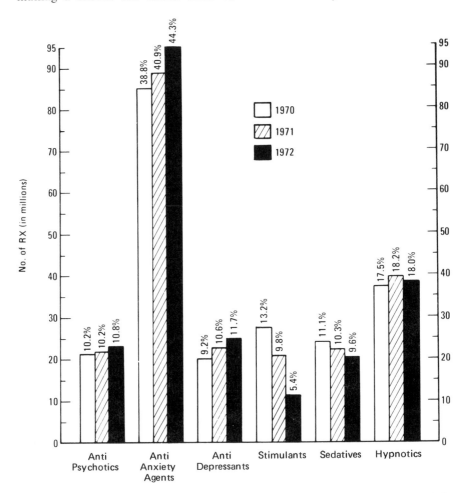

FIG. 13-1. Prescriptions for psychotropic drugs filled in American retail pharmacies (1970-1972). Total number of prescriptions and percentage of all psychotropic drug prescriptions are shown. (Kindly furnished by Dr. Mitchell Balter.)

TABLE 13-3. *Extent of use of selected antianxiety agents**

Drugs**	1970		1971		1972	
	Total prescriptions (% new)	Total cost	Total prescriptions (% new)	Total cost	Total prescriptions (% new)	Total cost
Benzodiazepines***	61.00 (32.9%)	$155.25	68.82 (34.5%)	$181.60	77.24 (35.1%)	$209.39
Meprobamate	16.79 (31.1%)	36.82	15.91 (37.9%)	36.24	13.90 (41.2%)	31.60
Phenobarbital	10.58 (44.5%)	8.80	10.95 (45.6%)	9.49	10.94 (43.4%)	9.70

*All figures are in *millions* and include only outpatient retail prescriptions. Quoted with permission from R.A. Gosselin and Co., Inc. (Ref. 2).
**Generic and trade-name prescriptions combined.
***Includes chlordiazepoxide, diazepam, oxazepam, chlorazepate (for further data see: JAMA 225:1637-1641, 1973).

patient, but also to "authorities"—the chief of medicine, the courts, the government—whose influence upon private practice becomes greater as time passes. No practitioner can be expected to make a truly rational choice of drugs if such a choice were to depend upon his own review of hundreds of published papers. The choice among benzodiazepines, meprobamate, barbiturates, and placebo exemplifies this dilemma. The purpose of this volume has been to provide a critical, concise, and complete literature review to assist the clinician in his "cost-benefit analysis" and rational choice of drug. As the medical literature becomes more voluminous and unwieldy, rational therapeutics will come to depend more and more upon similar impartial literature reviews—written as articles, monographs, or books—of other drugs and drug classes.

The third question touches the very foundations of free enterprise. Under the present system, private pharmaceutical firms expend vast capital and effort in developing new pharmacologic agents. Only rarely is a marketable new drug discovered. The firm responsible for developing the drug is rewarded with a patent, allowing the new agent to be marketed for a limited number of years without price competition. When drugs become as widely used as benzodiazepines, profits can be tremendous. In recent monumental action,[6-8] the British government declared that pharmaceutical profits from sales of diazepam and chlordiazepoxide were excessive. Sweeping price reductions were ordered, despite the manufacturer's claim that a significant proportion of the profits from sales of these drugs are used to defray cost of past and ongoing research.

The double-edged nature of this action was emphasized in the British medical literature.[9,10] The best of all possible pharmaceutical manufacture-and-delivery systems is the one that makes the largest number of quality pharmaceuticals available to those that need them at the lowest possible cost. Many believe that the private manufacture system currently operative in Britain and America is the "best of all possible." This is by no means proven. It is clear, however, that the free enterprise system is based upon reward-incentive. Governmental interference with these incentives, despite a beneficial short-term effect, has the potential to reduce the long-term efficiency and productivity of the entire system. Undoubtedly, similar disputes regarding profits and prices of these other drugs will arise in America. It is essential that the British experience be thoroughly studied before definitive action is taken.

REFERENCES

1. Siegelman S, et al. (eds): *1973 American Druggist Blue Book.* New York, The Hearst Corporation, 1973
2. *National Prescription Audit. Therapeutic Category Report.* Ambler, Pennsylvania, R.A. Gosselin and Co., Inc., December, 1972
3. Muller C: The overmedicated society: forces in the marketplace for medical care. Science 176:488-492, 1972
4. Benzodiazepines: use, overuse, misuse, abuse? Lancet 1:1101-1102, 1973
5. Kaufman A, Brickner PW, Varner R, Mashburn WJ: Tranquilizer control. JAMA 221:1504-1506, 1972
6. National health service. Chlordiazepoxide and diazepam prices. Lancet 1:876, 1973
7. Price of tranquillisers. Lancet 1:1069, 1973
8. Price of tranquillisers. Lancet 2:108, 1973
9. Unreasonable profit. Lancet 1:867, 1973
10. Profits from drugs. Brit Med J 2:132, 1973

Appendix 1
Bibliography of Synthetic Methods and Chemical Properties

Reviews

Archer GA, Sternbach LH: The chemistry of benzodiazepines. Chem Rev 68:747-784, 1968

Childress SJ, Gluckman MI: 1,4-benzodiazepines. J Pharmaceut Sci 53:577-590, 1964

Popp FD, Noble AC: The chemistry of diazepines. Adv Heterocycl Chem 8:21-82, 1967

Sternbach LH, Randall LO, Banziger R, Lehr H: Structure-activity relationships in the 1,4-benzodiazepines series. In, *Drugs Affecting the Central Nervous System,* Vol. 2. Edited by A Burger. New York, Marcel Dekker, Inc., 1968, pp 237-264

Sternbach LH, Randall LO, Gustafson SR: 1,4-benzodiazepines (chlordiazepoxide and related compounds). In *Psychopharmacological Agents,* Vol. I. Edited by M Gordon. New York, Academic Press, 1964, pp 137-224

Articles

Archer GA, Stempel A, Ho SS, Sternbach LH: Quinazolines and 1,4-benzodiazepines. Part XXIX. Synthesis of some 2,3-dihydro-5-pyridyl-1H-1,4-benzodiazepines. J Chem Soc [Org] 1031-1034, 1966

Archer GA, Sternbach LH: Quinazolines and 1,4-benzodiazepines. XVI. Synthesis and transformations of 5-phenyl-1,4-benzodiazepine-2-thiones. J Org Chem 29:231-233, 1964

Bell SC, Childress SJ: A rearrangement of 5-aryl-1,3-dihydro-2H-1,4-benzodiazepine-2-one 4-oxides. J Org Chem 27:1691-1695, 1962

Bell SC, Childress SJ: Additional rearrangements of 5-phenyl-1,4-benzodiazepines. J Org Chem 29:506-507, 1964

Bell SC, Gochman C, Childress SJ: Some analogs of chlordiazepoxide. J Med Pharmaceut Chem 5:63-69, 1962

Bell SC, Gochman C, Childress SJ: The rearrangement of 2-amino-5-phenyl-3H-1,4-benzodiazepine 4-oxides with acetic anhydride. J Org Chem 28:3010-3012, 1963

Bell SC, McCaully RJ, Childress SJ: A novel elimination-addition reaction of a diacylated hydroxylamine. Tetrahedron Lett 33:2889-2891, 1965

Bell SC, McCaully RJ, Childress SJ: A new synthesis of 7-chloro-1,3-dihydro-5-phenyl-2H-1,4-benzodiazepin-2-one 4-oxide. J Heterocyclic Chem 4:647-649, 1967

Bell SC, McCaully RJ, Childress SJ: 5-aryl-1,5-dihydro-2H-1,4-benzodiazepin-2-ones. J Med Chem 11:172-174, 1968

Bell SC, McCaully RJ, Gochman C, Childress SJ, Gluckman MI: 3-Substituted 1,4-benzodiazepin-2-ones. J Med Chem 11:457-461, 1968

Bell SC, Sulkowski TS, Gochman C, Childress SJ: 1,3-dihydro-2H-1,4-benzodiazepine-2-ones and their 4-oxides. J Org Chem 27:562-566, 1962

Blazevic N, Kajfez F: A new ring closure of 1,4-benzodiazepine. J Heterocyclic Chem 7:1173-1174, 1970

Blazevic N, Kajfez F: A new ring closure synthesis of 1,4-benzodiazepines. II. J Heterocyclic Chem 8:845-846, 1971

Carabateas PM, Harris LS: Analgesic antagonists. I. 4-substituted 1-acyl-2,3,4,5-tetrahydro-1H-1,4-benzodiazepines. J Med Chem 9:6-10, 1966

Castagnoli N, Sadee W: Mechanism of the reaction of a 1,4-benzodiazepine N-oxide with acetic anhydride. J Med Chem 15:1076-1078, 1972

Derieg ME, Fryer RI, Schweiniger RM, Sternbach LH: Quinazolines and 1,4-benzodiazepines. XXXIX. The synthesis of dihydroimidazo- and tetrahydropyrimido [1,2-a] [1,4] benzodiazepines. J Med Chem 11:912-913, 1968

Earley JV, Fryer RI, Winter D, Sternbach LH: Quinazolines and 1,4-benzodiazepines. XL. The synthesis of metabolites of 7-chloro 1-(2-diethylaminoethyl)-5-(2-fluorophenyl)-1,3-dihydro-2H-1,4-benzodiazepin-2-one. J Med Chem 11:774-777, 1968

Farber S, Wuest HM, Meltzer RI: Reaction of 6-chloro-2-chloromethyl-4-phenyl-quinazoline 3-oxide with dimethylamine. J Med Chem 7:235-237, 1964

Felix AM, Earley JV, Fryer RI, Sternbach LH: Quinazolines and 1,4-benzodiazepines. XLIII. Oxidation with ruthenium tetroxide. J Heterocyclic Chem 5:731-734, 1968

Field GF, Sternbach LH: Quinazolines and 1,4-benzodiazepines. XLII. Photochemistry of some N-oxides. J Org Chem 33:4438-4440, 1968

Field GF, Zally WJ, Sternbach LH: Quinazolines and 1,4-benzodiazepines. XXVI. 1,2-Dihydroquinazoline 3-oxides. J Org Chem 30:3957-3959, 1965

Field GF, Zally WJ, Sternbach LH: Quinazolines and 1,4-benzodiazepines. XXXI. Novel ring enlargements of 1,2-dihydroquinazoline 3-oxides. Tetrahedron Lett 23:2609-2613, 1966

Fryer RI, Archer GA, Brust B, Zally W, Sternbach LH: Quinazolines and 1,4-benzodiazepines. XXIII. Chromic acid oxidation of 1,4-benzodiazepine derivatives. J Org Chem 30:1308-1310, 1965

Fryer RI, Brust B, Earley J, Sternbach LH: Quinazolines and 1,4-benzodiazepines. XIX. N-alkyl derivatives of substituted 1,3,4,5-tetrahydro-5-phenyl-2H-1,4-benzodiazepin-2-ones. J Med Chem 7:386-389, 1964

Fryer RI, Brust B, Sternbach LH: Quinazolines and 1,4-benzodiazepines. Part XIV. The nitration products of 7-substituted 1,3-dihydro-5-phenyl-2H-1,4-benzodiazepine-2-ones. J Chem Soc 4977-4979, 1963

Fryer RI, Earley JV, Field GF, Zally W, Sternbach LH: A synthesis of amidines from cyclic amides. J Org Chem 34:1143-1145, 1969

Fryer RI, Earley JV, Sternbach LH: Quinazolines and 1,4-benzodiazepines. XXI. The nitration of 1,3,4,5-tetrahydro-5-phenyl-2H-1,4-benzodiazepin-2-ones. J Org Chem 30:521-523, 1965

Fryer RI, Earley JV, Sternbach LH: Quinazolines and 1,4-benzodiazepines. XLIV. The formation of isoindoles by the ring contraction of 1-alkyl-1,4-benzodiazepines. J Org Chem 34:649-654, 1969

Fryer RI, Schmidt RA, Sternbach LH: Quinazolines and 1,4-benzodiazepines. XVII. Synthesis of 1,3-dihydro-5-pyridyl-1,4-benzodiazepine derivatives. J Pharmaceut Sci 53:264-268, 1964

Fryer RI, Sternbach LH: Quinazolines and 1,4-benzodiazepines. XXII. A rearrangement of 5-phenyl-1,3-dihydro-2H-1,4-benzodiazepin-2-ones. J Org Chem 30:524-525, 1965

Garcia EE, Benjamin LE, Fryer RI, Sternbach LH: Quinazolines and 1,4-benzodiazepines. 55. Synthesis of two metabolites of demoxepam isolated from the dog. J Med Chem 15:986-987, 1972

Hester JB, Rudzik AD, Kamdar BV: 6-Phenyl-4H-s-triazolo[4,3-a][1,4]benzodiazepines which have central nervous system depressant activity. J Med Chem 14:1078-1081, 1971

Hester JB, Rudzik AD, Veldkamp W: Pyrrolo[3,2,1-jk][1,4]benzodiazepines and pyrrolo[1,2,3-ef][1,5]benzodiazepines which have central nervous system activity. J Med Chem 13:827-835, 1970

Inaba S, Hirohashi T, Yamamoto H: Benzodiazepines. III. A novel synthesis of a 1-cyclopropylmethyl-1,4-benzodiazepine derivative. Chem Pharm Bull 17:1263-1265, 1969

Ishizumi K, Inaba S, Yamamoto H: Benzodiazepines. VI. A rearrangement of 2-aminoacetanilides to anilinoacetamides. Chem Pharm Bull 20:592-596, 1972

Inaba S, Ishizumi K, Mori K, Yamamoto H: Benzodiazepines. V. A novel synthesis of a 7-nitro-1,4-benzodiazepine derivative. Chem Pharm Bull 19:722-729, 1971

Inaba S, Ishizumi K, Okamoto T, Yamamoto H: Benzodiazepines. VII. Pyrazino [1,2-a]indole-1(2H)-ones and their conversion to 2,3-dihydro-1H-1,4-benzodiazepines. Chem Pharm Bull 20:1628-1636, 1972

Inaba S, Ishizumi K, Yamamoto H: Benzodiazepines. IV. A new synthesis of 1-diethylaminoethyl-substituted 1,4-benzodiazepin-2-ones. Chem Pharm Bull 19:263-272, 1971

Kagei HH: Synthesis of 7-chloro-2,3-dihydro-1-methyl-5-phenyl-1H-1,4-benzodiazepine-5-14C hydrochloride. J Labelled Compounds 3:493-494, 1967

Lamdan S, Gaozza CH, Sicardi S, Izquierdo JA: Synthesis and structure-activity relationships of 1-alkoxyalkyl- and 1-aryloxyalkyl-1,4-ben-zodiazepin-2-ones. J Med Chem 13:742-744, 1970

Lemke TL, Hester JB, Rudzik AD: A new 2,6-diflurobenzodiazepinone. J Pharmaceut Sci 61:275-277, 1972

Loev B, Greenwald RB, Goodman MM, Zirkle CL: Benzazepinones. Synthesis of the monaza analog of diazepam, and the correct structure of the benzoylproprionanilide cyclization product. J Med Chem 14:849-852, 1971

Metlesics W, Silverman G, Sternbach LH: Quinazolines and 1,4-benzodiazepines. XII. Preparation and reactions of 2,3-dihydro-1H-1,4-benzodiazepine 4-oxides. J Org Chem 28:2459-2460, 1963

Metlesics W, Silverman G, Sternbach LH: Quinazolines and 1,4-benzodiazepines. XX. The formation of 3-phenylindole-2-carboxaldehydes from 2,3-dihydro-1H-1,4-benzodiazepine 4-oxides. J Org Chem 29:1621-1623, 1964

Metlesics W, Silverman G, Toome V, Sternbach LH: Quinzaolines and 1,4-benzodiazepines. XXVIII. Substituted 2(3H)-quinazolinones and -quinazolinethiones. J Org Chem 31:1007-1009, 1966

Metlesics W, Tavares RF, Sternbach LH: Quinazolines and 1,4-benzodiazepines. XXIV. Reaction of 1,4-benzodiazepin-2-ones with chloramine. J Org Chem 30:1311-1312, 1965

Miyadera T, Terada A, Fukunaga M, Kawano Y, Kamioka T, Tamura C, Takagi H, Tachikawa R: Anxiolytic sedatives. 1. Synthesis and pharmacology of benzo[6,7]-1,4-diazepino[5,4-b]oxazole derivatives and analogs. J Med Chem 14:520-526, 1971

Moffett RB, Rudzik AD: Central nervous system depressants. 9. Benzodiazepine sulfonamides. J Med Chem 14:588-593, 1971

Murphy MF: A study of the structure activity relationships of 1,4-benzodiazepines based upon molecular orbital calculations. Texas Rep Biol Med 28:404, 1970

Ott H, Hardtmann GE, Denzer M, Frey AJ, Gogerty JH, Leslie GH, Trapold JH: Tetrahydroisoquino[2,1-d][1,4]benzodiazepines. Synthesis and neuropharmacological activity. J Med Chem 11:777-787, 1968

Petersen JB, Lakowitz KH: New methods for the preparation of 1,4-benzodiazepinones, carbostyrils and indolo[2,3-c]quinolones. Acta Chem Scand 23:971-974, 1969

Sadee W, Garland W, Castagnoli N: Microsomal 3-hydroxylation of 1,4-benzodiazepines. J Med Chem 14:643-645, 1971

Schlager LH: Nitrone isomerization in the 1,4-benzodiazepine series. Tetrahedron Lett 51:4519-4520, 1970

Stempel A, Landgraf FW: Quinazolines and 1,4-benzodiazepines. IX. 2-carbobenzoxyglycylamidobenzophenones and their conversion to 1,4-benzodiazepines. J Org Chem 27:4675-4677, 1962

Stempel A, Reeder E, Sternbach LH: Quinazolines and 1,4-benzodiazepines.

XXVII. Mechanism of ring enlargement of quinazoline 3-oxides with alkali to 1,4-benzodiazepin-2-one 4-oxides. J Org Chem 30:4267-4271, 1965

Sternbach LH, Archer GA, Earley JV, Fryer RI, Reeder E, Wasyliw N, Randall LO, Banziger R: Quinazolines and 1,4-benzodiazepines. XXV. Structure-activity relationships of aminoalkyl-substituted 1,4-benzodiazepin-2-ones. J Med Chem 8:815-821, 1965

Sternbach LH, Archer GA, Reeder E: Quinazolines and benzodiazepines. XV. 7-Nitro- and 7-trifluoromethyl-2,3-dihydro-5-phenyl-1H-1,4-benzodiazepines and their transformations. J Org Chem 28:3013-3016, 1963

Sternbach LH, Fryer RI, Keller O, Metlesics W, Sach G, Steiger N: Quinazolines and 1,4-benzodiazepines. X. Nitro-substituted 5-phenyl-1,4-benzodiazepine derivatives. J Med Chem 6:261-265, 1963

Sternbach LH, Fryer RI, Metlesics W, Reeder E, Sach G, Saucy G, Stempel A: Quinazolines and 1,4-benzodiazepines. VI. Halo-, methyl-, and methoxy-substituted 1,3-dihydro-5-phenyl-2H-1,4-benzodiazepin-2-ones. J Org Chem 27:3788-3796, 1962

Sternbach LH, Fryer RI, Metlesics W, Sach G, Stempel A: Quinazolines and 1,4-benzodiazepines. V. o-Aminobenzophenones. J Org Chem 27:3781-3788, 1962

Sternbach LH, Kaiser S, Reeder E: Quinazoline 3-oxide structure of compounds previously described in the literature as 3,1,4-benzoxadiazepines. J Amer Chem Soc 82:475-480, 1960

Sternbach LH, Koechlin BA, Reeder E: Quinazolines and 1,4-benzodiazepines. (VIII). The photoisomerization of 7-chloro-2-methylamino-5-phenyl-3H-1,4-benzodiazepine 4-oxide. J Org Chem 27:4671-4672, 1962

Sternbach LH, Reeder E: Quinazolines and 1,4-benzodiazepines. IV. Transformations of 7-chloro-2-methylamino-5-phenyl-3H-1,4-benzodiazepine 4-oxide. J Org Chem 26:4936-4941, 1961a

Sternbach LH, Reeder E: Quinazolines and 1,4-benzodiazepines. II. The rearrangement of 6-chloro-2-chloromethyl-4-phenylquinazoline 3-oxide into 2-amino derivatives of the 7-chloro-5-phenyl-3H-1,4-benzodiazepine 4-oxide. J Org Chem 26:1111-1118, 1961b

Sternbach LH, Reeder E, Archer GA: Quinazolines and 1,4-benzodiazepines. XI. Synthesis and transformation of 7-chloro-2,3-dihydro (and 2,3,4,5-tetrahydro)-5-phenyl-1H-1,4-benzodiazepine. J Org Chem 28:2456-2459, 1963

Sternbach LH, Reeder E, Keller O, Metlesics W: Quinazolines and 1,4-benzodiazepines. III. Substituted 2-amino-5-phenyl-3H-1,4-benzodiazepine 4-oxides. J Org Chem 26:4488-4497, 1961

Sternbach LH, Reeder E, Stempel A, Rachlin AI: Quinazolines and 1,4-benzodiazepines. XVIII. The acetylation of chlordiazepoxide and its transformation into 6-chloro-4-phenyl-2-quinazolinecarboxaldehyde. J Org Chem 29:332-336, 1964

Appendix 2
Bibliography of Analytic Screening Techniques in Toxicology and Pharmaceutics

Bastos ML, Kananen GE, Young RM, Monforte JR, Sunshine I: Detection of basic organic drugs and their metabolites in urine. Clin Chem 16:931-940, 1970

Beckstead HD, Smith SJ: Detection of impurities in medicinal 1,4-benzodiazepines and related compounds by thin-layer chromatography. Arzneim-Forsch 18:529-535, 1968

Chafetz L, Gaglia CA: Stability assay for prazepam and related drugs. J Pharmaceut Sci 56:1681-1682, 1967

Comer JP, Comer I: Applications of thin-layer chromatography in pharmaceutical analysis. J Pharmaceut Sci 26:413-436, 1967

Davidow B. LiPetri N, Quame B: A thin-layer chromatographic screening procedure for detecting drug abuse. Amer J Clin Pathol 50:714-719, 1968

deSilva JAF, D'Arconte L: The use of spectrophotofluorometry in the analysis of drugs in biological materials. J Forensic Sci 14:184-204, 1969

de Zeeuw RA: Paper and thin-layer chromatographic techniques for separation and identification of barbiturates and related hypnotics. Progr Chem Toxicol 4:59-142, 1969

Finkle BS, Cherry EJ, Taylor DM: A GLC-based system for the detection of poisons, drugs, and human metabolites encountered in forensic toxicology. J Chrom Sci 9:393-419, 1971

Finkle BS, Taylor DM, Bonelli EJ: A GC/MS reference data system for the identification of drugs of abuse. J Chrom Sci 10:312-333, 1972

Jain NC, Kirk PL: Systematic applications of gas-liquid chromatography in toxicology. IV. The tranquilizers. Microchem J 12:256-264, 1967

Mulé SJ: Identification of narcotics, barbiturates, amphetamines, tranquilizers, and psychotomimetic drugs in human urine. J Chrom 39:302-311, 1969

Sohn D, Simon J: Rapid identification of psychopharmacologic agents in cases of drug abuse. Clin Chem 18:405-409, 1972

Street HV: Gas-liquid chromatography of submicrogram amounts of drugs. III. Analysis of alkaloids in biological media. J Chrom 29:68-79, 1967

Street RL, Perry WF: Rapid identification of common sedatives and stimulants by thin-layer chromatography. Clin Biochem 2:197-203, 1969

Thompson HL, Decker WJ: Analysis of blood. A simplified gas chromatographic approach for toxicologic purposes. Amer J Clin Pathol 49:103-107, 1968

Zingales I: Systematic identification of psychotropic drugs by thin-layer chromatography. Part I. J Chrom 31:405-419, 1967; Part II. J Chrom 34:44-51, 1968

Appendix 3
Bibliography of Uncontrolled Trials of Benzodiazepine Therapy in Emotional Disorders Published Since 1961

Chlordiazepoxide

Aivazian GH: Clinical evaluation of chlordiazepoxide. J Tennessee Med Assoc 54:115-119, 1961

Ayd FJ: A critical appraisal of chlordiazepoxide. J Neuropsychiat 3:177-180, 1962

Bambace F: Effects of chlordiazepoxide in severely disturbed outpatients. Amer J Psychiat 118:69-70, 1961

Barron AR, Rudy LH, Smith JA: Effect of drugs on "poor" treatment cases. Dis Nerv Syst 22:692-694, 1961

Barsa JA, Saunders JC: Comparative study of chlordiazepoxide and diazepam. Dis Nerv Syst 25:244-246, 1964

Batterman RC, Mouratoff GJ, Kaufman JE: Comparative treatment of the psychoneurotic reactive-type anxiety state with fluphenazine and chlordiazepoxide. J New Drugs 3:297-301, 1963

Boyle D, Tobin JM: Pharmaceutical management of behavior disorders. Chlordiazepoxide in covert and overt expressions of aggression. J Med Soc New Jersey 58:427-429, 1961

Bragan JH: Self-dosage in the psychiatric patient. Mind 1:21-24, 1963

Darling HF: A comparative study of diazepam and chlordiazepoxide in psychoneurotic patients. Dis Nerv Syst 24:501-503, 1963

Dunlop E: Anti-neurotic agents in office practice. Clin Med 68:2343-2346, 1961

Dye EN: Dual pharmacotherapy in grossly disturbed psychotic patients. Amer J Psychiat 118:548-549, 1961

Farb HH: Further experiences with chlordiazepoxide in a private psychiatric practice. J Newark Beth Israel Hosp 12:120-126, 1961

Ferner GN, Robertson MG: The treatment of anxiety. Report of a controlled trial. New Zealand Med J 61:592-595, 1962

Fishbein RE: Use of intravenous chlordiazepoxide in emergency room treatment. Curr Ther Res 3:345-350, 1961

Fishbein RE, Jones F: Use of chlordiazepoxide in general medicine. Int Rec Med 174:34-38, 1961

Jones TH: Chlordiazepoxide (Librium) and the geriatric patient. J Amer Geriat Soc 10:259-263, 1962

Kearney TR: Treatment of atypical depression with Librium and Parnate. Dis Nerv Syst 25:443-447, 1964

Kozlowski VL: Outpatient use of Librium in psychiatric disorders. J Michigan State Med Soc 60:906-908, 1961

Lapolla A: A controlled pilot study of tybamate in therapy of psychotic patients with chronic anxiety and psychoneurotic reactions. Int J Neuropsychiat 1:125-230, 1965

Matlin E: Use of chlordiazepoxide in obese patients. Clin Med 70:780-784, 1963

Pennington VM: A comparative clinical study of meprobamate and chlordiazepoxide. Med Times 90:841-846, 1962

Proctor RC: Chlordiazepoxide in the treatment of anxiety reactions. North Carolina Med J 22:224-226, 1961

Proctor RC: Industrial psychiatry. An evaluation of chlordiazepoxide in patients in an industrial setting. Med Times 89:1153-1158, 1961

Reiser P, Printz S, Harris SB, Robinson MS, Wainer D: The use of Librium in general practice. J Nat Med Assoc 54:244-247, 1962

Rosenstein IN: Parenteral administration of chlordiazepoxide: uses and limitations in internal medicine. J Amer Geriat Soc 10:969-974, 1962

Rosenstein IN, Silverblatt CW: Chlordiazepoxide as a broad-spectrum psychosedative. J Amer Geriat Soc 9:1003-1012, 1961

Sargant W: The treatment of anxiety states and atypical depressions by the monoamine oxidase inhibitor drugs. J Neuropsychiat 3(supp 1):s96-s103, 1962

Sargant W, Dally P: Treatment of anxiety states by antidepressant drugs. Brit Med J 1:6-9, 1962

Scherbel AL: Preliminary evaluation of chlordiazepoxide. Amer Pract Digest Treatm 12:275-281, 1961

Schopbach RR: Clinical report on methaminodiazepoxide (Librium). Amer J Psychiat 117:923-924, 1961

Settel E: Combined d-amphetamine and chlordiazepoxide therapy in the emotionally disturbed obese patient. Clin Med 70:1077-1088, 1963

Shackleford RW: Adjunctive use of chlordiazepoxide in general practice. Western Med 2:289-298, 1961

Slaughter I: Tybamate as an antineurosis drug in the treatment of emotional disorders. J New Drugs 5:177-180, 1965

Stanfield CE: Clinical experience with chlordiazepoxide (Librium). Psychosomatics 2:179-183, 1961

Vogt AH: Methaminodiazepoxide (Librium) in chronic refractory anxiety. Amer J Psychiat 117:743-745, 1961

Williams MW: Clinical impressions on the use and value of chlordiazepoxide in psychiatric practice. Southern Med J 54:922-926, 1961

Diazepam

Aivazian GH: Clinical evaluation of diazepam. Dis Nerv Syst 25:491-496, 1964

Barsa JA, Saunders JC: Comparative study of chlordiazepoxide and diazepam. Dis Nerv Syst 25:244-246, 1964

Beerman HM: A controlled study of diazepam in psychiatric outpatients. Amer J Psychiat 120:870-874, 1964

Blackman B: The adjunctive role of diazepam in the treatment of depression. Clin Med 70:1495-1500, 1963

Borelli N, Marjerrison G: Diazepam in long-term chronic schizophrenia. Amer J Psychiat 122:1292-1293, 1966

Bowes HA: The role of diazepam (Valium) in emotional illness. Psychosomatics 6:336-340, 1965

Burdine WE: Diazepam in a general psychiatric practice. Amer J Psychiat 121:589-592, 1964

Burnett RE, Holman RE: Experiences with Valium® in general practice. Med Times 93:56-60, 1965

Chesrow EJ, Kaplitz SE, Breme JT, Musci J, Sabatini R: Use of a new benzodiazepine derivative (Valium) in chronically ill and disturbed elderly patients. J Amer Geriat Soc 10:667-670, 1962

Cleckley HM: Use of diazepam as adjunctive therapy in psychiatric disorders. J South Carolina Med Assoc 61:1-4, 1965

Collard J: Clinical experience with diazepam in neuroses. J Neuropsychiat 3(supp 1):s157-s158, 1962

Constant GA, Gruver FA: Preliminary evaluation of diazepam in psychiatric disorders. Psychosomatics 4:80-84, 1963

Darling HF: A comparative study of diazepam and chlordiazepoxide in psychoneurotic patients. Dis Nerv Syst 24:501-503, 1963

Dorfman W: Some experiences in "total" treatment of patients with emotional illness. Psychosomatics 5:351-354, 1964

Dunlop E: The neurotic feeling of inferiority. J Neuropsychiat 3(supp 1):s79-s82, 1962

Feldman PE: An analysis of the efficacy of diazepam. J Neuropsychiat 3(supp 1):s62-s67, 1962

Galambos M: An interesting observation in the treatment of chronic psychiatric patients. Amer J Psychiat 121:273-274, 1964a

Galambos M: The long-term use of Valium. Amer J Psychiat 121:811, 1964b

Galambos M: Long-term clinical trial with diazepam on adult mentally retarded persons. Dis Nerv Syst 26:305-309, 1965

Gerzo HO: Severe depressive and anxiety states. Treatment with diazepam. Mind 1:235-238, 1963

Gillespe FA: The use of intravenous diazepam in stupor. Canad Psychiat Assoc J 16:445-446, 1971

Gold RL, Dribben IS: Diazepam therapy of depressed patients. J Neuropsychiat 5:366-369, 1964

Hegner HL: Diazepam in the treatment of myalgia, muscle spasm and the anxiety-tension state. Clin Med 71:1980-1988, 1965

Hirshleifer I, Kroger W: Benzodiazepines in the differentiation and treatment of anxieties. Clin Med 70:1673-1678, 1963

Holbrook AA: Experience with diazepam in internal medicine. Med Times 94:423-433, 1966

Hollister LE, Bennett JL, Kimbell I, Savage C, Overall JE: Diazepam in newly admitted schizophrenics. Dis Nerv Syst 24:746-750, 1963

Irvine BM, Schaechter F: "Valium" in the treatment of schizophrenia. Med J Aust 1:1387, 1969

Isham AD: Office evaluation of diazepam for psychoneurotic anxiety and depressive reactions. Int J Neuropsychiat 2:111-115, 1966

Kalina RK: Diazepam: its role in a prison setting. Dis Nerv Syst 25:101-107, 1964

Kelly JW: Management of psychiatric disorders with diazepam. Clin Med 69:1789-1802, 1962

Knapp JL: A multiple approach to the management of depression-tension states. Psychosomatics 6:166-170, 1965

Krakowski AJ: Long-term study of a new psychotropic drug in private psychiatric practice. Psychosomatics 4:44-51, 1963

Kramer JC: Treatment of chronic hallucinations with diazepam and phenothiazines. Dis Nerv Syst 28:593-594, 1967

Love J: Diazepam in treatment of emotional disorders. Dis Nerv Syst 24:674-677, 1963

Magyar I: Seduxen in neuropsychiatry. Ther Hung 16:123-130, 1968

McCray WE: Diazepam and combined treatment in outpatients with depressive symptoms. J Louisiana State Med Soc 117:232-238, 1965

Pignataro FP: Experience with chemotherapy in refractory psychiatric disorders. Amer J Psychiat 119:577-579, 1962

Pignataro FP: Experience with chemotherapy in refractory psychiatric disorders. Curr Ther Res 4:389-398, 1962

Proctor RC: The improved management of incapacitating anxiety states. J Neuropsychiat 3(supp 1):s151-s154, 1962

Rathbone R: The role of a psychotherapeutic drug in internal medicine. Med Times 91:1186-1191, 1963

Schuster TS, Winslow WW, Kellner R: A comparison of thioridazine and diazepam in non-psychotic anxiety-depression: a pilot study. Curr Ther Res 14:131-135, 1972

Spankus WH: Role of a new psychotropic drug in somatic disorders. Psychosomatics 5:153-156, 1964

Sprogis GR: Control of anxiety/depression in general practice. Curr Ther Res 8:490-493, 1966

Sussex JN, Linton PA, Herlihy CE: Anxiety and depression in "borderline" schizophrenic states—treatment with Valium, a Librium analog. Psychosomatics 2:256-260, 1961

Towler ML: The clinical use of diazepam in anxiety states and depressions. J Neuropsychiat 3(supp 1):s68-s72, 1962

Vilkin MI, Lomas JB: Clinical experience with diazepam in general psychiatric practice. J Neuropsychiat 3(supp 1):s139-s144, 1962

Youngblood BJ: Evaluation of diazepam in ambulatory psychotic and neurotic patients. Clin Med 71:2103-2108, 1964

Oxazepam

Armstrong ML: A sequential trial of oxazepam. Med J Aust 1:287, 1968

Gerz HO: A preliminary report on the management of geriatric patients with oxazepam. Amer J Psychiat 120:1110-1111, 1964

Gilbert MM: Clinical trial of a new drug, analog of chlordiazepoxide, for treatment of anxiety and tension. Int J Neuropsychiat 1:556-558, 1965

Halpern MM: The antianxiety activity of oxazepam in patients with multiple organic disorders. Clin Med 75:42-44, (July) 1968

Krakowski AJ: Suppression of anxiety with oxazepam in a private psychiatric practice. Psychosomatics 6:26-31, 1965

Merlin H: Management of anxiety in internal medicine with oxazepam. J Florida Med Assoc 53:397-400, 1966

Oosterbaan WM: Study of a new drug (oxazepam) in a large psychiatric institution. Psychiat Neurol (Basel) 153:153-165, 1967

Scasserra BB: Place of an anti-anxiety agent in general practice. Dis Nerv Syst 26:511-515, 1965

Thomas JCS: Clinical evaluation of oxazepam in an out-patient psychiatric clinic. Dis Nerv Syst 27:261-264, 1966

Warner RS: Management of the office patient with anxiety and depression. Psychosomatics 6:347-351, 1965

Zador I: Oxazepam in psychoneuroses and "anxiety bound" psychoses. Dis Nerv Syst 30:688-692, 1969

Medazepam

Brandsma M: Preliminary experience with medazepam (Nobrium) in the management of psychophysiologic reactions. Psychosomatics 11:197-200, 1970

Folkstuen T: Nobrium®, another benzodiazepine derivative. 29 months of experience. Int Pharmacopsychiat 3:130-135, 1970

Folkstuen T: Experiences with the benzodiazepine derivative Ro 5-4556. In, *The Present Status of Psychotropic Drugs. Pharmacological and Clinical*

Aspects. Edited by A Cerletti, FJ Bové. Amsterdam, Excerpta Medica Foundation, 1969, pp 506-507

Herlofsen HB: Brief report on a new benzodiazepin preparation Ro 5-4556/B-5. Acta Psychiat Scand (supp) 203:243-246, 1968

Krakowski AJ: Preliminary observations on the use of Ro 5-4556 in psychiatric disorders characterized by anxiety-tension. Psychosomatics 7:150-151, 1966

Lingjaerde O: Some clinical experiences with a new benzodiazepine. In *The Present Status of Psychotropic Drugs. Pharmacological and Clinical Aspects*. Edited by A Cerletti, FJ Bové. Amsterdam, Excerpta Medica Foundation, 1969, pp 517-518

Schopbach RR: A pilot study with Ro 5-4556 in the treatment of anxiety and depression. Int J Neuropsychiat 3:494-496, 1967

Lorazepam

Botter PA: Review of two years clinical experience with lorazepam. Curr Med Res Opin 1:282-284, 1973

Collard J: Initial psychopharmacological study of lorazepam (Wy 4036). Arzneim-Forsch 21:1091-1095, 1971

Deberdt R: Lorazepam in the treatment of severe anxiety and anxiety associated with psychotic symptoms. Curr Med Res Opin 1:296-300, 1973

Kudo Y: Clinical experiences with lorazepam in Japan. Curr Med Res Opin 1:301, 1973

van Groos GAK: The treatment of neurotic and psychotic anxiety with lorazepam. Curr Med Res Opin 1:288-290, 1973

Venema J: The use of lorazepam in psychiatric patients: a clinical assessment. Curr Med Res Opin 1:285-287, 1973

Other Benzodiazepines

Bethune HC, Burrell RH, Culpan RH, Ogg GJ: Preliminary notes on nitrazepam. New Zealand Med J 65:613-615, 1966

DiMascio A, Shader RI, Salzman C, Harmatz JS: An evaluation of isoquinazepon (SAH-1123). Curr Ther Res 9:517-521, 1967

Gallant DM, Bishop MP: SCH 12041: a new antianxiety agent. Curr Ther Res 13:107-110, 1971

Gallant DM, Guerrero-Figueroa R, Swanson WC: U-28,774 (ketazolam): an early investigation of a new antianxiety agent. Curr Ther Res 15:123-126, 1973

Gerz HO: A preliminary report on a new benzodiazepine in severe depressions. Amer J Psychiat 121:495-496, 1964

Kingstone E, Villeneuve A, Kossatz I: Prazepam in the treatment of anxiety and tension: a clinical study of a new benzodiazepine derivative. Curr Ther Res 8:159-163, 1966

Sakalis G, Pearson E, Kermani E, Gershon S: On the anti-anxiety properties of a new benzodiazepine, ORF 8063. Curr Ther Res 15:268-271, 1973

Appendix 4
The Benzodiazepines in Epilepsy:
Case Reports and Unselected Series

Baldwin RW, Kenny TJ, Gibbas D: Long term therapy of convulsive disorders with intramuscular diazepam. J Clin Pharmacol 9:343-344, 1969

Barsa JA, Saunders JC: Chlordiazepoxide in the treatment of psychotics with convulsive disorders. Dis Nerv Syst 23:106-108, 1962

Bercel N: Chlordiazepoxide (Librium) as a anticonvulsant. Dis Nerv Syst 22(July supp):17-19, 1961

Brock JT, Dyken M: The anticonvulsant activity of chlordiazepoxide and Ro 5-2807. Neurology (Minneap) 13:59-65, 1963

Brodie RE, Dow RS: Chlordiazepoxide in epilepsy. Northwest Med 61:513-516, 1962

Cohen NH, McAuliffe M, Aird RB: "Startle" epilepsy treated with chlordiazepoxide (Librium®). Dis Nerv Syst 22(July supp):20-27, 1961

Dyken PR: 'Half and half' seizures. Devel Med Child Neurol 11:94-95, 1969

Elian M: The long-term oral use of Valium (diazepam) in epilepsy. Epilepsia 10:487-493, 1969

Geller M, Christoff N: Diazepam in the treatment of childhood epilepsy. JAMA 215:2087-2090, 1971

Goddard P, Lokare VG: Diazepam in the management of epilepsy. Brit J Psychiat 117:213-214, 1970

Goldman D, Schynoll G: The effect of chlordiazepoxide on convulsive disorders. Dis Nerv Syst 25:52-58, 1964

Hernandez-Peon R, Rincon-Trujillo J, Chavez-Ibarra G: Effect of Valium on epilepsy and hypertonic muscular disorders. Acta Neurol Latinoamerica 9:372-385, 1963

Kaim SC, Rosenstein IN: Experience with chlordiazepoxide in the management of epilepsy. J Neuropsychiat 3:12-17, 1961

Lehmann HE, Ban TA: Studies with new drugs in the treatment of convulsive disorders. Int J Clin Pharmacol 1:231-234, 1968

leVann LJ: Chlordiazepoxide, a tranquillizer with anticonvulsant properties. Canad Med Assoc J 86:123-125, 1962

Liske E, Forster FM: Clinical study of a new benzodiazepine as an anticonvulsive agent. J New Drugs 3:241-244, 1963

Livingston S, Pauli L, Murphy JB: Ineffectiveness of chlordiazepoxide hydrochloride in epilepsy. JAMA 177:243-244, 1961

Merlis S, Turner WJ, Halpern S: Chlordiazepoxide as adjunctive therapy in convulsive disorders. Amer J Psychiat 119:575-576, 1962

Omar JB, Kumar V: Chlordiazepoxide in the treatment of epilepsy. J Assoc Physicians India 13:357-361, 1965

Peterson WG: Clinical study of Mogadon. A new anticonvulsant. Neurology (Minneap) 17:878-880, 1967

Sansoy OM, Whorton D: Chlordiazepoxide hydrochloride in treatment of convulsive disorders. A three year retrospective study. Rocky Mountain Med J 63:56-58, (Dec) 1966

Trolle E: Diazepam (Valium) in the treatment of epilepsy. A report of fifty cases. Acta Neurol Scand 41(supp 13):535-539, 1965

Watson CW, Bowker R, Calish C: Effect of chlordiazepoxide on epileptic seizures. JAMA 188:212-216, 1964

Appendix 5
The Benzodiazepines in Status Epilepticus and Intractable Seizures

Bailey DW, Fenichel GM: The treatment of prolonged seizure activity with intravenous diazepam. J Pediat 73:923-927, 1968

Calderon-Gonzales R, Mireles-Gonzales A: Management of prolonged motor seizure activity in children. JAMA 204:544-546, 1968

Chokroverty S, Mayo CM, Ouyang R: Intravenous chlordiazepoxide (Librium) in status epilepticus. Clin Electroenceph 1:143-152, 1970

Chokroverty S, Rubino FA: Treatment of status epilepticus with intravenous chlordiazepoxide (Librium). (Abstract). Electroenceph Clin Neurophysiol 31:287, 1971

Gastaut H, Naquet R, Poire R, Tassinari CA: Treatment of status epilepticus with diazepam (Valium). Epilepsia 6:167-182, 1965

Gordon NS: Treatment of status epilepticus with diazepam. Devel Med Child Neurol 8:668-672, 1966

Henriksen PB: Acute treatment of epileptic seizures with diazepamum (Valium®). Acta Neurol Scand 43 (supp 31):168-169, 1967

Howard FM, Seybold ME, Reiher J: The treatment of recurrent convulsions with intravenous injection of diazepam. Med Clin NA 52:977-987, 1968

Lalji D, Hosking CS, Sutherland JM: Diazepam ("Valium") in the control of status epilepticus. Med J Aust 1:542-545, 1967

Little SC, Green J: The intravenous use of diazepam in focal status epilepticus. Southern Med J 62:381-385, 1969

Lombroso CT: Treatment of status epilepticus with diazepam. Neurology (Minneap) 16:629-634, 1966

McMorris S, McWilliam PKA: Status epilepticus in infants and young children treated with parenteral diazepam. Arch Dis Child 44:604-611, 1969

Naquet R, Soulayrol R, Dolce G, Tassinari CA, Broughton R, Loeb H: First attempt at treatment of experimental status epilepticus in animals and spontaneous status epilepticus in man with diazepam (Valium). (Abstract). Electroenceph Clin Neurophysiol 18:427, 1965

Nicol CF, Tutton JC, Smith BH: Parenteral diazepam in status epilepticus. Neurology (Minneap) 19:332-343, 1969

Oller-Daurella L: Advantage of benzodiazepines in the treatment of epileptic crises. In, *The Present Status of Psychotropic Drugs. Pharmacological and Clinical Aspects.* Edited by A Cerletti, FJ Bové. Amsterdam, Excerpta Medica Foundation, 1969, pp 441-442.

Parsonage MJ, Norris JW: Use of diazepam in treatment of severe convulsive status epilepticus. Brit Med J 3:85-88, 1967

Prensky AL, Raff MC, Moore MJ, Schwab RS: Intravenous diazepam in the treatment of prolonged seizure activity. New Eng J Med 276:779-784, 1967

Sawyer GT, Webster DD, Schut LJ: Treatment of uncontrolled seizure activity with diazepam. JAMA 203:913-918, 1968

Smith BT, Masotti RE: Intravenous diazepam in the treatment of prolonged seizure activity in neonates and infants. Devel Med Child Neurol 13:630-634, 1971

Tutton JC: New treatment for old neurologic disease. Status epilepticus treatment with diazepam. NY State J Med 70:2425-2428, 1970

Wilson PJE: Drugs for status epilepticus. Brit Med J 1:239, 1967

Wilson PJE: Treatment of status epilepticus in neurosurgical patients with diazepam ('Valium'). Brit J Clin Prac 22:21-24, 1968

Appendix 6
Bibliography of Reviews

Alps BJ, Harry TVA, Southgate PJ: The pharmacology of lorazepam, a broad-spectrum tranquillizer. Curr Med Res Opin 1:239-261, 1973

Anxiety and investigations. Brit Med J 2:377, 1970

Appleton WS: Psychoactive drugs: a usage guide. Dis Nerv Syst 32:607-616, 1971

Archer GA, Sternbach LH: The chemistry of benzodiazepines. Chem Rev 68:747-784, 1968

Ban TA: Clinical pharmacology of psychotropic drugs. Appl Ther 9:366-371, 1967

Ban TA: The benzodiazepines—Part II. Appl Ther 9:677-680, 1967

Ban TA: Methodological problems in the clinical evaluation of anxiolytic drugs. In, *Advances in Neuro-Psychopharmacology.* Edited by O Vinar, Z Votava, PB Bradley. Amsterdam, North-Holland Publishing Co., 1971, pp 211-224

Barry H, Buckley JP: Drug effects on animal performance and the stress syndrome. J Pharmaceut Sci 55:1159-1183, 1966

Becker CE, Scott R: The treatment of alcoholism. Rational Drug Ther 6:Oct 1972

Benor D, Ditman KS: Tranquilizers in the management of alcoholics: a review of the literature to 1964. Part I. J New Drugs 6:319-337, 1966

Benor D, Ditman KS: Tranquilizers in the management of alcoholics: a review of the literature to 1964. Part II. J Clin Pharmacol 7:17-25, 1967

Berger FM: The similarities and differences between meprobamate and barbiturates. Clin Pharmacol Ther 4:209-233, 1963

Boissier J-R, Simon P: Evaluation of experimental techniques in the psychopharmacology of emotion. Ann NY Acad Sci 159:898-914, 1969

Brett EM: Diazepam—the new wonder drug? Devel Med Child Neurol 12:655-659, 1970

Brophy JJ: Suicide attempts with psychotherapeutic drugs. Arch Gen Psychiat 17:652-657, 1967

Carter S, Gold AP: The critically ill child: management of status epilepticus. Pediatrics 44:732-733, 1969

Cazzullo CL: Pharmacologic and clinical differences in the actions of sedative-hypnotic tranquilizers and neuroleptic drugs. Differences in neuropathology. In, *Neuro-Psycho-Pharmacology*. Edited by H Brill. Amsterdam, Excerpta Medica Foundation, 1966, pp 124-129

Childress SJ, Gluckman MI: 1,4-Benzodiazepines. J Pharmaceut Sci 53:577-590, 1964

Cohen IM: The benzodiazepines. In, *Discoveries in Biological Psychiatry*. Edited by FJ Ayd, B Blackwell. Philadelphia, JB Lippincott, 1970, pp 130-141

Conney AH: Pharmacological implications of microsomal enzyme induction. Pharmacol Rev 19:317-366, 1967

Cook L, Catania AC: Effects of drugs on avoidance and escape behavior. Fed Proc 23:818-835, 1964

Cook L, Kelleher RT: Effects of drugs on behavior. Ann Rev Pharmacol 3:205-222, 1963

Coon WW, Willis PW: Some aspects of the pharmacology of oral anticoagulants. Clin Pharmacol Ther 11:312-336, 1970

Davis JM, Bartlett E, Termini BA: Overdosage of psychotropic drugs: a review. Dis Nerv Syst 29:157-164, 246-256, 1968

Davis JM: Efficacy of tranquilizing and antidepressant drugs. Arch Gen Psychiat 13:552-572, 1965

Domino EF: Behavioral and electrophysiological aspects of antianxiety agents. In, *Advances in Neuro-Psychopharmacology*. Edited by O Vinar, Z Votava, PB Bradley. Amsterdam, North-Holland Publishing Co., 1971, pp 147-154

Domino EF: Human pharmacology of tranquilizing drugs. Clin Pharmacol Ther 3:599-664, 1962

Downing RW, Rickels K: The prediction of placebo response in anxious and depressed outpatients. In, *Psychopharmacology and the Individual Patient*. Edited by JR Wittenborn, SC Goldberg, PRA May. New York, Raven Press, 1970, pp 160-188

Downing RW, Rickels K, Wittenborn JR, Mattsson NB: Interpretation of data from investigations assessing the effectiveness of psychotropic agents. In, *Principles and Problems in Establishing the Efficacy of Psychotropic Agents*. Edited by J Levine, BC Schiele, L Bouthilet. Washington, DC, USPHS Publication #2138, 1971, pp 321-369

Dundee JW, Haslett WHK: The benzodiazepines. A review of their actions and uses relative to anaesthetic practice. Brit J Anaesth 42:217-234, 1970

Dundee JW, Keilty SR: Diazepam. Int Anaesth Clin 7:91-121, 1969

Fisher S: Nonspecific factors as determinants of behavioral response to drugs. In, *Clinical Handbook of Psychopharmacology*. Edited by A DiMascio, RI Shader. New York, Science House, 1970, pp 17-39

Flurazepam (Dalmane), a new hypnotic. Med Lett Drugs Ther 12:89-90, 1970

Foreman PA: Intravenous diazepam in general dental practice. New Zealand Dent J 65:243-253, 1969

Garattini S, Marcucci F, Mussini E: Benzodiazepine metabolism in vitro. Drug Metab Rev 1:291-309, 1972

Garattini S, Mussini E, Marcucci F, Guaitani A: Metabolic studies on benzodiazepines in various animal species. In, *The Benzodiazepines.* Edited by S Garattini, E Mussini, LO Randall. New York, Raven Press, 1973, pp 75-97

Greenblatt DJ, Greenblatt M: Which drug for alcohol withdrawal? J Clin Pharmacol 12:429-431, 1972

Greenblatt DJ, Shader RI: Acute poisoning with psychotropic drugs. In, *Psychotropic Drug Side Effects: Clinical and Theoretical Perspectives.* By RI Shader, A DiMascio, and associates. Baltimore, Williams and Wilkins, 1970, pp 214-234

Greenblatt DJ, Shader RI: Meprobamate: A study of irrational drug use. Amer J Psychiat 127:1297-1303, 1971

Greenblatt DJ, Shader RI: The clinical choice of sedative-hypnotics. Ann Intern Med 77:91-100, 1972

Hartmann E: Pharmacological studies of sleep and dreaming: chemical and clinical relationships. Biol Psychiat 1:243-258, 1969

Hartmann E: The biochemistry and pharmacology of the D-state (dreaming sleep). Exp Med Surg 27:105-120, 1969

Hayman M: The effects of Librium in psychiatric disorders. Dis Nerv Syst 22(July supp):60-69, 1961

Himwich HE, Morillo A, Steiner WG: Drugs affecting rhinencephalic structures. J Neuropsychiat 3(supp 1):s15-s26, 1962

Hinton J: Sedatives and hypnotics. Practitioner 200:93-101, 1968

Hollis DA: Diazepam: its scope in anaesthetic practice. Proc Roy Soc Med 62:806-807, 1969

Hollister LE: Clinical use of psychotherapeutic drugs: current status. Clin Pharmacol Ther 10:170-198, 1969

Hollister LE: Methodological considerations in evaluating antianxiety agents. J Clin Pharmacol 10:12-18, 1970

Hollister LE: Clinical use of psychotherapeutic drugs. II. Antidepressant and antianxiety drugs and special problems in the use of psychotherapeutic drugs. Drugs 4:361-410, 1972

Hollister LE: Drug therapy. Mental disorders—antianxiety and antidepressant drugs. New Eng J Med 286:1195-1198, 1972

Hollister LE: The prudent use of antianxiety drugs. Rational Drug Ther 6:March, 1972

Hollister LE: Uses of psychotherapeutic drugs. Ann Intern Med 79:88-98, 1973

Honigfeld G: Non-specific factors in treatment. I. Review of placebo reactions and placebo reactors. Dis Nerv Syst 25:145-156, 1964

Honigfeld G: Non-specific factors in treatment. II. Review of social-psychological factors. Dis Nerv Syst 25:225-239, 1964

Horovitz ZP, Babington RG: Differences in effects of sedatives, tranquilizers, and neuroleptics on the electrical activity of the brain in animals and man. In, *Neuro-Psycho-Pharmacology.* Edited by H Brill. Amsterdam, Excerpta Medica Foundation, 1966, pp 94-100

Hughes G: Diazepam in the dental surgery. Ann Royal Coll Surg England 48:38-39, 1971

Irwin S: Anti-neurotics: practical pharmacology of the sedative-hypnotics and minor tranquilizers. In, *Psychopharmacology: A Review of Progress 1957-1967.* Edited by DH Efron. Washington DC, USPHS publication #1836, 1968, pp 185-204

Irwin S: A rational framework for the development, evaluation, and use of psychoactive agents. Amer J Psychiat 124(Feb supp):1-19, 1968

Janke W, Debus G: Experimental studies on antianxiety agents with normal subjects: methodological considerations and review of the main effects. In, *Psychopharmacology: A Review of Progress 1957-1967.* Edited by DH Efron. Washington DC, USPHS publication #1836, 1968, pp 205-230

Kales A, and discussants: Drug dependency. Investigations of stimulants and depressants. Ann Intern Med 70:591-614, 1969

Kales A, Kales J: Evaluation, diagnosis, and treatment of clinical disorders related to sleep. JAMA 213:2229-2235, 1970

Katz RL: Drug therapy. Sedatives and tranquilizers. New Eng J Med 286:757-760, 1972

Kehoe MJ: I. Minor tranquilizers. Southern Med J 64:366-369, 1971

Kellner R: Drugs, diagnoses, and outcome of drug trials with neurotic patients. J Nerv Ment Dis 151:85-96, 1970

King CD: The pharmacology of rapid eye movement sleep. Adv Pharmacol Chemother 9:1-91, 1971

Kissin B, Gross MM: Drug therapy in alcoholism. Amer J Psychiat 125:31-41, 1968

Koch-Weser J, Sellers EM: Drug interactions with coumarin anticoagulants. New Eng J Med 285:487-498, 547-558, 1971

Lader M: The nature of anxiety. Brit J Psychiat 121:481-491, 1972

Lader MH: Anxiolytic drugs. Brit J Clin Prac 9:79-82, 1973

Lasagna L: The controlled clinical trial: theory and practice. J Chronic Dis 1:353-367, 1955

Lasagna L: The pharmacological basis for the effective use of hypnotics. Pharmacology for Physicians 1:1-4, (Feb) 1967

Laties VG, Weiss B: A critical review of the efficacy of meprobamate (Miltown, Equanil) in the treatment of anxiety. J Chronic Dis 7:500-519, 1958

Librium and Valium. Med Lett Drugs Ther 11:81-84, 1969

Link RE: The relation of drug trials to chlordiazepoxide and diazepam. Appl Ther 7:978-987, 1965

Loew DM: Methods of evaluation of anxiolytics. In, *Advances in Neuro-Psychopharmacology.* Edited by O Vinar, Z Votava, PB Bradley. Amsterdam, North-Holland Publishing Co., 1971, pp 155-166

Margules˙DL, Stein L: Neuroleptics vs. tranquilizers: evidence from animal behavior studies of mode and site of action. In, *Neuro-Psycho-Pharmacology.* Edited by H Brill. Amsterdam, Excerpta Medica Foundation, 1966, pp 108-120

Marks J: Methaminodiazepoxide (Librium): a new psychotropic drug. Chemother Rev 1:141-144, 1960

Mattson RH: The benzodiazepines. In, *Antiepileptic Drugs.* Edited by DM Woodbury, JK Penry, RP Schmidt. New York, Raven Press, 1972, pp 497-518

Miller RR, DeYoung DV, Paxinos J: Hypnotic drugs. Postgrad Med J 46:314-317, 1970

Norris W: The quantitative assessment of premedication. Brit J Anaesth 41:778-784, 1969

O'Reilly RA, Aggeler PM: Determinants of the response to oral anticoagulant drugs in man. Pharmacol Rev 22:35-96, 1970

Oswald I: Drugs and sleep. Pharmacol Rev 20:274-303, 1968

Overall JE, Hollister LE, Kimbell I, Shelton J: Extrinsic factors influencing responses to psychotherapeutic drugs. Arch Gen Psychiat 21:89-94, 1969

Overton DA: Dissociated learning in drug states (state dependent learning). In, *Psychopharmacology: A Review of Progress 1957-1967.* Edited by DH Efron. Washington DC, USPHS publication #1836, 1968, pp 918-930

Park LC, Imboden JB: Clinical and heuristic value of clinical drug research. J Nerv Ment Dis 151:322-340, 1970

Parkes MW: The pharmacology of diazepam. In, *Diazepam in Anaesthesia.* Edited by PF Knight, CG Burgess. Bristol, John Wright and Sons, 1968, pp 1-7

Pearlman CA, Greenberg R: Medical-psychological implications of recent sleep research. Psychiatry in Medicine 1:261-276, 1970

Pletscher A, daPrada M, Foglar G: Differences between neuroleptics and tranquilizers regarding metabolism and biochemical effects. In, *Neuro-Psycho-Pharmacology.* Edited by H Brill. Amsterdam, Excerpta Medica Foundation, 1966, pp 101-107

Popp FD, Noble AC: The chemistry of diazepines. Adv Heterocyclic Chem 8:21-82, 1967

Randall LO: Pharmacology of chlordiazepoxide (Librium). Dis Nerv Syst 22(July supp):7-15, 1961

Randall LO, Schallek W: Pharmacological activity of certain benzodiazepines.

In, *Psychopharmacology: A Review of Progress 1957-1967*. Edited by DH Efron. Washington, DC, USPHS publication #1836, 1968, pp 153-184

Randall LO, Kappell B: Pharmacological activity of some benzodiazepines and their metabolites. In, *The Benzodiazepines*. Edited by S Garattini, E Mussini, LO Randall. New York, Raven Press, 1973, pp 27-51

Reggiani G, Hurlimann A, Theiss E: Some aspects of the experimental and clinical toxicology of chlordiazepoxide. In, *Proceedings of the European Society for the Study of Drug Toxicity*. Vol 9. *Toxicity and Side-Effects of Psychotropic Drugs*. Edited by SBD Baker, JR Boissier, W Koll. Amsterdam, Excerpta Medica Foundation, 1968, pp 79-97

Rickels K: Antineurotic agents: specific and non-specific effects. In, *Psychopharmacology: A Review of Progress 1957-1967*. Edited by DH Efron. Washington DC, USPHS publication #1836, 1968, pp 231-247

Rickels K: Drug use in outpatient treatment. Amer J Psychiat 124(Feb supp):20-31, 1968

Rickels K (ed): *Non-specific Factors in Drug Therapy*. Springfield, Illinois, Charles C Thomas, 1968

Rushworth G: Skeletal muscle spasm and some speculations on the mode of action of diazepam. Ann Phys Med supp:1-2, 1964

Schallek W, Schlosser W, Randall LO: Recent developments in the pharmacology of the benzodiazepines. Adv Pharmacol Chemother 10:119-183, 1972

Schreiber EC: The metabolic alteration of drugs. Ann Rev Pharmacol 10:77-98, 1970

Schwartz MA: Pathways of metabolism of the benzodiazepines. In, *The Benzodiazepines*. Edited by S Garattini, E Mussini, LO Randall. New York, Raven Press, 1973, pp 53-74

Schweigert BF, Mackewicz DW: Diazepam anticonvulsant properties. Hosp Formulary Management 7:20-22, (Jan-Feb) 1972

Shader RI: Antianxiety agents: a clinical perspective. In, *Clinical Handbook of Psychopharmacology*. Edited by A DiMascio, RI Shader. New York, Science House, 1970, pp 71-77

Shapiro AK: Iatroplacebogenics. Int Pharmacopsychiat 2:215-248, 1969

Sternbach LH: Chemistry of 1,4-benzodiazepines and some aspects of the structure-activity relationship. In, *The Benzodiazepines*. Edited by S Garattini, E Mussini, LO Randall. New York, Raven Press, 1973, pp 1-26

Sternbach LH: 1,4-Benzodiazepines. Chemistry and some aspects of the structure-activity relationship. Agnew Chem (Internat Edit) 10:34-43, 1971

Sternbach LH, Randall LO, Banziger R, Lehr H: Structure-activity relationships in the 1,4-benzodiazepine series. In, *Drugs Affecting the Central Nervous System,* Vol 2. Edited by A Burger. New York, Marcel Dekker Inc., 1968, pp 237-264

Sternbach LH, Randall LO, Gustafson SR: 1,4-Benzodiazepines (chlordiazepoxide and related compounds). In, *Psychopharmacological Agents,* Vol I. Edited by M Gordon. New York, Academic Press, 1964, pp 137-224

Sternbach LH, Randall LO: Some aspects of the structure-activity relationship in psychotropic agents of the 1,4-benzodiazepine class. In, *CNS Drugs.* Edited by GS Sidhu et al. New Delhi, Council of Scientific Research, 1966, pp 53-69

Stille G, White T: Correlation between pharmacology and clinic. In, *Advances in Neuro-Psychopharmacology.* Edited by O Vinar, Z Votava, PB Bradley. Amsterdam, North-Holland Publishing Co., 1971, pp 167-177

Svenson SE, Gordon LR: Diazepam: a progress report. Curr Ther Res 7:367-391, 1965

Svenson SE, Hamilton RG: A critique of overemphasis on side effects with the psychotropic drugs: an analysis of 18,000 chlordiazepoxide-treated cases. Curr Ther Res 8:455-464, 1966

Swash M: Status epilepticus. Brit J Hosp Med 8:269-272, 1972

Szobor A: Classification of somatogenic neuroses and their prolonged treatment with diazepam (Seduxen). Ther Hung 17:17-21, 1969

Today's drugs. Hypnotics. Brit Med J 2:409-411, 1968

Turner P: Drugs and the special senses. Seminars in Drug Treatment 1:335-352, 1971

Uhlenhuth EH, Lipman RS, Chassan JB, Hines LR, McNair DM: Methodological issues in evaluating the effectiveness of agents for treating anxious patients. In, *Principles and Problems in Establishing the Efficacy of Psychotropic Agents.* Edited by J Levine, BC Schiele, L Bouthilet. Washington DC, USPHS publication #2138, 1971, pp 137-161

Uphold JD: The benzodiazepines. Texas Medicine 69:83-88, (June) 1973

Viamontes JA: Review of drug effectiveness in the treatment of alcoholism. Amer J Psychiat 128:1570-1571, 1972

Valzelli L: Drugs and aggressiveness. Adv Pharmacol 5:79-108, 1967

Way WL, Trevor AJ: Sedative-hypnotics. Anesthesiology 34:170-182, 1971

Wheatley D: Chlordiazepoxide in the treatment of the domiciliary case of anxiety neurosis. In, *Proceedings of the Fourth World Congress of Psychiatry.* Edited by JJL Ibor. Amsterdam, Excerpta Medica Foundation, 1968, pp 2034-2037

Wittenborn JR: *The Clinical Psychopharmacology of Anxiety.* Springfield, Illinois, Charles C Thomas, 1966

Wittenborn JR: The design of clinical trials. In, *Principles and Problems in Establishing the Efficacy of Psychotropic Agents.* Edited by J Levine, BC Schiele, L Bouthilet. Washington DC, USPHS publication #2138, 1971, pp 227-262.

Zbinden G, Randall LO: Pharmacology of benzodiazepines: laboratory and clinical correlations. Adv Pharmacol 5:213-291, 1967

INDEX

A

Acetaminophen, 45
Acetophenazine, 82
Addiction. *See* Chlordiazepoxide,
  habituation; Diazepam, habituation
Adenosine monophosphate (AMP),
  110, 159
Adenosine triphosphate (ATP), 110
Adrenocorticotropic hormone
  (ACTH), 129, 174-175
Alcoholism, 5, 6, 33, 219-223, 240
γ-Aminobutyric acid, 108
Amiphenazole, 232
Amitriptyline, 79, 82, 150, 235
Amobarbital, 75, 146, 158, 186-188,
  190, 247
Amphetamines, 46, 51-52, 64, 174,
  217, 245-246
Analeptic drugs, 107-108
Antipyrine, 247
Anxiety, 2, 62, 68-69, 84-85, 141,
  157-158, 183-184, 245
  and cardiac disease, 146-147
  and gastrointestinal disorders,
  150-151
  measurements of, 70-71, 84,
  150, 157, 176
Anxiety neurosis, 1, 4, 5, 6, 44,
  62-65, 67, 72-79, 80-81, 160-161,
  241
Anxiolytics, 43, 47-48, 75. *See also*:
  Barbiturates, Hydroxyzine,
  Meprobamate
Atropine, 67, 142, 151, 201
Auditory flutter fusion (AFF), 178

B

Barbiturates, 1, 75, 109, 148, 149,
  151, 178, 186, 190, 206,
  224, 232, 247
  and amphetamines, 46
  anxiety, treatment of, 88
  avoidance response, 44, 49

cardiovascular and respiratory
  effects, 130, 145, 160, 178,
  203, 204, 232, 247
disinhibitory effect, 43, 48
hypnotic, 184, 185, 189
status epilepticus, treatment of,
  121, 129
withdrawal syndromes, 217, 219
See also: Amobarbital, Butabarbital,
  Pentobarbital, Phenobarbital,
  Secobarbital
Bell, S. C., 7
Belladonna, 202
Benzodiazepines. *See* Bromazepam,
  Chlordiazepoxide, Clonazepam,
  Demoxepam, Desmethyldiazepam,
  Diazepam, Flunitrazepam, Flurazepam, Lorazepam, Medazepam, Nitrazepam, Oxazepam, Prazepam, Temazepam. *See also*: Benzodiazepines
  in the treatment of children; Screening procedures and analyses
Benzodiazepines in the treatment of
  children,
  cerebral palsy, 86, 122
  dentistry, 209
  emotional disorders, 87-88
  enuresis, 87-88, 191
  epilepsy, 33, 132
  facial tics, 127-128
  hyperkinesis, 87
  infantile spasms, 132
  neurosis, 87
  pavor nocturnus, 191
  premedication, 207-208
  psychosis, 88
  seizures, 129
  somnambulism, 191
  tetanus, 127
  withdrawal from opiates, 223
Benzotamine, 78-79

295